INTRODUCTION TO ADDICTIVE BEHAVIORS

INTRODUCTION TO
ADDICTIVE
BEHAVIORS

FIFTH EDITION

DENNIS L. THOMBS
CYNTHIA J. OSBORN

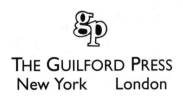

THE GUILFORD PRESS
New York   London

Library of Congress Cataloging-in-Publication Data

Names: Thombs, Dennis L., author. | Osborn, Cynthia J., author.
Title: Introduction to addictive behaviors / Dennis L. Thombs, Cynthia J.
    Osborn.
Description: Fifth edition. | New York : The Guilford Press, [2019] |
    Includes bibliographical references and index.
Identifiers: LCCN 2018041447 | ISBN 9781462539222 (hardback)
Subjects: LCSH: Substance abuse—Etiology. | Substance abuse—Treatment. |
    BISAC: PSYCHOLOGY / Psychopathology / Addiction. | MEDICAL /
Psychiatry / General. | SOCIAL SCIENCE / Social Work. | PSYCHOLOGY /
Psychotherapy / Counseling.
Classification: LCC RC564 .T55 2019 | DDC 362.29—dc23
LC record available at *https://lccn.loc.gov/2018041447*

About the Authors

Dennis L. Thombs, PhD, FAAHB, is Professor and Dean of the School of Public Health at the University of North Texas Health Science Center in Fort Worth. The focus of his scholarship is addictive behaviors, with special interests in the epistemology of addiction, and in alcohol and drug use during the period of emerging adulthood. In recent years, Dr. Thombs's research has focused on analyzing drinking practices and their consequences in natural settings. He is a past president and Fellow of the American Academy of Health Behavior.

Cynthia J. Osborn, PhD, LPCC-S, LICDC, is Professor of Counselor Education and Supervision at Kent State University. Her clinical background is in treatment of adults with co-occurring disorders (substance use disorders and mental illness). Dr. Osborn's teaching, supervision, and scholarship focus on addictions counseling, particularly evidence-based practices such as motivational interviewing. She is a member of the Motivational Interviewing Network of Trainers and has extensive experience in the clinical supervision of counselors-in-training and professional counselors.

Preface

This book was written for practicing health and human services professionals with no formal training in the prevention and treatment of substance use disorder and for undergraduate and graduate courses on addictive behaviors. The book has two primary goals. The first is to challenge and strengthen the reader's understanding of addiction by exploring how others in the field have come to know it. We hope that this will enable the reader to create a clear and logically consistent perspective on addiction. The second goal is to show the reader how theory and research are important to both the prevention and treatment of substance abuse. This information should provide the reader with an array of strategies for addressing substance abuse problems and help make him or her an effective practitioner.

A number of good books are currently available on substance abuse and dependence. For the most part, however, these books either are written at an advanced level for the sophisticated practitioner or researcher or focus on a limited set of theoretical orientations. The present text is unique in that it attempts to present a comprehensive and thoughtful review of theory and research with the front-line practitioner and student in mind. Exposure to complex and divergent theories of addictive behavior has often been neglected in the preparation and training of health and human services professionals, including substance abuse or addictions counselors, public health practitioners, prevention specialists, social workers, psychologists, and nurses. Some of these practitioners are familiar with one or more of the disease models, but even here they often have not had the opportunity to examine propositions critically. This book assumes virtually no preexisting knowledge in the biological and behavioral sciences, medicine, or public health. In each chapter, a careful attempt is made to explain the conceptual underpinnings of the theories and approaches described therein, as well as the research supporting these frameworks.

The fifth edition of *Introduction to Addictive Behaviors* has been revised to appeal to a broad audience of practitioners and students. The primary purpose of the first two editions was to provide a multidisciplinary foundation for addiction treatment. The third edition was revised to include a theoretical and research foundation for substance abuse *prevention* as well. The fourth edition was expanded to include three new chapters: "The Controversial Science of Behavioral Addiction," "Promoting Motivation and Autonomy for Personal Change," and "Linking Theory, Evidence, and Practice." The fifth edition has been extensively updated and includes new research, such as that on the genetics of addiction, which can be found in Chapter 2, "The Disease Models." Chapter 9, "Social and Cultural Foundations," has been extensively rewritten to include new sections on addiction stigma and a comprehensive overview of the current opioid epidemic. For the fifth edition, other chapters from the fourth edition have been updated, examples are provided throughout, and revised Review Questions appear at the end of each chapter.

Special thanks are in order to those who helped us complete the fifth edition. We are grateful to The Guilford Press, and especially to Jim Nageotte and Jane Keislar, for their encouragement and assistance in preparing this edition. Several anonymous reviewers provided feedback that also was extremely helpful in steering the direction of the book.

DENNIS L. THOMBS
University of North Texas
Health Science Center at Fort Worth

CYNTHIA J. OSBORN
Kent State University

Acknowledgments

We thank the publishers of the following works, who have generously given us permission to use extended quotations or paraphrases and to reprint or adapt tables and figures:

"Principles of Alcoholism Psychotherapy" by S. Zimberg, 1978, in S. Zimberg, J. Wallace, and S. Blume (Eds.), *Practical Approaches to Alcoholism Psychotherapy*, New York: Plenum Press. Copyright 1978 by Springer Science and Business Media.

"Dual Diagnosis: A Review of Etiological Theories" by K. T. Mueser, R. E. Drake, and M. A. Wallach, 1998, *Addictive Behaviors, 23*, 717–734. Copyright 1998 by Elsevier.

"Self-Determination Theory and the Facilitation of Intrinsic Motivation, Social Development, and Well-Being" by R. M. Ryan and E. L. Deci, 2000, *American Psychologist, 55*, 68–78. Copyright 2000 by the American Psychological Association.

Addiction and Change: How Addictions Develop and Addicted People Recover by C. C. DiClemente, 2003, New York: Guilford Press. Copyright 2003 by The Guilford Press.

Motivating Substance Abusers to Enter Treatment: Working with Family Members by J. E. Smith and R. J. Meyers, 2004, New York: Guilford Press. Copyright 2004 by The Guilford Press.

Motivational Interviewing: Helping People Change (3rd ed.) by W. R. Miller and S. Rollnick, 2013, New York: Guilford Press. Copyright 2013 by The Guilford Press.

"The Experiences of Affected Family Members: A Summary of Two Decades of Qualitative Research" by J. Orford, R. Velleman, A. Copello, L. Templeton, and A. Ibanga, 2010, *Drugs: Education, Prevention and Policy, 17*(Suppl. 1), 44–62. Copyright 2010 by Taylor & Francis.

Contents

CHAPTER 1

Conceptualization of Addictive Behavior and the Need for Informed Practice

Why a book on theories of addictive behavior? For at least the last 200 years in U.S. history, substance misuse (primarily alcohol) has been viewed as an immoral or sinful activity and addiction as a somewhat mysterious, or at least nonspecific, condition frequently referred to as a disease. These views remain prominent today in the legal and correctional system, as well as in the treatment community. For many years, it also was believed that the sole or preferred qualification to work as an addictions counselor was to be a recovering addict. Knowledge of addiction thus was based mostly on one's personal recovery experiences, and invariably addiction was understood as a primary and involuntary disease and nothing else. Many still endorse this belief. Indeed, disease models remain the foundation of much of the addiction treatment provided in the United States today.

Disease models clearly have facilitated the adoption of more humane public policies, such as medical insurance provisions, and have helped a large number of persons who have sought treatment. However, as judged by the very large number who avoid or refuse treatment, drop out of treatment, and/or relapse, it reasonably can be asserted that these particular models are not a "good fit" for many (perhaps most) individuals. It is imperative that practitioners consider a wider range of prevention and treatment models, especially for populations and individual clients who cannot work within a disease model. Doing so would likely expand the reach of prevention and treatment services, identifying a greater number of

1

individuals who could benefit from such services but so far have purpose-fully stayed away for reasons such as monetary cost and/or insistence on abstinence.

There is not just one way to explain addiction. Results of scientific investigations; social, cultural, and political events throughout U.S. his-tory; and firsthand accounts of people who have experienced and been affected by addiction support this contention. Addiction is an extremely complex condition arising from multiple pathways and manifesting itself in innumerable ways. It thus defies a simple and absolute definition. It may be convenient to narrowly define the problem as a "brain disease," but this term is insufficient and possibly misleading. Addiction also is not just a bad habit that can be stopped through willpower. Furthermore, it is not only (or even) a character or spiritual defect, although many fiercely defend the use of these descriptors. Addiction is more than any one of these characteriza-tions. In many ways, addiction remains a puzzle, a mystery, a conundrum. Those who insist on a singular, absolute, and all-encompassing explana-tion of addiction are either ill-informed or championing a specific (social, political) cause, or both. For students of addiction etiology, understanding its complexity requires reliance on multilevel analyses and the capacity to examine the problem through different lenses.

Credentialing requirements for drug and alcohol counselors, preven-tion specialists, and other professional practitioners now include educa-tion in a range of theories of addiction, including science-based theories that describe addiction as a learned and adaptive behavior. Unfortunately, training in theories of addictive behavior does not translate automati-cally—if at all—to theoretically informed practice. All too often, practitio-ners rigidly cling to a favorite theory, in many cases without fully under-standing its concepts and implications. At the same time, other theories may be callously disregarded. As noted by Webb, Sniehotta, and Michie (2010), many practitioners use interventions not informed by, or linked to, a specific theory—or, when they are, the connection is not clear. There is a similar disconnect with respect to research and practice, discussed later in this chapter and throughout the remaining chapters. As professionals, we should possess the flexibility to work with different communities and clients, and tailor our approaches to their needs. This is the meaning of *individualized* or *customized care*.

As in previous editions of this book, the threefold purpose of this edi-tion remains to expose students and practitioners to a range of theories of addictive behavior, to review longstanding and current scientific research that has tested these theories, and to help make theories of addictive behav-iors and their research relevant for contemporary prevention and treatment services. Although idealistic, we hope that in a small way the book helps to bridge the gap that exists between theory and research on one side and practice on the other. We also hope students and in-service professionals will find the review of theory and research to be provocative enough to cause them to reconsider their conceptions of addiction.

WHAT EXACTLY IS A THEORY?

The popular understanding of the term *theory* is that it is a belief or set of beliefs distinguished from and in opposition to practice, science, and certainty or fact. Many of us have heard someone retort, "Oh, that's just a theory." This offhand remark suggests several things: theory is a spontaneous idea, the result of informal brainstorming; a cerebral invention of one or a select few persons isolated from mainstream thinking; and something to be minimized and not trusted. It also implies that theory is mere speculation, lacking substantiation or verification. Although there is a tendency to equate theory with things that are impractical or devoid of common sense, all of us rely on theory to function in our relationships with family members, friends, professional colleagues, and others. In most cases, these theories are crude and not explicit; nonetheless, they exist, if only in our minds. Thus, to dismiss theory as useless is to fail to recognize its universal application, both in science and in everyday life.

In the behavioral sciences, the term *model* is often used in place of *theory*. According to West and Brown (2013), a model describes or represents something, such as an object, a set of events, or a narrow aspect of some behavior. Unlike a theory, however, a model is not well developed and does not necessarily explain anything. Models "fall short of being theories" because they often are isolated from other models and may remain somewhat ambiguous (Ryan & Deci, 2017, p. 6). Throughout this book, we use the terms *model* and *theory* interchangeably, and we distinguish between the two periodically.

The word *theory* is derived from Greek for viewing or serving as a spectator. Theory thus is an observation. It not only describes what has been observed; it speculates about the meaning of or explains that observation. In this sense, theories should offer new perspectives for understanding a certain body of knowledge, predict new possibilities, and, at the very least, provide a means for experimentation (Cottone, 1992). Although theory should not be thought of as "truth" or "fact," Cottone (1992) argued that theory implies a scientific ideal or a rational construction representing some form of reality. Think of theory as an explicit, comprehensive, and comprehensible account or explanation of something that has happened or continues to happen. This something can be a singular event (e.g., a solar eclipse) or a series of events (e.g., businesses closing in a local community). It also can be human behavior that is exhibited rarely (e.g., an acute psychotic episode) or repeatedly (e.g., smoking tobacco daily) by a few or a vast number of persons. These events, behaviors, and experiences are the observable phenomena that theory seeks to describe and explain. In so doing, an attempt is made to regulate these phenomena.

Theories are not predetermined by nature or data, or any other orderly process; they rest largely on a theorist's prior knowledge and creativity. Theory is understood further as a coherent and consistent body of knowledge (Prochaska & Norcross, 2018; Ryan & Deci, 2017) that, when applied to addiction, helps explain human behavior and change mechanisms. The function of theory is thus to organize and impose order and meaning on a collection of isolated observations, data, or facts (Ryan & Deci, 2017). In this respect, theories attempt to make sense of dissimilar findings and to explain relationships among variables of interest. In the study of addictive behavior, theory helps us understand its etiology and points to possible intervention strategies.

A theory is a tentative approximation of "the truth" (Prochaska & Norcross, 2018) and is provisional (i.e., it does not explain a phenomenon in absolute or final terms). It therefore is inappropriate to characterize it as "true" or "false" (Feist & Feist, 2009). Instead, it is best to describe a theory as "useful" or "not useful" (Hall, Lindzey, & Campbell, 1998), as well as relevant or irrelevant. A theory's utility and relevance can be assessed by its ability to (1) explain certain events in a cogent and cohesive manner and (2) generate ideas and concepts that enhance understanding. These two functions go hand in hand. A useful and relevant theory explains an observation and generates alternative explanations for new observations. This means that a useful and relevant theory is never permanent or impervious to change. Quite the contrary: It remains tentative and subject to revision; it is constantly in flux, depending on how it is tested. And by tested we mean its application over time to explain new developments, such as findings from scientific investigations.

The application of theory to science does not mean findings from research studies can "prove" or "disprove" a theory. Also, research findings, particularly from one or a handful of studies, do not "confirm" or "refute" a theory. This kind of thinking confuses the separate, though related, constructs of theory (i.e., abstraction) and empiricism (i.e., observation). Theory guides and explains observation, and observation guides theory development. Both are needed to enhance understanding of addictive behavior; they are complementary, and therefore one cannot dismiss the other. Although "the link between theory and data is extremely tenuous" (West & Brown, 2013, p. 28), it is important that persons devoted to understanding and changing addictive behavior (practitioners, family members, researchers, politicians, and community leaders) consult both sources of information: theories of addiction and empirical research. This book showcases both.

ATTRIBUTES AND FUNCTIONS OF A GOOD THEORY

Given the importance of a theory, it is worth considering what makes a good theory. What is it about a theory that makes it relevant and useful in practice? What criteria should a practitioner use to determine whether a particular theory is worth selecting to guide clinical decision making and plan interventions?

Theorists and researchers in the social and behavioral sciences (e.g., Ryan & Deci, 2017), including the addictions (e.g., West & Brown, 2013), have proposed that a good theory has at least eight attributes. Although enumerated in the following listing, they are not presented in any order of priority. Each describes the function of a good theory, that is, what a good theory should be able to do to be useful in practice. A good theory:

1. *Explains a related set of observations.* The explanatory function of a theory is crucial. More than simply describing a collection of observations (as a model does), a good theory explains the meaning or purpose of those observations by seeing beyond the visible to underlying connections. A good theory not only answers the question, "*What* is happening?" it goes further by attempting to answer the question, "*Why* is this happening?" A good theory thus is speculation about how and why a set of observations are related. It helps to make sense of observations by proposing connections that are not obvious, such as why a person who was surrounded by a strong support system and had been sober and in active recovery from drug use for 15 consecutive years would overdose and die from injecting heroin. Pursuing explanations for unconventional occurrences or complex phenomena is not a simple or convenient task. It can be arduous, and it requires patience and persistence. Doing so renders meaning and a sense of order to the set of observations.

2. *Is coherent and cohesive.* The connections that a theory comprises should logically "stick together." For example, a theory of social skills development in humans should account for both verbal and nonverbal forms of expression, not just one; it also should explain how these two forms of communication are connected. This makes a good theory internally consistent. It also helps explain to clients in a group session, for example, what makes a certain behavior effective, such as the social skill of refusing an offer to use a drug (i.e., not only *what* is verbalized, but *how* the message is conveyed nonverbally). A coherent and cohesive theory is solid rather than shaky and tight rather than loose.

3. *Is comprehensible.* A good theory is readily understandable. This means that its propositions can be clearly described and easily communicated. Ideally, theory will lift a cloud of confusion and replace it with clarity. A good theory represents a common language for researchers and

practitioners (Ryan & Deci, 2017). It makes it possible for professionals to communicate with one another observations that are made across settings and populations, and to anticipate and even predict certain events (e.g., relapse). Questions about how the propositions of a theory coalesce or fit together no longer need to be raised.

4. *Is explicit*. Precision is a chief characteristic of a good theory. Important theoretical concepts must be capable of being defined operationally. That is, concepts must be measurable with a high degree of reliability. Autonomous behavior is one such concept in self-determination theory (Ryan & Deci, 2017). It can be measured on the Index of Autonomous Functioning (Weinstein, Przybylski, & Ryan, 2012; also see *www. selfdeterminationtheory.org*), which has demonstrated acceptable reliability. Theories that rely on vague, ill-defined, or difficult-to-measure concepts cannot be checked against clear referents in the real world (Stefflre & Burks, 1979). For example, the popular terms *codependency* and *chemical imbalance* purport to explain certain aspects of addiction. However, neither has been operationalized or subjected to rigorous scientific study. They remain poorly defined concepts. Indeed, the "chemical imbalance" hypothesis as an explanation for depression has been refuted (Schultz, 2015) and has even been called a hoax (Carey, 2016).

5. *Involves no more concepts or elements than are necessary.* A good theory explains phenomena in a relatively simple and straightforward manner. It is concise and to the point; it is parsimonious. This means a good theory encompasses only essential ingredients; extraneous material is discarded as unnecessary. Describing addiction as a "brain disease" or a "chronic relapsing disease" comparable to diseases such as diabetes or hypertension (see Heilig, 2015) is one example of a parsimonious theory. It is straightforward and can be conveyed easily to and understood by others (e.g., clients in group counseling). Its premise and explanatory function, however, remain in question (Lewis, 2015, 2017; Peele, 2016). A theory that can explain behavioral events in innumerable ways is suspect. A theory that "overexplains" something may be creative, but it may also be fiction; it may not accurately reflect reality.

6. *Is comprehensive.* Although a good theory does not attempt to explain everything, it can be applied to many individuals in many different situations. A theory is not useful if it is isolated to only one occurrence at one point in time. A good theory should be able to explain events that extend across a variety of time periods, geographic areas, sociopolitical and sociocultural contexts, and sociodemographics (e.g., gender, race/ethnicity, religion). This function also speaks to a theory's relevance.

7. *Generates predictions that can be tested.* For a theory to remain relevant over time, it must be able to generate questions and offer predictions

that can be tested. Theories are always "under construction." A good theory is one that is responsive to feedback from empirical studies. This means theories must adapt to new observations or discoveries, such as recent empirical findings that mindfulness meditation improves emotion regulation and decreases drug use (Tang, Tang, & Posner, 2016). A good theory has a history of generating research findings (i.e., data) that support or are consistent with its concepts and further its enhancement. Theories that have little or no empirical support are less useful than those that have considerable data driving further investigation of their propositions.

8. *Is not contradicted by empirical evidence.* West and Brown (2013) maintain that for a theory to develop, mature, and endure, it must not be "overruled" by a competing theory; it must be able to stand alone. This attribute and function of a theory is necessary so as to eliminate nonuseful, opportunistic, and ephemeral theories. Subject to ongoing testing, a good theory must be able to explain "big observations" so as to exert its utility over time and across populations. Theories that persist despite overwhelming evidence to the contrary (i.e., existence of strong counterexplanations) may continue to serve as an important historical foundation for the study of addictive behavior, but they should be challenged and in most cases should not serve as conceptual frameworks for contemporary practice.

THEORY AS A ROAD MAP

Some time ago, Stefflre and Burks (1979) aptly summarized the attributes and functions of a good theory by likening it to a road map. Just as maps necessarily change to reflect alterations of the terrain, so too must theories change to account for new discoveries. In this way, a good theory not only explains what is known; it is revised based on new data and ideas. A good theory thus is sturdy *and* fluid, solid *and* malleable. It remains relevant by harnessing its dialectical functions of explanation and proposition. In a sense, a good theory is perpetually reinventing itself. And as it does, it serves to point practitioners and researchers in a direction that is clear and helpful. As Stefflre and Burks stated, "A theory is always a map that is in the process of being filled in with greater detail. We do not so much ask whether it is true, but whether it is helpful" (p. 9).

CONCEPTIONS OF ADDICTION IN U.S. HISTORY

Notable events in U.S. history have shaped today's conceptions of substance use and addiction. A review of these conceptions provides insight into how we have come to understand addiction in three distinct ways: as (1) immoral conduct, (2) disease, or (3) maladaptive behavior. In this section, you are encouraged to critically evaluate the historical conceptions of addiction by applying the eight attributes and functions of a good theory presented earlier. For example, for each perspective of addictive behavior mentioned in U.S. history, how clear, comprehensible, and parsimonious is it? Has the concept been contradicted by subsequent empirical evidence?

The Incongruent Views of Addiction

For most of American history, habitual drunkenness and drug use have been viewed as both sinful conduct and disease. In recent decades, they also have been considered maladaptive behavior or debilitative behavior that is "overlearned." Today, some insist that addiction evolves from all three sources: It is a *disease* in which people *learn* to act in *immoral* ways.

This incongruent view of addiction has a long history. Only in recent years, however, has this history been studied in a systematic way (Nathan, Conrad, & Skinstad, 2016; White, 2014). Addiction to alcohol has been the primary concern over time. However, the use of drugs other than alcohol (e.g., opiates, cocaine, marijuana) also has a lengthy history in the United States. Nevertheless, historical analysis of alcohol problems has garnered more attention in recent years, owing in part to the emergence of interest in the era of National Prohibition and the lessons it may provide in today's debate about the size and scope of the federal government. This historical review therefore emphasizes conceptions of alcoholism more so than other drug addictions.

Colonial Period and Reformation

In the United States, the conception of addiction to alcohol has been evolving since the colonial period (roughly 1607–1776). During that time, alcohol consumption in the populace was high (by today's standards), and inebriety was quite common (Burns, 2004). There was little concern about excessive drinking and drunkenness, and those who engaged in these behaviors were regarded simply as "distractions" from more important events (Weinberg, 2005). Even after the Revolutionary War and into the 19th century, Americans—having only recently gained their freedom from British rule—generally had a high tolerance for social deviance, and thus they were mostly indifferent to the problems caused by heavy drinking. Alcohol was used as a beverage, as medicine, as barter, and as a social lubricant. The town tavern was at the center of social and political life. Workers often drank throughout the day, and some employers actually supplied them with free liquor. Okrent (2010) reported that by 1830 each adult, on average, was consuming the equivalent of 1.7 bottles of 80 proof liquor per week, or roughly seven gallons of pure ethanol per year!

During the 17th century and for most of the 18th century, alcohol was not seen as an addictive substance, and habitual drunkenness was not viewed as a disease or a medical condition (Edwards, 2010). Moreover, frequent, heavy drinking was not understood to be a compulsion involving a so-called loss of control, nor was it considered a progressive, deteriorative disorder. Although most Americans considered excessive drinking to be of little importance, some prominent figures did warn about and chastise drunkenness. In these instances, it often was defined as a vice, as immoral behavior. In sermons, Puritan ministers warned that drunkards faced eternal suffering in hell, and although Cotton Mather referred to alcohol as the "good creature of God," he also described drunkenness as "this engine of the Devil" (Mather, 1708). In the 1760s, John Adams proposed restrictions on taverns, Benjamin Franklin described these establishments as "pests to society," and President George Washington labeled as traitors the "Whiskey Boys," who rebelled against the 1791 congressional tax on whiskey and other liquors (Gately, 2008; Rorabaugh, 1976).

With the dawn of the Enlightenment period and the Age of Reason in the United States (roughly the mid- to late 18th century), habitual drunkenness became a focus of concern and systematic inquiry. This was also true during the Georgian period in Britain, when England was ruled by four successive King Georges (1714–1830). The introduction of cheap distilled spirits to the working class and poor in England in the early 1700s led to an increase in public intoxication and diseases, a time in British history known as the "gin craze" (Warner, 2003). Although it was deemed immoral, the habit of drunkenness also came to be viewed as a type of disease state. It would be erroneous, however, to equate the very early understanding of *disease* with how it is often understood today—as a distinct pathology (Edwards, 2010). According to Porter (1985), *disease* in 18th-century Britain was understood as *dis-ease*—a state of discomfort or an imbalance in the human constitution (and relating primarily to bodily fluids) attributable to a lack of wholesome diet and proper exercise. In the late 1700s and early 1800s, the disease state of habitual drunkenness referred to the behavior itself, to the act of drinking in excess, and this behavior was only a concern because of the medical complications it caused, such as gout, jaundice, and depression. Thus, habitual drunkenness 200 years ago was not considered a medical condition or a disease in its own right. It was a disease by association only—that is, by the dysfunctions, disabilities, or diseases that it caused.

The first American to write extensively about habitual drunkenness as a type of disease state was Dr. Benjamin Rush, considered the father of American psychiatry (Brodsky, 2004). He was a Philadelphia physician, a signer of the Declaration of Independence, a Christian reformer, and surgeon general of the Continental Army who, in 1784, authored a pamphlet titled *An Inquiry into the Effects of Ardent Spirits on the Human Mind and Body*. In this work, Rush challenged the conventional view that habitual drunkenness was an innocuous activity. He did not condemn alcohol use per se, but rather its excessive consumption and drunkenness. Rush also confined his commentary to the excessive use of distilled spirits or hard liquor (specifically "grog" or rum, and "toddy"), not fermented alcohol (i.e., beer and wine), which he viewed as "generally innocent" and even having a "friendly influence upon life and health" when consumed in moderation (1790/1814/1943, p. 325). Rush acknowledged that "drunkenness resembles certain hereditary, family and contagious diseases" (p. 327), but he also inferred that the condition is actively acquired (i.e., becomes customary practice) and is not beyond the individual's control. For example, he described a gradual process of "contracting a love for distilled liquors by accustoming the stomach to their stimulus" (p. 333). He also categorized the death that results from habitual drunkenness as suicide, implying that intoxicated "self-murderers" (p. 329) were able to exert some measure of control over their circumstances. Furthermore, he believed that the "condemnation" received "at the day of judgment" (p. 329) would be far greater for those who died from habitual drunkenness than those who died from using opium (a substance he deemed to be "less injurious to the body and mind" than distilled alcohol).

Levine (1978, p. 152) contended that Benjamin Rush contributed to a new understanding of habitual drunkenness that included the contemporary understanding of alcoholism as a "loss of control" over drinking behavior and that its only "cure" was complete abstinence. A close review of Rush's writings, however, does not reveal a clear articulation of the involuntary nature of habitual drunkenness, and abstinence from all hard liquor is only one of 12 "remedies" that he identified to prevent further drunkenness. These remedies can be categorized as "religious, metaphysical, and medical" (p. 338) and included obeying Christian doctrine, feeling guilt and shame, eating vegetables, temporarily substituting beer or wine when abstaining from hard liquor (to assuage craving and withdrawal), and engaging in alternative behaviors on the days and times when one would customarily drink.

White (2014) agrees that Benjamin Rush is not to be credited with formulating "a fully developed disease concept of alcoholism" (p. 3), a concept that did not emerge in the United States until the 1870s. White argues, however, that "Rush's writings stand as the first articulation of a disease concept of alcoholism by an American physician" (p. 3). Levine (1978) stated that Rush is to be credited specifically with alerting Americans to the dangers of unrestrained drinking, or to what Rush referred to as the "evils produced by ardent spirits" (p. 329). Rush emphasized that alcohol misuse contributed to an array of social problems: disease, poverty, crime, insanity, and broken homes. In this regard, habitual drunkenness was a public health issue necessitating a comprehensive and multifaceted approach extending beyond the purview of medicine.

At about the same time as Benjamin Rush, Thomas Trotter, a recently retired British physician to the Royal Navy, proposed that "the habit of drunkenness" was a "disease of the mind," similar to delirium and mania. His 1804 *An Essay, Medical, Philosophical and Chemical, on Drunkenness and its Effects on the Human Body* was "a pioneering text and the first book-length treatise on what is today referred to as 'alcoholism' to appear in any language" (Vale & Edwards, 2011, p. 156). It earned him recognition as "the first scientific investigator of drunkenness" (Harrison, 1971, p. 92). Although Trotter may not have been the first British physician to refer to excessive alcohol consumption as a "disease" (according to Porter's [1985] historical review), his treatise appeared at a time when psychiatry was a nascent profession. He may be credited, therefore, with prioritizing medical and specifically psychiatric interventions for habitual drunkenness, more so than moral reform. According to Edwards (2010), Trotter challenged the medical community to assume ownership for the issue of habitual drunkenness, whereas Benjamin Rush appealed to Christian clergy to champion its fight. Over the course of history, however—in the United States and in Britain—both the medical and religious communities have been instrumental in defining alcohol misuse and its remedies, and this included their involvement in temperance societies.

The writings of Benjamin Rush and Thomas Trotter (and those before them; see Porter, 1985) contributed to the process of redefining "habitual drunkenness" from an exclusively immoral condition to one also influenced by physiological and mental dysfunctions and reflecting a medical disorder. This paradigm shift, however, took place over almost 150 years, and it was not until the late 1800s that excessive drinking was specifically referred to as a treatable disease. According to Tracy (2005, 2007), the shift in understanding habitual drunkenness is evident in four distinct terms that each held prominence in the American medical community at different times from 1870 to 1920: intemperance, dypsomania, inebriety, and alcoholism. *Intemperance* was the earliest of these terms that referred to problematic alcohol use as primarily an immoral condition. This was followed for a short period by the term *dypsomania,* a heritable medical condition similar to insanity that primarily affected the middle and upper classes. *Inebriety* then became the preferred descriptor, and it referred to an involuntary yet habituated condition, reflecting both medical and moral characteristics. The latest of these terms was *alcoholism,* which by its very name attributed the medical condition for the first time to the substance, alcohol, rather than to the behavior of the drinker. Although practitioners today may regard some or all of these terms as crass, Tracy (2007) proposed that all four terms "actually reflected a sophisticated understanding of alcoholism's etiology—one that acknowledged heredity, environmental circumstance, and individual temperament" (p. 88).

It is important to note that the different views of substance use throughout U.S. and British history are the direct result of changes in economic, political, religious, scientific, and other social conditions. Addictive behavior—then and now—cannot be studied and understood apart from these factors; it is not an isolated phenomenon. Substance use was therefore not the sole focus of reform efforts during the 18th, 19th, and into the 20th centuries in America and Britain. Economic development, governmental structure and political party formation, religious freedom, the institution of formal education, and public health and safety were all the essential ingredients of nation building. Although Rush addressed the issue of habitual drunkenness, his work also focused on education, abolition, the humane treatment of criminals and the insane, and an extensive array of physical illnesses. As a Christian reformer, physician, and politician, Rush produced work and writings that were instrumental to the Temperance movement in the United States, the largest campaign of the 19th century for moral and social reform.

Temperance Movement and Prohibition Period

The first Temperance Society was formed in 1808. Three years later a number of independent groups united, and in 1826 the American Society for the Promotion of Temperance (later renamed the American Temperance Society) was founded. Consistent with the views of Dr. Rush, the initial objective of the society was to promote moderation, not prohibition. To accomplish this objective, the society organized itself into local units that sent lecturers out into the field, distributed information, and served as a clearinghouse for movement information.

By the mid-1830s, over 500,000 Americans had joined the Temperance movement *and* made a pledge to abstain from all alcoholic beverages (Levine, 1978). In the 5 years after the 1840 founding of the non-Christian temperance fraternity, the Washingtonians, approximately 600,000 had pledged to refrain from any alcoholic beverages, including wine and cider (Tracy, 2005). The emphasis on moderation gave way to the necessity of abstinence for all citizens. Thus, the *temperance* movement became a *prohibitionist* movement, and increasingly habitual drunkenness or intemperance was seen as immoral conduct. Famous American huckster P. T. Barnum, who later founded the Barnum and Bailey Circus, was one of the most popular and outspoken campaigners for prohibition at this time. He drew crowds to his American Museum in New York City, which included "moral plays in a moral manner," with one act featuring an extreme case of alcohol-induced delirium and seizures (delirium tremens, or DTs) intended to scare the public into abstaining from all alcohol (Okrent, 2010). After the Civil

War (1861–1865), this view was also applied to opium and morphine, as well as to cocaine, which were all subsequently viewed as inherently addicting poisons.

Those in the Temperance Society worked hard to proselytize others, and to an extent they were successful. Employers stopped supplying alcohol to their employees on the job. Politicians were more restrained in their relations with alcohol producers and distributors. In many areas, local legislation was passed to regulate taverns—an outcome of lobbying by the society. Goode (1993) reported that between 1830 and 1840, annual alcohol use dropped from 7.1 gallons per person (age 15 and older) to 3.1 gallons. Support for temperance waned, however, during and after the Civil War (Tracy, 2005): The United States Brewers' Association was established 1 year after the war began, and the amount of alcohol consumed increased by 300% from 1850 to 1870.

It was not until the late 1800s that the Temperance movement experienced resurgence, most notably under the leadership of women, many of whom had experienced the debilitating effects (e.g., loss of family income and home; domestic violence) of the excessive drinking of their husbands and other male family members. The Women's Christian Temperance Union (WCTU) was founded in Cleveland, Ohio, in 1874 on the platform of "protection of the home" against the "ravages of alcohol." Although their efforts may have been to help reform the "habitual drunkard" through the Christian gospel and "moral suasion," members of the WCTU launched a strident "do everything possible" national campaign that included shutting down drinking establishments, supporting newly developed "cures" for inebriety, advocating against the use of alcohol in medical interventions, and changing workforce policies and practices.

For Frances Willard, the second and most famous president of the WCTU, habitual drunkenness was both a moral and a medical condition—the former, however, remained more important for her and her followers. The priorities or values of the WCTU are evident in the ordering of the words that comprise its name: It was first and foremost a women's organization "born of Christ's Gospel and cradled at His altars," whose purpose was "to help forward the coming of Christ" by prohibiting the traffic of "intoxicating drinks" (despite its use of the word *temperance*) and mobilizing "the total abstinence agenda" (excerpts from Frances Willard's speeches, cited in Gordon, 1898, pp. 131, 133, 139). The WCTU regarded "the drunkard as one who commits a crime against society" and therefore favored legal intervention and custody so as to imprint upon "the drunkard . . . the displeasure of the community in which he moves about as a perpetual danger" (see Gordon, 1898, p. 175). Given the WCTU's vehemently moralistic approach to habitual drunkenness, it is no wonder that Tracy (2007) declared it as "one of the most visible and powerful critics of the disease concept" (p. 88).

John B. Gough (1881), another prominent temperance lecturer, said that he considered "drunkenness as sin, but I consider it also disease. It is a physical as well as moral evil" (p. 443). These mixed medical–moral conceptualizations of inebriety were actually consistent with those expressed by physicians at the time. In her review of the history of alcoholism in America during the late 1800s and early 1900s, Tracy (2005) reported that upon the recommendation of Dr. B. N. Comings, a Civil War surgeon, the American Medical Association (AMA) adopted a resolution in June 1876 that inebriety was both a vice and a disease, even though one member contended that the moral failing was actually the disease. It is evident that the muddled conceptions of alcoholism that exist today have a long history.

In 1870, the American Association for the Cure of Inebriates (AACI) was founded in the United States. AACI members identified themselves more as scientists than as temperance leaders. Their main goal was to "reveal that [inebriates] were victims of a curable condition, worthy of public sympathy and medical care rather than punishment" (Tracy, 2005, p. 3). Four of their eight principles were:

1. Intemperance is a disease.
2. It is curable in the same sense that other diseases are.
3. Its primary cause is a constitutional susceptibility to the alcoholic impression.
4. This constitutional tendency may be either inherited or acquired.

These principles may have inspired Dr. Leslie E. Keeley, a surgeon for the Union Army during the Civil War, to boastfully proclaim in 1879 that "drunkenness is a disease and I can cure it." He proceeded to market a tonic to treat inebriety and also to open up over 100 institutions for its treatment, settings wherein male residents could experience camaraderie (similar to that experienced in taverns, minus the alcohol) to restore their dignity. Although Keeley was regarded as a charlatan by many in the medical community, he is credited with convincing the public that inebriety was a treatable condition. The opening of various state inebriate asylums in Massachusetts, Connecticut, Minnesota, and Iowa in the mid- to late 1800s also served to medicalize intemperance and spawn a new medical specialty.

It also was at this time that problems associated with the use of narcotics (e.g., morphine and other opiates) were more noticeable. Musto (1999) cited a committee report of the American Pharmaceutical Association that from 1898 to 1902 importation of cocaine and opiates (opium and morphine) had risen 40% to almost 600%, respectively, even though the American population had increased by only 10% in that time period. The invention of the hypodermic needle led to an increase in morphine addiction in the late 1800s. It was generally believed that physicians were the primary cause of their patients' drug addiction in their efforts to treat such maladies as cholera and dysentery, as well as obstetrical and gynecological problems. This form of physician-assisted addiction is known as *iatrogenic addiction*. Iatrogenic addiction has received renewed scrutiny in the midst of the current opioid epidemic in the United States. As Beauchamp, Winstanley, Ryan, and Lyons (2014) noted, "Physicians undoubtedly, and in most cases unknowingly, contributed significantly to recent increases in opioid-related morbidity and mortality" (p. 2023).

The dangers of morphine and other opiates were balanced by their effective treatment of physical ailments, most notably in reducing pain and calming nervous conditions. The iatrogenic explanation for drug addiction, however, applied only to the wealthy and upper middle class, those who had access to and could afford medical services and whose "innocent" or "accidental" addiction could therefore be excused because of negligent physicians or "dope doctors." A "social contagion" explanation for drug addiction applied to the poor and the working class because of their involvement in prostitution, gambling, and other deviant and illegal behaviors. To address the concerns of drug addiction, Campbell (2010) reports that state and local government bodies and private philanthropic foundations funded research initiatives and established treatment facilities in the late 1800s, including the New York City Narcotic Clinic.

Despite these attempts to define and treat addiction as a medical condition in the 1800s and early 1900s, the moral campaign—or "moral contagion" (Clark, 2017, p. 5)—gained the upper hand. Physicians were not united in their belief that drug addiction (including its withdrawal syndrome) was an organic disease (Musto, 1999), and many believed that addicts who frequented their medical offices were troublesome and could not be trusted. The Harrison Narcotic Act, passed by Congress in 1914 and implemented in 1915, gave authority to the Internal Revenue Service to tax—and therefore to regulate—opiates, derivatives of the coca plant, and other drugs. Specifically, it forbade the purchase of narcotics by unlicensed persons and prevented the refilling of prescriptions containing narcotics (Kolb, 1928).

The Harrison Narcotic Act may have provided further momentum to the cause of alcohol prohibitionists, even though at the time alcohol and drugs, such as narcotics, were not viewed by many as equal vices. As Clark (2017, p. 6) writes: "The two groups—pathetic drunkards and dangerous dope fiends—supposedly had little in common." The increased consumption of alcohol at the turn of the century may have been reason enough for alcohol reformers to forge ahead. According to Okrent (2010), consumption of alcoholic beverages "exploded" in the late 1800s: it increased from 36 million gallons in 1850 to 855 million gallons in 1890. And from 1900 to 1913, per capita consumption of both beer and liquor increased by one-third (Blocker, 2006). Although the United States Brewers' Association in 1866 attributed domestic troubles, poverty, crime, and disease to the use of hard liquor, it referred to its own product—beer—as "liquid bread."

Temperance and prohibition leaders had reason to be concerned. The Anti-Saloon League (ASL), established in 1893 in Oberlin, Ohio, assumed the reins of the Temperance and Prohibition movements by maintaining an anti-alcohol focus. The ASL appealed to clergy (including popular evangelist and former professional baseball player Billy Sunday), engaged in inventive political maneuvering, and published and distributed mass propaganda (with messages conveying its moral authority). References to people and localities as either "wet" or "dry" signaled the transition from a goal of moderate and nonproblematic alcohol use to one of zero tolerance. This dichotomous thinking also promoted further divides—between poor and rich, black and white, native and immigrant. Although the inebriety of European immigrants (e.g., Irish) had been a concern for some time, World War I heightened specifically anti-German sentiment in the United States. This sentiment extended to those whose names were *Pabst, Anheuser,* and *Busch,* even though their brewery businesses were already well established. An ASL argument was that breweries were using grain that should be targeted for more wholesome purposes, such as food for U.S. soldiers. Interestingly, the ASL's efforts did not appear to blame men for the alcohol problem in as pronounced a manner as other reform groups did. Perhaps it was because the prohibitionist and the suffrage movements joined forces at this time to achieve their respective goals in 1920: National Prohibition became law (the Eighteenth Amendment to the U.S. Constitution) and women gained the right to vote (the Nineteenth Amendment to the U.S. Constitution).

The federal ban on all production, transportation, and sale of "intoxicating liquors" had a profound effect on how addiction was—and still is—understood and treated. Even though prohibitionists located the culprit of alcohol addiction in its "poisonous" beverage, the person who "allowed" himself or herself to become victim to excessive alcohol consumption (whether it was beer, wine, or distilled alcohol) still was viewed by the majority of the populace as morally depraved and deserving punishment. This was particularly true during a time when alcohol was not supposed to be readily available, a time that Blocker (2006) notes essentially "wiped out" a collective and successful industry (breweries and distilleries in particular; wineries less so). Granted, the habitual drunkard could still find alcohol. What he or she could not find was help when needed because most of the inebriate asylums had closed and mutual aid societies had dissolved. Clark (2017, pp. 4–5) cites a 1922 study that reported that approximately 80% of pre-Prohibition treatment facilities had by that time disappeared, closed, or begun treating other conditions. Only 27 inebriety treatment providers remained. Therefore, the moral victory achieved during Prohibition essentially "extinguished America's collective memory of the early movement to medicalize alcoholism" (Tracy, 2005, p. 275).

This included the memory of physicians. In 1917, the AMA adopted a resolution stating that medicinal alcohol lacked any scientific value. Only 5 years later (and only 2 years into Prohibition), the AMA essentially reversed itself by declaring that any restriction on the medicinal use of alcohol represented an interference with medical practice. Okrent (2010) reports that during Prohibition, physicians increasingly prescribed alcohol for various ailments, including asthma, cancer, diabetes, and even old age. Add to that the increased acquisition of sacramental wine (its production was exempted in the Eighteenth Amendment) by rabbis and priests during Prohibition. Prohibition thus served to showcase more than ever before Americans' conflicted attitudes toward alcohol and addiction.

Post-Prohibition and the Medicalization of Addiction

Blocker (2006) contends that the Great Depression of the 1930s was largely responsible for repeal of the Eighteenth Amendment in 1933. Widespread economic hardship—due in small part to the loss of tax revenue on beer and liquor manufacturing and sale—replaced alcohol as the explanation for human travails. Furthermore, Prohibition had been unsuccessful in eliminating alcohol consumption, and it was only moderately successful in reducing drinking: According to Okrent (2010, p. 148), the best estimates of authoritative scholars are that use decreased by 30% in the first decade of Prohibition. Blocker argues, however, that Prohibition did succeed in keeping drinking rates below pre-Prohibition levels until the 1970s. Even during World War II, when the federal government did not enforce stringent restrictions on the alcohol industry, drinking rates remained relatively low. Kolb (1928) claimed that drug addiction "decreased rapidly" during Prohibition. It could be said, therefore, that Prohibition was "partly successful as a public health innovation" (p. 241). But credit for decreased alcohol consumption also must be extended to the economic strain of the Great Depression, state (rather than local or federal) liquor control policies, ongoing labor reform, the founding of the Research Council on Problems of Alcohol in 1937 (financed by the alcohol beverage industry), and the founding in 1935 of what now is considered the largest and most successful self-help group in the world: Alcoholics Anonymous (AA). That a physician (Dr. Bob Smith) and an unemployed stock broker (Bill Wilson) would join forces, after a chance meeting in Akron, Ohio, to establish a fellowship based on Christian principles that would embrace and become synonymous with the disease concept of addiction symbolizes, quite profoundly, the enigmatic tapestry of addiction.

Although prohibitionists and members of AA were united in their efforts to prevent the destructive effects of alcohol, this was their only similarity. Prohibitionists believed that anyone could become an alcoholic, whereas AA members identified themselves as compulsive drinkers who had a unique constitution that prevented them from drinking "normally." Their problems stemmed from a yet undefined condition within themselves rather than from the pharmacological properties of ethanol. This condition was a type of "allergy" that induced excessive drinking. Dr. William Silkworth, a New York physician, proposed the "allergy" theory adopted by AA. In the AA's view, this distinctive condition set alcoholics apart from other drinkers. Furthermore, AA was established primarily to rehabilitate "drunkards" by welcoming them into a morally supportive fellowship of other—and recovering—drunkards, not by humiliating them or subjecting them to punitive measures. Such a welcoming community that offered a message of hope through personal testimonials was just the balm many habitual drunkards needed at the time, particularly those still scarred by their treatment as immoral outcasts during the self-righteous Prohibition movement. Publication in 1939 of AA's "Big Book" that outlined its founders' views on alcoholism brought further attention to AA. But the *Saturday Evening Post* cover story of AA in March 1941 is widely considered the primary reason AA membership quadrupled from 2,000 to 8,000 that year (Weinberg, 2005).

Scientific interest in chronic inebriety also increased after Prohibition, supported financially by the liquor industry (which was interested in diverting causation of alcoholism away from alcoholic beverages to the drinker) and by notable industrialists (e.g., John D. Rockefeller, Jr. and Andrew Carnegie) who favored alcohol taxation for their own financial gain. The Research Council on Problems of Alcohol was established in 1937, and the Yale Center of Alcohol Studies soon followed in 1941. Although these early, private research institutes did not support AA's adoption of the allergy theory of alcoholism, and AA was "quite cavalier about the relevance of science to their own work" (Weinberg, 2005, p. 58), these separate movements needed each other to promote their own interests. As Weinberg noted, the scientific community benefited from the popularity of AA because more research dollars were solicited from private foundations to study a condition that afflicted the middle class (not just "skid row bums") and was potentially curable (i.e., worth the investment). In turn, AA benefited from the scientific community's legitimization of alcoholism as a disease, albeit a heretofore nonspecific and elusive medical disorder that included certain characteristics within the drinker, chiefly "loss of control."

Due to the effects of the 1915 Harrison Narcotic Act and America's involvement in World War II and then the Vietnam War, drug addiction remained a focus of scientific inquiry. Prisons had become overcrowded with convicted narcotic users in the 1920s, and two penitentiaries or "narcotic farms" were established in the 1930s to relieve this burden: one in

Lexington, Kentucky; the other in Fort Worth, Texas. Placed under the federal jurisdiction of the Public Health Service, these facilities laid the groundwork for medicalizing drug addiction (Musto, 1999). Dr. Lawrence Kolb was the first medical director of the Lexington, Kentucky, facility and later worked for what would become the National Institutes of Health in Washington, DC. He proposed that drug addiction resulted primarily from preexisting psychopathology (e.g., "abnormal nervous makeup," neurosis, psychopathy; Kolb, 1928), whether or not addicts began their use "accidentally" to satisfy pleasure (classified as "pure dissipators") or to treat a medical condition, for which narcotics or amphetamines were prescribed. Although Kolb was criticized for what Weinberg (2005) described as "the veiled moralism of his own theories" (p. 67), he advocated for a medical approach to the treatment of drug addiction rather than punishment. This approach was challenged from 1935 to 1960 when anticommunist sentiment and fear of any efforts to undermine nationalistic fervor or patriotism contributed to an escalation in criminalization for drug use and drug-related behaviors. Ironically, it was during this same time that pharmaceutical companies were in their heyday developing and marketing a wide range of amphetamines for mental health conditions, such as depression (see Rasmussen, 2008). It was in 1953 that Narcotics Anonymous was founded in Southern California.

The civil rights movement in the United States and the counterculture of the 1960s represented a slight shift in tide toward drug addiction and also showcased a greater variety of addictive substances, namely, hallucinogens and marijuana, and in the 1980s, cocaine. This generated expanded considerations about the nature and causes of addiction. Although federally funded research on drug and alcohol dependence had been under the purview of the National Institute of Mental Health since its inception in 1948, it was only with the founding in the early 1970s of federal agencies devoted specifically to substance use issues that addiction research, treatment, and prevention gained prominence. Harold Hughes, a self-described recovering alcoholic and a member of AA, was elected in Iowa to the U.S. Senate in 1968 and was instrumental in passing through Congress the act that established the National Institute on Alcohol Abuse and Alcoholism (NIAAA) in 1970. According to Weinberg (2005), this legislation effectively "institutionalized the disease concept of alcoholism" (p. 62). The National Institute on Drug Abuse was established in 1973 and, in partial contrast to NIAAA, promoted the concept of drug addiction as a form of deviant behavior (Campbell, 2010). This sociological emphasis allowed researchers and policymakers to consider environmental factors (e.g., poverty, urban decline) more so than biological factors when explaining addiction. There is logic to a predominant focus on biological mechanisms (including genetic predisposition) to explain addiction when only one substance—alcohol—is considered. When a wide variety of substances classified under the nebulous heading "drugs" is the focus, however, explanations for addiction beyond "disease" are necessarily entertained.

The difficulty is that addiction as "disease" is not and never was confined to a biological or medical condition. Psychoanalytic or psycho-dynamic explanations of addiction in the 1940s and well into the 1960s included references to character malformation and deficits, such as having an infantile or immature and narcissistic ego incapable of accurate self-assessment. Clark (2017) describes the common psychiatric view of addic-tion at that time as "the expression of an underlying, individual psychologi-cal disturbance caused by insufficient psychosexual development" (p. 63). Alcoholics and addicts thus were viewed as infants who needed a type of "rebirth" that was overseen by persons in authority (e.g., professionals, recovering addicts) who provided so-called loving, yet firm, guidance. They also were branded as "liars" who were "in denial" about their addiction, and so treatment approaches necessarily included confrontation to "break through" their strong defense mechanisms. (Chapter 5 provides further dis-cussion of a psychoanalytic understanding of addiction.)

These characterizations persisted into the counterculture of the 1960s and 1970s, a time of great societal change in the United States. It also was during this time that prominent psychotherapies (e.g., Gestalt therapy, reality therapy, rational-emotive behavior therapy) endorsed direct and confrontational approaches (e.g., disputing "irrational thinking") to pro-mote client catharsis. It was believed that recovery from addiction could occur only by first uncovering "deeply rooted" and repressed beliefs and feelings and then encouraging clients to vent in dramatic fashion. Psycho-therapists and other helping professionals were not alone in adopting this approach; so did laypersons or paraprofessionals working in treatment programs.

One such treatment program was Synanon, founded in the late 1950s in Ocean Park, California, by Charles "Chuck" Dederich, a recovering alcoholic and former oil salesman. Dederich had benefited from AA but thought its nonjudgmental practice of sharing testimonials "was too gentle to affect heroin addicts hardened by criminal careers, underworld asso-ciations, and socially unacceptable substance choice" (Clark, 2017, p. 11). Like AA, Synanon was group-based and peer-led. Unlike AA, Synanon was a residential treatment program that operated according to strict rules and prioritized intense aggressive and confrontational tactics, including ridicule. Sessions focused on challenging residents to come face to face with their moral failings, substituting their ineffective defenses with new, healthy habits. Few viable treatment alternatives were available at that time, and science-based evidence was in its infancy. Unfortunately, despite the growth of evidence-based practices today, remnants of Synanon phi-losophy and practices persist in many U.S. addiction treatment facilities. Although confrontational practices now are more subtle compared to the outright confrontational methods of 60 or 70 years ago, nonetheless various forms of coercion remain.

Current Views of Addiction

Throughout U.S. history, addiction to alcohol or other drugs has consistently been viewed as a "hybrid medical–moral affliction" (see Tracy, 2005, p. 26). This remains true today. Despite 65 years of the American Psychiatric Association's recognition of substance-related conditions as mental disorders and the American Society of Addiction Medicine's definition of addiction as "a primary, chronic disease" (*www.asam.org*), advances in neurobiology and biochemistry, and findings from sophisticated behavioral and social science research (e.g., behavioral economics) that implicate conditioning and environmental factors (e.g., poverty) in the initiation and maintenance of addiction, the person who has become addicted to a substance is still often regarded as blameworthy and consequently is treated as a criminal in modern society.

Federal policies and practices have promoted this form of public excoriation of alcoholics and drug addicts. For example, the 1986 Anti-Drug Abuse Act signed into law by President Reagan drastically cut funding for treatment and research, while dramatically increasing funding for law enforcement to "fight drugs" and implement a "zero tolerance" policy. This moralistic and punitive view of addiction still guides alcohol and drug control policies today. For instance, drug courts "sentence" offenders to "treatment": Driving while intoxicated offenders are required to participate in treatment and/or attend AA meetings, employers make workers' continued employment contingent on seeking treatment, and some medical centers may not accept for liver transplantation individuals diagnosed with alcoholic liver disease. Such practices tend to impede progress toward developing widely shared social norms about acceptable and unacceptable substance use, and they spur acrimonious debates about public drug control policy. Peele's (1996) description of the "disease law enforcement model" is reminiscent of practices more than a century old, and it still applies today: "When public figures in the United States discuss drug policy, they generally veer between these two models, as if the debate is over whether we should imprison or treat drug addicts. The contemporary U.S. system has already taken this synthesis of the law enforcement approach to drug abuse and the disease approach almost as far as it can go" (p. 204).

Americans remain conflicted about alcohol and other drug use (e.g., marijuana) and perhaps increasingly about specific behaviors that can become addictive (e.g., gambling, video gaming). This ambivalence is likely due to the futility—or more precisely, the impossibility—of isolating a singular and direct cause of addiction. With respect to substance addictions, Kalant (2009) offers the following observation: "Addiction is not produced by a drug, but by self-administration of a drug; the difference is of funda-mental importance" (p. 781). He proposes a comprehensive, complex, and integrative approach to understanding substance addiction rather than the frequently used approach known as *biological reductionism*. Kalant con-tends that addiction can only be explained by considering multilevel factors from the molecular to the societal. This view is shared by Lewis (2015, 2017), who proposed a *developmental learning model* of addiction that highlights the brain's neuroplasticity as part of the process of learning—the learning of addiction and the learning of recovery. His model is discussed briefly in a later section of this chapter.

The American conception of addiction, particularly alcoholism, has for too long been defined by incongruous assumptions involving disease and morality. Neither perspective has supplanted the other, probably due, at least in part, to various interest groups seeing benefit in maintaining the incongruent medical–moral addiction model. For example, municipal court and common pleas court judges who oversee drug court programs routinely "sentence" "offenders" to drug treatment for a certain length of time (e.g., 1 year), and sentencing may include mandated attendance at mutual aid societies, such as AA. A more sophisticated debate about the nature of addiction, one free of moral overtones and disease labels, may be too controversial and uncomfortable. We believe it is necessary none-theless. In 2017, the peer-reviewed scholarly journal *Neuroethics* devoted one entire issue to the controversial topic of whether addiction is a brain disease. The 17 original articles in that issue present a sophisticated debate.

In practice settings, however, there does not seem to be much inter-est in entertaining the more complex perspective that addiction represents maladaptive behavior—behavior arising from interactions between char-acteristics of the individual and their environmental conditions. Such an analysis would include examining poverty, inadequate education, lack of employment, racism and other forms of oppression, and access to services. The prospects for this type of comprehensive analysis gaining traction are not bright, except perhaps in academic and scientific circles. Attempts to define addiction continue to stumble when challenged by the entanglements of personal responsibility and blameworthiness, reward seeking and brain circuitry, and disease and suffering. They intersect and are entwined by myriad contemporary social conditions, including (1) the politics of spe-cial interest groups, such as Mothers Against Drunk Driving; (2) relentless attempts to medicalize human behavior whereby pharmaceutical compa-nies and medical professionals benefit; (3) growing opposition to regulating economic markets and concerns about restrictions on personal liberties, such as the continued efforts to legalize cannabis use in the United States; and (4) persistent poverty coupled with growing income inequality and increasing health disparities. Much disagreement and confusion about the nature of addiction remain.

THEN AND NOW: THREE BROAD PERSPECTIVES ON THE NATURE OF ADDICTION

The preceding historical review of conceptions of substance use and addiction in U.S. history highlights three broad perspectives on the nature of addiction that remain "alive and well" today. These perspectives regard addiction as (1) immoral conduct, (2) disease, or (3) maladaptive behavior. All three of these perspectives, to varying degrees, were evident from the early Temperance days and into Prohibition, and they continue to be prominent today in public attitudes and professional circles.

Addiction as Immoral Conduct

The first set of beliefs maintains that addiction represents a refusal to abide by some ethical or moral code of conduct. Excessive drinking and drug use are considered freely chosen behaviors that are at best irresponsible and at worst evil. By classifying addictive behavior as sinful, one does not necessarily ascribe the same level of "evilness" to it as one would to rape, larceny, or murder. Nevertheless, in this view it remains a transgression, a wrong.

Note that this broad perspective assumes that alcohol and drug misuse (and other non-substance-related behaviors, e.g., gambling) are freely chosen. In other words, with respect to this sphere of human conduct, people have autonomy and are free agents: They have decision-making capacity and are able to control or regulate their behavior. Those who struggle with alcohol or drug use or gambling, for example, are not considered "out of control"; rather, they *choose* to use substances or to engage in activities in such a way that they create suffering for others (e.g., family members) and for themselves. Thus, they can be blamed justifiably for their addiction.

Because addiction results from a freely chosen and morally wrong course of action, the logical way to "treat" the problem is to punish the person, who is often referred to pejoratively as an alcoholic, addict, or offender. From this perspective, legal sanctions such as jail sentences, fines, and other punitive actions are seen as most appropriate. The addict is not thought to be deserving of care or help. Rather, addicts must face the natural (or societal) consequences of their actions. More often than not, this means punishment to rectify past misdeeds and to prevent further substance use or addictive behavior. Relapse is considered evidence of lingering evil in the addict; therefore, punishment is again needed to correct "slipping" or backsliding.

In the United States today, this perspective on alcohol and other drug use is typically advocated by politically conservative groups, law enforcement organizations, and some zealous religious factions. During political campaigns, candidates frequently appeal to this sentiment by proposing tougher legal penalties for possession and distribution of illicit drugs and for drunken driving. As is apparent in the historical review presented at the beginning of this chapter, U.S. history is marked by repeated (and failed) government efforts to eliminate addiction with such legal sanctions. The crackdown on Chinese opium smokers in the 1800s and the enactment of National Prohibition in 1920 are two noteworthy examples.

The addiction-as-sin perspective has several advantages as well as disadvantages. One advantage is that it is straightforward and clear; it is parsimonious (refer to the fifth attribute and function of a good theory mentioned earlier in this chapter). There is little ambiguity or murkiness associated with this stance. Furthermore, it is absolute; there is no need for theorizing or philosophizing about the nature of addiction. It is simply misbehavior, and as such it needs to be confronted and punished. Scientific investigation of the problem is believed to be unnecessary because that which must be done to correct it (i.e., implementing sanctions) is already well understood. From this perspective, society's inability to adequately address the problems of addiction reflects widespread moral decay. Proponents of the addiction-as-sin perspective typically call for a return to "traditional" or "family" values as the way to ameliorate the problem. This was the case in the campaign of the WCTU in the late 1800s and early 1900s, a campaign that continues today (see *www.wctu.org*).

The perspective that addiction is immoral, a sin, has at least three disadvantages. First, science suggests that addiction is anything but a simple phenomenon. Addictive behaviors have multiple origins, stemming from pharmacological, biological, economic, psychological, and social factors. The apparent complexity of addiction is underscored by the variety of diverse theories seeking to explain it (many of which are described in subsequent chapters of this book). Moreover, as science has begun to shed light on various aspects of addictive behaviors, it is clear that much still remains to be learned. The genetic vulnerability hypothesis (see Chapter 2), expectancy theories (see Chapter 7), and the purported stabilizing effects of alcohol use on family structure (see Chapter 8) are all cases in point.

Another disadvantage of the perspective that addiction is immoral conduct is that it is not at all clear that addiction is freely chosen. The disease models (see Chapter 2) maintain that exactly the opposite is the case. That is, excessive drinking or drug use represents being "out of control" or having impaired self-control (see Tang, Posner, Rothbart, & Volkow, 2015). In either case, the individual does not freely choose addictive behavior. Repeatedly engaging in compulsive behavior is not voluntary. A further point of departure is offered by the social and behavioral sciences, where, at least from several theoretical perspectives, a high rate of drug self-administration is understood to be under the control of social or environmental contingencies. These contingencies are usually external to the person struggling with substance use and are not under their personal control. Thus, both the disease models and the social and behavioral sciences challenge the notion that addiction is willful misconduct.

A third disadvantage of the addiction-as-sin position is that, as history suggests, punishment is an ineffective means of reducing the prevalence of addictive problems in the population. Aside from the issue of inhumane sanctions (which is a real possibility if a political majority adopts the moral view of addiction), a reasonably strong case can be made, based on historical precedents, that striking back at those who struggle with addiction via governmental authority simply does not work over an extended period of time. Law enforcement crackdowns often have the unintended effects of strengthening organized crime networks, creating underground markets, bolstering disrespect for the law, clogging court dockets, and overloading local jails and prisons (at substantial cost to taxpayers).

Addiction as Disease

The second broad perspective on addiction contends that excessive consumption of alcohol or drugs is the result of an underlying disease process (Detar, 2011). The disease process is thought to cause excessive drinking or drug use; the high rate and volume of use are merely the manifest symptoms of an existing illness. The exact nature of the illness is not fully understood at this point, but many proponents of disease models believe that it has genetic origins. For these reasons, it is hypothesized that individuals cannot drink or drug themselves into alcoholism or drug addiction. If the disease (possibly arising from a genetic vulnerability) is not present, then substance use disorders cannot develop, no matter how much of the substance is ingested.

The addiction-as-disease conception maintains that persons struggling with their substance use are victims of an illness. The afflicted individual is not evil or irresponsible; the person is ill or sick. And the illness or sickness is endogenous, which explains the reference to addiction as a *dispositional* disease (Miller, Forcehimes, & Zweben, 2011). Thus, substance use and behavioral addictions are not freely chosen. Excessive drinking, drugging, and gambling, for example, change the brain's neurochemistry, resulting in compromised decision-making capability and increased reliance on extrinsic sources for motivation and reward. The ability to self-regulate (e.g., delay gratification, not act on impulse) is jeopardized. A common feature of the disease conception is loss of control. This mechanism involves cravings that rob addicts of personal control. The power to resist temptation has disappeared (see West & Brown, 2013, p. 96).

Because alcoholics and addicts are seen as suffering from an illness, the logical conclusion is that they deserve compassionate care. And because the condition is considered a disease, medical treatment is appropriate.

Competent treatment, then, especially on an inpatient basis, is physician-supervised. Traditionally, treatment based on the disease models emphasized the management of medical complications (e.g., liver disease, stomach ulcer, anemia), as well as patient education about the disease concept and recovery.

Five groups of persons or organizations strongly advocate for the disease models of addiction: the (1) medical profession, (2) treatment industry, (3) pharmaceutical industry, (4) alcohol industry, and (5) recovery movement. For quite some time, critics have indicated that physicians have a vested interest in convincing society that addiction is a disease. As long as it is considered such, they can admit patients to treatment programs, bill insurance companies, and collect fees. This also is true for nonmedical treatment providers, such as counselors and social workers. Unless addiction is endorsed as a disease, many argue, professional treatment will wane. The pharmaceutical industry also strongly advocates for the disease models of addiction. If addiction is a disease similar to hypertension and diabetes, it is logical to assume that pharmacological interventions would be recommended to treat its symptoms (e.g., cravings) and stabilize the condition. The pharmaceutical industry has taken full advantage of this logic, with support from the medical profession. Although extremely unsettling, it is unfortunately not surprising that the increase in overdose deaths in the United States between 1999 and 2010 directly corresponded to the dramatic increases in the sale of opioid pharmaceuticals in those same years (Beauchamp et al., 2014). To add salt to the wound, these same pharmaceutical producers now manufacture medications to counter the negative side effects of their opioid medications, such as opiate-induced constipation. This seems a cruel cycle.

Another group that endorses addiction, specifically alcoholism, as disease is the alcohol industry (i.e., the brewers, distillers, and winemakers). As long as it is a disease suffered by only 10% of all drinkers, then government entities will not take serious steps to restrict the manufacture, distribution, sale, and consumption of alcoholic beverages. Note that the alcohol industry wants the public to believe that the problem lies in the alcoholic (i.e., consumer), and not in their alcohol products.

The final group that strongly supports addiction as disease is the recovery movement, composed of individuals and families in recovery, including members of AA and other 12-step mutual aid societies. From this group's perspective, calling addiction a disease makes it more respectable than labeling it a moral problem or a mental disorder. It also can serve to reduce possible guilt or shame about past misdeeds, thereby allowing recovering individuals to focus on the work they need to do to establish and maintain a healthy life.

The disease models have several advantages. Most importantly, addiction is taken out of the moral realm, and its victims are helped rather than scorned and punished. In addition, society is more willing to allocate resources to help those who have a disease than to individuals who are merely wicked. It also is clear that the disease models have helped hundreds of thousands of alcoholics and addicts return to healthy living. Thus, its utility in assisting at least a large subset of addicts is beyond question.

The disease models have a number of disadvantages as well, only a few of which are discussed here. (Chapter 2 includes a more extensive discussion of them.) Briefly, several of the key concepts have not held up under scientific scrutiny. For example, the loss of control hypothesis, the supposedly progressive course of alcoholism, and the belief that a return to controlled drinking is impossible are all propositions that have been seriously challenged by scientific investigations. Within the scientific community, it is acknowledged that these assumptions are not well supported by empirical evidence. And many have argued that the disease models of addiction do not refer to a condition that is strictly biomedical in etiology and treatment (Lewis, 2015, 2017; Tracy, 2007). Unfortunately, substantial segments of the prevention, treatment, and recovery communities do *not* appear to use research as a guide for practice.

Addiction as Maladaptive Behavior

The third broad perspective on addiction is that it is a form of maladaptive behavior. This means that addictive behavior is shaped by the same laws that shape all human behavior. Essentially, addiction is learned. And this learning takes place not only at a cognitive level; it also occurs neurologically or neurochemically. Lewis (2015, 2017) maintains that engaging in rewarding behaviors (whether addictive or nonaddictive) results in the formation of new synapses (known as synaptogenesis) as well as the depletion of synapses (known as pruning). This change in brain circuitry is a form of learning, and, in the instance of addictive behaviors, this learning is maladaptive in that it is not healthy or beneficial. Lewis (2017) describes addiction as "the repeated pursuit of highly attractive goals and the brain changes that condense this cycle of thought and behavior into a well-learned habit" (p. 12).

Addiction as a "well-learned habit" is neither sinful (as the moral model purports) nor out of control (as the disease models purport). Instead, from a maladaptive perspective, addiction is seen as an inability to adjust to healthy living conditions, a maladjustment that consequentially presents significant environmental, family, and social stressors. Furthermore, as in the disease models, individuals with an addiction are considered victims, though not victims of a disease. From the maladaptive perspective, the "victimhood" of addiction results from the destructive living and learning conditions in which persons find themselves, such as early childhood trauma and impoverished and crime-ridden neighborhoods. Addictive behavior as maladaptive behavior is, for the most part, not freely chosen, although some social and behavioral science theories (e.g., social-cognitive theory) do assert that addicts retain some degree of control over their problem behaviors and that addiction is a failure of self-regulation in a challenging environment.

It is important to understand the value placed on objectivity in the social and behavioral sciences. When addiction is described as a *maladaptive behavior,* this is very different from describing the condition as *misbehavior* (a moral perspective). Social and behavioral scientists retain a neutral stance and avoid passing judgment on the "rightness" or "wrongness" of addiction. *Maladaptive* is used to convey a behavior pattern or habit that is thought to have harmful or destructive consequences for persons struggling with an addiction, their families, and society. It does not imply that addicts are bad, sinful, or irresponsible persons.

In the social and behavioral sciences, both preventive efforts and treatment interventions are based on learning principles, and both attempt to help individuals modify their lifestyle by enhancing behavioral skills, such as improving healthy decision making and delaying gratification. Change mechanisms also target the social conditions in which they live, and formats for doing so can be group- and family-based, as well as individual. Multilevel interventions combine individual-level change strategies with those that seek to change conditions in neighborhoods, business practices, workplaces, and communities. Policy interventions also are key components of multilevel interventions. Professionals in the social and behavioral sciences (including public health) are most heavily involved in these approaches to prevent and treat addiction.

Interventions attempting to influence the social environment and the behavior of individuals are labor-intensive and evaluation-focused. Thus, professional practice ideally should be theoretically informed, data-driven, and subject to frequent modification. Although these characteristics are consistent with today's emphases on efficiency and accountability, many prevention and treatment programs are slow to adopt this kind of empirical approach (Miller, 2009). Today, facilitating the adoption of evidence-informed practice is variously described as *research translation, technology transfer,* and *diffusion of innovation.* Each phrase has somewhat different meanings, but they all refer to processes by which new products and services are moved from research settings to practice settings and consumer markets.

EVIDENCE IN SUPPORT OF PREVENTION AND TREATMENT

A major problem in U.S. drug control policy today is the lack of awareness, among both the general public and political leaders, that comprehensive and competently administered prevention programming and addiction treatment are effective in addressing problematic substance use; that is, prevention and treatment do "work." This is true for universal school-based prevention programs that focus on a combination of social competence and social influence and not on knowledge about drugs. These types of school-based programs have been found to reduce any drug use, including marijuana (Faggiano, Minozzi, Versino, & Buscemi, 2014). Furthermore, Swensen (2015) calculated that for each 10% increase in the number of treatment facilities in the United States, mortality is lowered by 2%. Despite these and other findings that prevention and treatment services reduce substance misuse and its consequences (including death), federal funding to control illegal drug use remains invested in law enforcement and interdiction first, followed by treatment and prevention (U.S. Office of National Drug Control Policy, 2016).

Why advocate for drug abuse prevention? Since 1989, a number of well-controlled preventive interventions have identified effective approaches to deterring tobacco, alcohol, and illegal drug use among youth. Among these seminal studies are those that found support for school-based interventions (Botvin, Baker, Dusenbury, Botvin, & Diaz, 1995; Ellickson, Bell, & McGuigan, 1993) and community-based approaches with parent and school components (Pentz et al., 1989; Perry et al., 1996). Some of the lessons learned from these early trials that remain true today are that positive program outcomes decay over time and, as a result, ongoing "booster sessions" are essential to maintain gains. Of course, such additional services require resources, commitment, and collaboration among communities, schools, and parents. Another finding of the studies from this era that remains important today is that perceived peer norms mediate between program activities and outcomes. Prevention programming appears to be effective to the extent that it can instill conservative norms about substance use. Stated in another way, if youth are influenced to perceive that substance use is uncommon (not prevalent) and is socially unacceptable among their peers, they are less likely to initiate or continue substance use.

Existing research also provides a strong rationale for greater public support of substance abuse treatment programs (Cao, Marsh, Shin, & Andrews, 2011; Carroll et al., 2011). In 1999, the National Institute on Drug Abuse established the National Drug Abuse Treatment Clinical Trials Network (CTN) to bring together clinical practitioners and researchers to identify ways to increase the relevance of research in practice and to foster the adoption and dissemination of evidence-based treatment practices (see *www.nida.nih.gov/ctn*). By 2017, CTN had completed 50 trials testing pharmacological, behavioral, and integrated treatment strategies involving more than 24,500 clients. In one study, Ball and colleagues (2007) tested a brief motivational enhancement therapy (MET) treatment against a brief counseling as usual (CAU) control condition in a multisite randomized clinical trial. A total of 461 outpatient clients were treated in five outpatient programs by 31 treatment practitioners. The study found no retention differences between the two brief intervention conditions. The results indicated that both three-session treatment conditions produced decreases in substance use during the 4-week treatment phase. However, MET produced sustained reductions over the subsequent 12-week period compared to the CAU condition, which was associated with significant increases in substance use during this follow-up period. Further examination of the findings revealed that MET produced more sustained substance use reductions among primary alcohol users than among primary drug users. Overall, the results showed that brief MET is an effective strategy for helping clients with substance abuse problems. Further studies of MET are discussed in Chapter 11.

In another CTN study, Petry and colleagues (2005) examined the efficacy of an abstinence-based contingency management intervention in eight community-based outpatient treatment programs. The 415 clients were cocaine or methamphetamine users who were randomly assigned to a usual care control condition or a usual care plus abstinence-based incentives treatment condition for a 3-month period. Those assigned to the treatment condition were provided with opportunities to win prizes for submitting drug-free urine samples. The lottery was set up such that those who achieved continuous abstinence increased their chances of winning prizes. Compared to clients in the control condition, those in the treatment condition (1) stayed in treatment significantly longer, (2) were more likely to submit stimulant-free and alcohol-free samples, and (3) were more likely to achieve 4 to 12 weeks of continuous abstinence (Petry et al., 2005). The study documents the viability and efficacy of using motivational incentives in community-based treatment settings. Free resources describing this intervention, including a video depicting its implementation in practice settings, are available at *www.bettertxoutcomes.org*.

For some time, treatment for substance-related addictions has been found to be cost-effective. The Rand Corporation (1994), for example, found that for every dollar spent on treatment, $7 was saved on crime-related costs and lost workplace productivity. A subsequent Rand study found that treatment was more cost-effective than either conventional law enforcement or mandatory minimum drug sentences in reducing both cocaine consumption and related violence (Caulkins, Rydell, Schwabe, & Chiesa, 1997). More recently, standard outpatient therapy supplemented by computer-assisted training in cognitive–behavioral therapy was found to be cost-effective in the outpatient treatment of substance dependence (Olmstead, Ostrow, & Carroll, 2010). Another study found that a one-session motivational intervention designed to assist alcohol-involved youth treated in a hospital emergency department, costing $170–$173, was found to save $8,795 per quality-adjusted life year in societal costs (Neighbors, Barnett, Rohsenow, Colby, & Monti, 2010).

The outcomes of the major prevention and treatment studies described here represent a small number of the evidence-based practices that have been validated by researchers. Although much remains to be learned, particularly about how to efficiently transfer research findings to community practice settings on a broad scale, it is clear that the approach and methods used in behavioral and social interventions make an important difference. Thus, a major challenge facing the addictions field is implementing evidence-based practices into in-service and formal training programs needed to prepare highly competent practitioners for the future. Chapter 12 addresses this challenge in more detail.

CHAPTER SUMMARY

Advances in scientific research and technology, recent and further changes to health care policy, and economic instability at the state and federal levels necessitating funding restrictions, have all helped to shape contemporary views of addiction and the design of interventions. Although the relationship between empiricism or science and theory is tenuous, as West and Brown (2013) suggest, it is clear that this relationship is symbiotic. This means that social, economic, and political conditions influence perspectives of addiction and, in turn, views or theories of addiction influence these trends and events. A prominent example in U.S. history is National Prohibition. Fueled by a Christian crusade of moral reform, the Temperance movement quickly turned into a political force that changed the U.S. Constitution and had a powerful effect on conceptions of alcoholism and the resources used to address the problem.

Because addiction is a complex condition, there are multiple explanations for its etiology, prevention, and treatment. Three broad perspectives, traced through the past 200 years of U.S. history, can help professionals frame and further develop their understanding of addiction. These perspectives see addiction as (1) immoral conduct, (2) disease, or (3) maladaptive behavior. In the subsequent chapters of this book, we discuss various theories of addiction associated with each of these three broad perspectives. In so doing, we present pertinent research to alert practitioners to the possible shortcomings and strengths of these theories, and we provide recommendations for prevention and treatment. We hope the theories presented herein serve as a useful guide for implementing effective intervention strategies in the prevention and treatment of addiction and, more broadly, addictive behaviors.

REVIEW QUESTIONS

1. How does theory contribute to (a) new knowledge, (b) science, and (c) practice?

2. What is the purpose of theory?

3. What are the attributes and functions of a good theory?

4. What have been the incongruent views of addiction in American history? To what extent has the conception of addiction changed over time? What views of addiction today are parallel to those earlier in American history?

5. What are the characteristics of the three perspectives on addiction that make them distinctive and logically exclusive of one another? What are the advantages and disadvantages of each view?

6. How are the interests of different groups of persons or organizations aligned with the different views of addiction?

7. Which broad view of addiction has received less attention in scientific and treatment circles and among the general public than the other two broad views? What explains this?

CHAPTER 2

The Disease Models

In the United States today, the predominant model for understanding alcoholism and other addictions is the view that these disorders are diseases (Barnett, Hall, Fry, Dilkes-Frayne, & Carter, 2017). This view is particularly strong within the treatment community and within self-help fellowships or mutual aid societies such as Alcoholics Anonymous (AA) or Narcotics Anonymous (NA). The vast majority of treatment programs rely on the disease (or medical) models for a conceptual base (McLellan, Lewis, O'Brien, & Kleber, 2000); it shapes the selection of treatment options and focuses the content of patient and family education. Thus, most treatment programs in this country require AA or NA attendance, advocate abstinence, teach that the disorder is a chronic condition, and so forth. To the credit of the treatment community, these efforts have lessened the stigma associated with addiction. Compared to 75 or more years ago, those experiencing substance abuse problems today are less likely to be scorned and more likely to be offered help.

However, it should be recognized that controversy has surrounded the disease concept of addiction. Some legal authorities insist that the use and abuse of drugs and alcohol are intentional acts that deserve punishment (Sessions, 2017). In such a view, substance abuse results from a lack of self-restraint and self-discipline. Herbert Fingarette (1988), a philosopher, maintained that the disease models are a myth that endures because it fulfills the economic or personal needs of some groups (i.e., the medical community and recovery groups, respectively). He strongly supported helping alcoholics or addicts but believed that the "disease myth" limited treatment options for many needy individuals. For many years, behavioral and social science researchers have questioned the validity of the models (e.g., Lewis, 2015, 2017; Peele, 1985, 2016) and have described them as patently unscientific (e.g., Alexander, 1988).

Confusion and disagreement about the nature of addiction persist today. This becomes most evident following revelations of addiction problems among public figures, such as celebrities in the entertainment industry, politicians, or sports stars. Such disparate views are not likely to be resolved in the near future. To evaluate these arguments and counterarguments knowledgeably, it is essential to understand exactly what is meant by addiction as a disease. Only then can the utility of this model be intelligently weighed and articulated in a clear manner.

DIFFERENT DISEASE CONCEPTIONS

Before the core concepts of the disease models are reviewed, it should be noted that there is not just one disease model. Over the past 40 years or so, a number of proponents of the models, though not necessarily in disagreement, have emphasized different elements. The differences can be striking. For instance, in the 1980s, V. E. Johnson's (1980) description of the dynamics of alcoholism progression differed from that described by Milam and Ketcham (1983), and later Vaillant (1990) provided yet another perspective. Disease models differ with respect to the importance placed on physical, psychological, and spiritual factors in the etiology of alcoholism. These different emphases are probably related to the authors' personal experience with alcoholism (i.e., whether or not they are recovering alcoholics) and their professional training (i.e., whether they are physicians, psychiatrists, or psychologists).

Peele (1996) provided a useful distinction for thinking about the different disease models that remains highly relevant. He suggests that there are relatively distinct *susceptibility* and *exposure* constructions. The susceptibility variant emphasizes that genetic factors play an important role in the development of substance dependence. These factors influence the individual's *vulnerability* to the disorders. In contrast, the exposure position holds that chemicals and their actions on the brain are the primary causes of addiction. This position asserts that addiction is a *brain disease*. Here, risk for the disease is determined by the extent to which the brain is exposed to drugs of abuse. These two disease models are not in conflict with one another; they simply represent different emphases. Each is discussed in detail in this chapter.

Also, it should be noted that the disease model favored by AA differs somewhat from that espoused by the medical community. The AA disease model stresses the importance of spirituality in the etiology of, and recovery from, alcoholism. Indeed, many AA members report that they are recovering from a "spiritual disease." Although many outsiders to AA consider "spiritual disease" an oxymoron (i.e., a figure of speech that is a contradiction in terms), many recovering persons feel that it accurately describes their drinking problems. AA encourages its members to find a "Higher Power" and to turn their will and life over to a supernatural being. These spiritual conversions are considered crucial to recovery.

In contrast, the medical community tends to point to the significance of biological factors in addiction. Physicians often emphasize the role of genetic susceptibilities, increasing tolerance, withdrawal symptoms, liver disease, brain abnormalities, and so forth. Of course, this biomedical approach is consistent with their training. It is not that they ignore spiritual elements; rather, they tend to give such factors less weight than, for example, laboratory test results.

There is another difference between the disease model of AA and that of the medical community. It is a subtle difference, and it is closely related to the dichotomy of spirituality versus science. In AA, members often use the disease concept in a metaphorical sense; that is, they describe their alcohol problems as being "like" a disease. In many cases, recovering individuals do not intend (or perhaps even care) to convey that they literally have a disease. They simply are attempting to express the idea that the experience of compulsive chemical use feels like having a disease. It is characterized by feelings of loss of control and hopelessness, conditions familiar to the victims of other diseases (cancer, heart disease, emphysema, etc.).

Most often, physicians do not use the term *disease* as a metaphor. They tend to use the term in a literal sense—that is, "Alcoholism *is* a disease." Consider the following statement by a physician who directed a chemical dependency rehabilitation program some time ago:

> Whether you become an alcoholic or not depends on genetic predisposition. We know the reason the compulsivity exists is because of a change in the endorphin and cephalin systems in a primitive portion of the brain. The reason for this disturbance in the biochemistry of the primitive brain is a predisposition. Nobody talks any longer about becoming an alcoholic. You don't become an alcoholic—you are born an alcoholic. (Talbott, 1989, p. 57)

As this discussion illustrates, the disease models are not a unitary framework for understanding addiction. However, despite nuances and ambiguities, certain concepts have traditionally represented the disease model of addiction. Let us examine these concepts in light of the current scientific literature.

TOLERANCE AND WITHDRAWAL

The two clinical features of substance dependence that are commonly viewed as disease symptoms are tolerance and withdrawal. Drug *tolerance* is the need to use increasingly greater amounts of a substance to obtain the desired effect. With regular use, tolerance develops to most of the commonly abused psychoactive drugs, including alcohol, cocaine, heroin, and LSD. Although some substance users may initially take pride in their ability to consume large amounts of a drug, increasing tolerance is regarded as an early symptom of dependence (Wessel, Martino-McAllister, & Gallon, 2009).

Acute drug *withdrawal* results when blood or body tissue concentrations of a substance decline following a period of prolonged heavy use (American Psychiatric Association, 2000). The duration, symptoms, and severity of withdrawal vary across drugs and according to the amount of the substance being consumed prior to cessation (Crevecoeur, 2009). Alcohol withdrawal, in particular, varies significantly in both its symptoms and severity (McKeon, Frye, & Delany, 2008). Clinical manifestations in alcohol withdrawal can range from insomnia to severe conditions such as delirium tremens (DTs) and possibly even death.

Prolonged use of most psychoactive drugs can produce a withdrawal syndrome (Crevecoeur, 2009). These include opiates, heroin, barbiturates, cocaine, and a variety of other substances. The exceptions are several of the commonly abused hallucinogens (LSD, psilocybin, and mescaline). The unpleasant symptoms of withdrawal provide motivation for the person to self-administer more of the drug to relieve or even to avoid discomfort.

The more contemporary view of addiction is that tolerance and withdrawal are not required for diagnosis of a substance use disorder (American Psychiatric Association, 2013). Tolerance and withdrawal are but two of the possible diagnostic criteria that need to be considered within the past 12-month period. The diminished emphasis placed on tolerance and withdrawal has occurred because a compelling body of research has shown that in both clinical and general population samples, substance abuse and substance dependence are not distinct disorders. Instead, their criteria are intermingled and exist on a single severity continuum (American Psychiatric Association, 2013). In many cases, the presence of withdrawal represents a more severe form of addiction. However, withdrawal symptoms (and tolerance) are not necessary for addiction to be diagnosed by a clinical practitioner.

GENETIC ORIGINS OF ADDICTION: THE SUSCEPTIBILITY MODEL

There is compelling evidence for the familial transmission of substance use disorders (e.g., Verhulst, Neale, & Kendler, 2015; Volkow & Baler, 2014). This familial transmission occurs via gene–environment interactions. The genetic factors probably operate through their effects on brain development, specific neurotransmitter systems, drug metabolism, tolerance, epigenetic processes, and other effects (Benowitz, St. Helen, Dempsey, Jacob, & Tyndale, 2016; Hart, Lynch, Farrer, Gelernter, & Kranzler, 2016; Volkow & Baler, 2014; Xu et al., 2016; Xu, Wang, Kranzler, Gelernter, & Zhang, 2017). The accompanying environmental influences are numerous and may include harmful home environments, inadequate parental monitoring and supervision, child–parent modeling processes, marital discord, social stress, and childhood trauma (Ajonijebu, Abboussi, Russell, Mabandla, & Daniels, 2017; Patterson, 1996). Thus, the clustering of substance abuse in families is determined by the confluence of genetic and environmental variables.

As noted in Chapter 1, the idea that alcoholism, in particular, has genetic origins can be traced back to the 19th century (Levine, 1978). More recently, scientists also have examined the role of genetic influence on other drugs of abuse. Interest in the general field of behavioral genetics has grown for three reasons. First, there is a large body of research showing hereditary influence on animal behavior. Second, the methodologically sound twin studies conducted since the 1980s have consistently found that genes contribute to the development of complex disorders, such as alcoholism. Third, and perhaps of greatest importance, there is a considerable amount of evidence indicating that genes and the environment jointly determine human behavior—particularly addictive behavior (Ajonijebu et al., 2017; Vanyukow, 2009).

Genotype and Phenotype

The study of genetics deals with characteristics that are transmitted from parents to their offspring via biological mechanisms. These characteristics are not acquired as a result of learning, modeling, socialization, or other postnatal experiences; they are hereditary or inborn. Such human characteristics as eye color and blood type are determined by genetic factors.

Genes provide the information that directs human cellular activity. They constitute the functional units of DNA that form the human genome. Research on the human genome has discovered that, on average, the DNA sequences of any two people are about 99.9% identical (Collins & Mansoura, 2001; Kwok, Deng, Zakeri, Taylor, & Nickerson, 1996). Nevertheless, the remaining 0.1% variation in sequences is extremely important because it represents approximately three million differences in the nearly three billion base pairs of DNA sequence. These differences in DNA sequence account for the many variations in visible traits, such as skin color and height, as well as for many unseen traits, such as susceptibility to addiction (Sankar & Cho, 2002).

Each person shares 50% of the genes of each parent in a unique arrangement that is different from that of both parents. This assemblage of genes is the person's "genotype." During both pre- and postnatal development, the individual is exposed to a variety of environmental influences. This interaction between genotype and environment generates an enormous number of individual traits and characteristics, which are referred to as the person's "phenotype." The phenotype, then, is the outcome of the interaction between genes and environment. It should be noted that fetal exposure to alcohol or other drugs is an environmental influence on the phenotype; fetal alcohol syndrome and related conditions among newborns are not genetic disorders.

Concerns about Genetic Determinism

During the last 20 years or more, advances made in the field of behavioral genetics have generated evidence to support claims that heredity plays a role in a wide range of human behavior. The popular press sometimes distorts these findings, with superficial reports describing an "intelligence gene" and a "violence gene" (Guo, Roettger, & Cai, 2008; Nisbett et al., 2012; Weiss, 2006). Too often, the magnitude of the genetic influence is exaggerated, or relevant environmental factors are unduly minimized, often as a result of ignorance about the interactive nature of each (Wilde, Bonfiglioli, Meiser, Mitchell, & Schofield, 2011). This lack of understanding also has fueled the mistaken belief in "genetic determinism." Clearly, for complex human traits, genes are not destiny but parameters of risk as well as protection. According to Kenneth Kendler, a behavioral genetics researcher, "genes and environment loop out into each other and feed back on each other in a complex way that we have just begun to understand" (Mann, 1994, p. 1687). More recently, Sellman (2009) has described the interaction of genetic and environmental factors this way: "Genes and environment are no longer viewed as separate entities, but interconnected intimately as a continuum in the mysterious dance of life" (p. 7). The important point is that genes operate in a probabilistic manner in addictive behavior (Vanyukov, 2009). They are not deterministic factors.

Addiction as a Polygenetic Disorder

Some disorders, such as sickle cell anemia and cystic fibrosis, are caused by mutations or errors in a single gene (De Boeck et al., 2006; Fitzsimmons, Amin, & Uversky, 2016). In these diseases, the presence of a single mutation predicts the presence of the disorder regardless of the environmental conditions to which a person is exposed. However, most common diseases such as cancer, diabetes, and heart disease are polygenetic, involving variations in multiple genes, as well as the influence of environmental exposures, all of which contribute to a person's overall level of risk or protection (Vink, 2016). In these cases, mutations elevate risk, or one's liability, for developing disease; that is, the presence of a mutation may increase the likelihood of disease occurrence but not determine its outcome with certainty (Krammer et al., 2017). Addiction is an example of one of these complex health disorders that are produced by an interaction of multiple genetic and environmental factors.

SNPs

Single-nucleotide polymorphisms (SNPs—usually pronounced "snips") are the most common form of genetic variation in human beings (National Institutes of Health, 2017). The human genome is made up of approximately 10 million SNPs. They are studied because they can be used to mark the genes associated with disease. Sometimes SNPs are located in a gene or in a regulatory region near a gene. In these situations, they may play a role in disease occurrence by affecting the function of the gene. Researchers also use SNPs to track the inheritance of risk genes within families. Genomewide association studies (GWAS) and whole genome sequencing are advanced technologies used today to identify linkages between sets of genes and a disorder.

Epigenetics

Epigenetics is the study of changes in organisms caused by environmental alterations of gene expression rather than by changes in the genetic sequence itself (Nestler, 2014). The postconception exposures that humans have to a wide range of physical and social conditions in the environment can actually transform the DNA structure at the cellular level or even at the level of the whole organism. In other words, the dynamic environment in which a human is located can modify the expression of genetic information without changing their fixed DNA coding sequence. From an evolutionary perspective, epigenetic processes exist to meet the need of multicellular organisms, including humans, to adapt to their environment without depending on slow genetic mutations that might require multiple generations (Volkow & Baler, 2014). Not only can epigenetic processes have negative impacts on human health, they can also influence the expression of traits passed down to children. Research has shown that the damage caused by substance abuse is not restricted to the user. The substance use can "mark" genes that increase the addiction susceptibility of the user's children. According to Ajonijebu and colleagues (2017), "Epigenetic signatures, early life experience and environmental factors, converge to influence gene expression patterns in addiction phenotypes and consequently may serve as mediators of behavioural trait transmission between generations" (p. 2735). Thus, both genetic and environmental factors are important in addiction etiology, and their respective contributions cannot be easily teased apart.

EFFECTS OF DRUGS ON BRAIN STRUCTURE AND FUNCTION: THE EXPOSURE MODEL

Cell Activity of the Human Brain

Cells of the brain are known as *neurons*. Figure 2.1 illustrates the structural features of a presynaptic and postsynaptic neuron. It should be noted that this figure depicts only two neurons and thus is quite simplistic. In the brain, each neuron forms synapses with many other neurons and, in turn, receives synaptic connections from an equally large number of neurons.

The brain's signaling functions are primarily conducted by the neurons of the brain. There are approximately 86 *billion* neurons in the human brain (Azevedo et al., 2009) that provide the capacity for sensation, movement, language, thought, and emotion. Although neurons in different parts of the brain vary in size, shape, and electrical properties, most share the common features that appear in Figure 2.1. The cell body containing the nucleus holds the cell's genetic information. Dendrites are the treelike projections that integrate information from other neurons. Many neurons have a single axon that conducts electrical signals away from the cell body. At the end of each axon, branches terminate at a microscopic, fluid-filled gap known as the *synapse*. Thus, this electrochemical system consists of neurons that are separated by very small synaptic gaps (see Figure 2.2).

Vesicles located at presynaptic axon terminals release brain chemicals, known as *neurotransmitters,* into the synapse in response to electrical

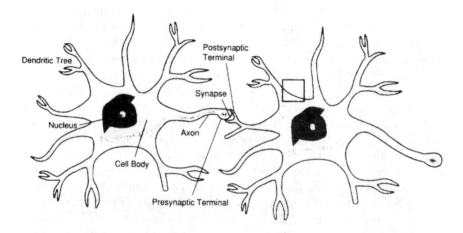

FIGURE 2.1. Structural features of presynaptic and postsynaptic neurons. This schematic drawing depicts the major components of neuronal structure, including the cell body, nucleus, dendritic trees, and synaptic connections. From National Institute on Alcohol Abuse and Alcoholism (1997).

stimuli. Homeostatic mechanisms attempt to maintain the appropriate concentration or balance of particular neurotransmitters in the synapse. One mechanism involves the action of enzymes that break down available neurotransmitters. (*Enzymes* are specialized proteins that serve as a catalyst for a specific chemical reaction.) When the concentration of a neurotransmitter becomes too great, enzymatic activity in the synapse increases to reduce it. A second mechanism is known as *reuptake*. Here, presynaptic "pumps" draw neurotransmitter molecules back into vesicles located at presynaptic terminals. This reabsorption process intensifies when the concentration of neurotransmitter in the synapse becomes too great. In tandem, the processes of enzymatic activity and reuptake work to maintain optimal neurotransmitter concentration.

Postsynaptic axon terminals (see Figure 2.2) receive and respond to the particular neurotransmitter they are designed to operate. There are target areas for the neurotransmitter molecule at the postsynaptic terminals. These target areas are known as *receptor sites* or just *receptors*. Typically, each neurotransmitter has an affinity for a specific type of receptor, and their relationship has often been described as akin to that of a key (the neurotransmitter) to its lock (the receptor). In some cases, a receptor may recognize more than one chemical. Nevertheless, the design of the receptor is such that it usually responds only to the specific molecular structure of its neurotransmitter. The postsynaptic terminals respond to the diffusion

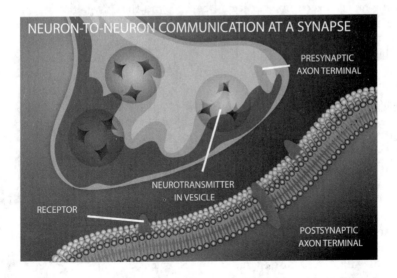

FIGURE 2.2. A typical synapse in the human brain showing the presynaptic and postsynaptic axon terminals of two neurons. Adapted from the News Image Bank of the National Institutes of Health (available at *https://imagebank.nih.gov*).

of neurotransmitters across the synapse by sending an electrical signal toward their cell body. In this way, the neurons "communicate" or relay information to one another in a highly rapid manner.

Mesolimbic Dopamine Pathway: The Brain's Reward Center

Many drugs stimulate reward circuitry in the brain known as the *mesolimbic dopamine pathway* (Lingford-Hughes, Watson, Kalk, & Reid, 2010; Pierce & Kumaresan, 2006). This pathway extends through several regions of the brain and is composed of a system of neurons that operates primarily on a type of neurotransmitter known as *dopamine*. From an evolutionary perspective, the forces of natural selection are thought to have fostered development of this reward circuitry to reinforce those behaviors most necessary for survival, such as eating food and having sex. The mesolimbic system can be considered the neurobiological substrate that produces pleasure. Unfortunately, many drugs also commonly stimulate reward centers in this system. Thus, the mesolimbic dopamine system is implicated in addiction. Other chemical pathways, using serotonin and glutamate, also are implicated in the reinforcing effects of particular drugs, but these are not reviewed here.

As can be seen in Figure 2.3, the mesolimbic system arises in the ventral tegmental area in the brainstem and projects to the nucleus accumbens in the ventral striatum and the frontal cortex. The system then consists of the nucleus accumbens, frontal cortex, and the amygdala. The nucleus accumbens is implicated in the expectation and pursuit of rewards, such as the "high" accompanying drug use. The frontal cortex supports the human abilities to evaluate stimuli, weigh the pleasure produced by an action, and activate impulse control. The amygdala is responsive to the intensity of pleasure and pain, and is involved in the human ability to associate pleasurable experiences with neutral environmental stimuli.

Most drugs of abuse directly or indirectly alter the brain's reward circuitry by flooding it with the neurotransmitter known as dopamine. The pleasure associated with dopamine release reinforces the act of drug self-administration, that is, drinking, smoking, injecting, and so on. Thus, without thinking about it, users want to repeat taking a drug because they quickly learn that pleasure will follow. Over time, this motivation to use a drug strengthens while interest in other natural rewards weakens. For these reasons, addiction can be thought of as an overlearned behavior or activity driven by dopamine release.

Elevated levels of dopamine in the nucleus accumbens are associated with the rewarding effects of all common drugs of abuse, with the possible exception of the benzodiazepines (Koob & Le Moal, 2001). In the ventral striatum, the euphoric effects of stimulants are associated with dopamine increases (Volkow, Fowler, & Wang, 2003). Elevated dopamine levels

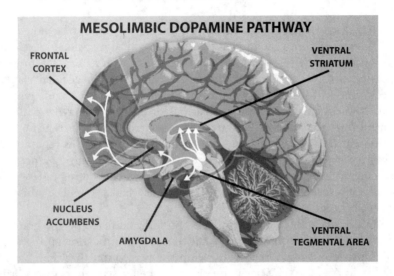

FIGURE 2.3. The mesolimbic pathway transmits dopamine from the ventral tegmental area to other regions of the brain. This pathway is activated by many drugs of abuse and by some non–substance-related behaviors such as pathological gambling. Adapted from the News Image Bank of the National Institutes of Health (available at *https://imagebank.nih.gov*).

have also been observed in relation to nicotine and alcohol use, but these findings are not consistent (Boileau et al., 2003; Montgomery, Lingford-Hughes, Egerton, Nutt, & Grasby, 2007).

The Neurobiological Basis for Development of Tolerance

In nonaddicts, repeated drug exposure is associated with elevated levels of dopamine, which make the mesolimbic reward pathway more sensitive, that is, effective at producing euphoria (Boileau et al., 2003). However, in a chronic addictive state, dopamine levels gradually decrease over time, making the mesolimbic system less sensitive and thereby producing deficient rewards. The user often responds by attempting to increase his or her dopamine release by using larger and larger doses of the drug, which only exacerbates the addiction. This is the process of increasing tolerance. These changes in reward circuitry sensitization may be the neurobiological basis for addicts "wanting," but no longer "liking," the effects of a drug (Berridge & Robinson, 2016; Blum, Gardner, Oscar-Berman, & Gold, 2012).

The biological purpose of the mesolimbic system probably is to mediate reward and pleasure and to create motivation to engage in life-sustaining tasks (e.g., eating and reproduction). However, it should be noted that motivation has both cognitive and emotional dimensions. Cognitive expectations in the form of anticipated reinforcement arise from previous life experiences and influence motivation. It is likely not an accident that our expectations of future events are formed in the prefrontal cortex, which is linked to the nucleus accumbens. Previous drug "highs" may be preserved as memories, and they may motivate the user to engage in repeated self-administration of a euphoric substance. Furthermore, as this region of the brain becomes increasingly exposed to excess dopamine during a period of substance abuse, its natural production may decline, resulting in fewer and less sensitive receptors for the neurotransmitter. This is one mechanism for the development of drug tolerance.

As a result of these changes to the brain, the addicted person gradually relies more and more on the drug as the source of gratification and pleasure. In this process, addicts tend to develop the perception that they have an inability to regulate their desire for the drug (i.e., perceived loss of control). As interest in nondrug activities diminishes, involvement in drug-related behaviors increases. Drug seeking, intoxication, and recovering from the deleterious effects (e.g., hangover) typically become the central activities in the addict's life.

HISTORICAL DISEASE CONCEPTS

Addiction as a Primary Disease

In primary care medicine, addiction, especially alcoholism, is still described as a "primary disease" (G. D. Carr, 2011); that is, it is not the result of another condition. This is usually taken to mean that the disease is not caused by heavy drinking or drug use, stress, or psychiatric disorders; rather, it is thought to be the cause of these very conditions. In other words, heavy drinking/drug use, stress, psychiatric disorders, and so forth are secondary symptoms or manifestations of an underlying disease process known as addiction. If the drinking or drug use is stopped, it is believed that the symptoms will, for the most part, disappear (G. D. Carr, 2011).

This view is contrary to popular conceptions of addiction, especially of alcoholism. To take alcoholism as an example, many laypeople (even those who view alcoholism as a disease) feel that alcoholism results from abusive drinking, which in turn stems from irresponsibility, stress, or emotional problems. The disease models, properly understood, dispute these ideas (G. D. Carr, 2011). The models propose that alcoholics are not responsible for contracting their disease; the disease itself causes or drives the heavy drinking. Furthermore, a long-held belief in some recovery circles is that those drinkers who lack genetic susceptibility to the disease cannot drink themselves into alcoholism (Milam & Ketcham, 1983). This belief is consistent with research indicating that genetic factors may protect some individuals from alcohol dependence (Webb et al., 2011).

However, various lines of research have developed data that contradict the primary-disease concept for all alcoholics. For example, in clinical research circles, it has become widely accepted that multiple types of alcoholism exist (Johnson, 2010). Some early-onset types may be strongly associated with genetic factors, whereas late-onset forms may be triggered by stressful life events and problems in living. Furthermore, individuals with alcohol and/or drug problems fulfill the criteria for antisocial personality disorder at a much higher rate than what would be expected by chance (Fenton et al., 2012; Grant et al., 2006; Schuckit, 1989). This finding suggests that severe antisocial life problems may cause alcohol and drug addiction in some individuals.

Findings such as these suggest that the causes of addiction are multiple and mediated by both genetic and environmental factors. For each person with an addiction, a relatively unique combination of forces probably led to the development of his or her problem. Some cases may be strongly influenced by genetic factors; others may be mediated solely by environmental ones. In the future, the concept of "primary" disease is likely to be further restricted as various types of addictive disorders continue to be identified and their comorbidity with other psychiatric disorders is recognized to be a common phenomenon (see Chapter 4).

Loss of Control

Loss of control is a longstanding and central premise of the traditional disease model of alcoholism. Indeed, Step 1 of AA's "12 steps" is an admission that alcoholics are "powerless over alcohol" (Alcoholics Anonymous, 1981). It is asserted that the alcoholic's loss of control stems from some unknown defect or abnormality. This abnormality is described as a compulsion or an intense craving (Milkman & Sunderwirth, 1987). More rigorous examinations of drug urges and cravings have been conducted in cognitive psychology (see Chapter 7).

In the traditional disease model, the exact nature of the abnormal craving for alcohol is not claimed to be well understood, but the "Big Book" of AA teaches as follows: "We are equally positive that once he takes any alcohol whatever into his system, something happens, both in the bodily and mental sense, which makes it virtually impossible for him to stop. The experience of any alcoholic will abundantly confirm this" (Alcoholics Anonymous, 1976, pp. 22–23). As this passage indicates, the notion of loss of control is consistent with the subjective experience of many alcoholics. Why, then, do so many of the leading alcoholism researchers reject the concept?

Logical Inconsistency

Some time ago, Fingarette (1988) pointed out that the classic loss-of-control concept is illogical. This concept maintains that after a minimal amount of alcohol enters the body, all ability to control drinking disappears. If this were actually the case, an alcoholic would have no desire, cravings, or compulsion to drink when sober. Abstention from drinking and recovery from alcoholism would actually be quite easy. Fingarette observed:

> If the loss of control is triggered by the first drink, then the only hope for an alcoholic is to refrain from that first drink, that is, total abstention. But if loss of control is triggered only after the first drink, and not before, why should the alcoholic have any special difficulty mustering the self-control to simply avoid that first drink? Why should abstinence pose any special problem? (p. 34)

Long ago, practitioners recognized that many alcoholics would terminate use of disulfiram (Antabuse) in order to resume drinking several days later (Merry, 1966). Behavior of this type suggests that the loss-of-control construct is invalid because, at least among some alcoholics, the intention to drink is formed prior to any consumption. In such situations, binge drinking may not be impulsive at all but actually planned for a future point in time. Why is the hypothesis maintained that control is lost after consumption has begun? One can only speculate, but it may be related to the alcoholic's need to blame the drug (alcohol) or some unknown biological mechanism. If the hypothesis did not first require alcohol to be introduced into the body, the only possible explanations would be psychological or behavioral in nature. Proponents of the traditional disease model typically prefer to avoid nonbiological explanations.

Laboratory Experiments

For more than 30 years, evidence has shown that chronic alcoholics (including those who have previously experienced alcohol withdrawal sickness) can drink in a controlled manner in laboratory settings (Pattison, Sobell, & Sobell, 1977). A 1977 review of the alcoholism research literature found that in almost 60 laboratory studies, some involving experiments lasting as long as 2 months, alcoholics demonstrated no loss of control (Pattison et al., 1977). Fingarette (1988) points out that the amount of alcohol consumed by alcoholics is a function of the "costs and benefits perceived by the drinker—an observation that radically contradicts the idea of some overpowering inner drive that completely overwhelms all reason or choice" (p. 36). The contingencies (i.e., rewards and punishers) attached to drinking (as perceived by the drinker) appear to control the amount consumed. The arrangement of contingencies in three different studies involving alcoholics (Bigelow & Liebson, 1972; Cohen, Liebson, Fallace, & Allen, 1971; Cohen, Liebson, Fallace, & Speers, 1971) was summarized by Fingarette:

> One research team was able, by offering small payments, to get alcoholics to voluntarily abstain from drink even though drink was available, or to moderate their drinking voluntarily even after an initial "priming dose" of liquor had been consumed. (The larger the "priming dose," the less moderate the subsequent drinking, until a modest increase in the amount of payment offered prompted a resumption of moderation.) In another experiment, drinkers were willing to do a limited amount of boring work (pushing a lever) in order to earn a drink, but when the "cost" of a drink rose (i.e., more lever pushing was asked of them) they were unwilling to "pay" the higher price. Still another experiment allowed alcoholic patients access to up to a fifth of liquor, but subjects were told that if they drank more than five ounces they would be removed from the pleasant social environment they were in. Result: Most of the time subjects limited themselves to moderate drinking. (p. 36)

A common counterargument to these findings is that the drinking occurred in artificial or unnatural drinking environments (i.e., hospital units or laboratories), and thus the data have little relevance for understanding typical alcoholic drinking. In other words, drinking in a clinic under the observation of investigators radically affects an alcoholic's self-control and drinking behavior. This counterargument is faulty and does not adequately address deficiencies in the loss-of-control hypothesis. If it is proposed that the social setting or observation by others affects alcoholic drinking, it cannot be argued that loss of control stems from the effects of alcohol or some biological abnormality. Thus, even though the experimental settings may have been anomalous, the findings indicate that frequency and quantity of drinking among alcoholics are not determined solely, or even in a significant way, by ethanol or endogenous mechanisms.

Addiction as a Progressive Disease

In the classic disease model, addiction is believed to follow a "progressive" course (Talbott, 1989). That is, if alcoholics or addicts continue to engage in substance abuse, their condition will deteriorate further and further. Marital, family, work, and medical problems only worsen over time; they do not get better with continued use. Life becomes increasingly unmanageable.

Johnson (1980) put forth a widely adopted model of alcoholism that described the progression of alcoholism in terms of the alcoholic's emotional relationship to the drug. His scheme relied on four phases. The first two phases represent "normal" drinking, whereas the third and fourth are typical of alcoholic drinking. Johnson identified these four phases as

(1) learning the mood swing, (2) seeking the mood swing, (3) harmful dependence, and (4) drinking to feel normal.

In Phase 1, learning the mood swing, the drinker is initiated into the use of alcohol. In our culture, it usually occurs at a relatively young age. The drinking is associated with pleasant feelings. There are no emotional "costs" as a result of the consumption. In Phase 2, seeking the mood swing, the drinker purposely drinks to obtain euphoria. The amount of alcohol increases as intoxication becomes desired; however, in this phase, there are still no significant emotional costs or adverse consequences. In Phase 3, harmful dependence, an "invisible line" is crossed (Johnson, 1980, p. 15). In this first stage of alcoholic drinking, the individual still finds euphoria in excessive consumption, but there is a price to pay. Following each drinking episode, there are consequences (e.g., hangovers, damaged relationships, arrests for driving while intoxicated). Despite such problems, the alcoholic continues to drink excessively. In the last phase, the alcoholic's condition has deteriorated to the point that he or she must drink just to feel "normal." When the alcoholic is sober, he or she is overwhelmed by feelings of remorse, guilt, shame, and anxiety (Johnson, 1980); the natural tendency is to drink to block out these feelings. Johnson describes the alcoholic in this last phase as being at risk for premature death.

At about the same time, Milam and Ketcham (1983) described the progression of alcoholism in somewhat different terms. Their scheme focused more on physiological deterioration than on the emotional relationship with the chemical. It consists of three stages: (1) the adaptive stage, (2) the dependent stage, and (3) deterioration. The chief characteristic in the adaptive stage is increasing tolerance to the drug. Alcoholics believe that they are blessed to have such a capacity for alcohol because they experience no negative symptoms. They typically do not appear to others to be grossly intoxicated; thus, there is no apparent behavioral impairment. However, physiological changes associated with increasing tolerance are occurring, but the drinker is not aware of these changes (Milam & Ketcham, 1983).

The chief characteristic of the dependent stage is physical withdrawal. These symptoms build gradually during this stage. Initially, they are not recognized as withdrawal symptoms but are confused with symptoms of a hangover. To manage these symptoms "effectively," many alcoholics fall into a "maintenance drinking" pattern in which they drink relatively small amounts at frequent intervals to avoid withdrawal sickness. They usually avoid gross intoxication out of a fear of having their problem exposed to others (Milam & Ketcham, 1983).

The last stage, deterioration, is characterized by major medical problems. Various organs are damaged as a result of long-term heavy drinking. In addition to the liver, the brain, the gastrointestinal tract, the pancreas, and even the heart may be affected. These pathological organ changes will cause death if an alcoholic does not receive treatment (Milam & Ketcham, 1983).

Johnson's (1980) and Milam and Ketcham's (1983) cogent descriptions of the progression of alcoholism (and possibly other addictions) were not consistent with epidemiological findings, however. Studies in the 1980s and 1990s that examined large populations, rather than just those alcoholics who present themselves for treatment, indicated that alcoholism and other addictions do not follow a predictable sequence of stages in which the user inevitably deteriorates (National Institute on Alcohol Abuse and Alcoholism, 1990). On the contrary, so-called *natural remission* (disappearance of an alcohol problem without treatment) is not uncommon among men as they move into older age categories (Fillmore, 1987a). Furthermore, it appears that among males there is a relationship between dependence problems and alcohol-related social problems, on the one hand, and age, on the other. Generally, by the time men reach their 40s, alcohol problems have declined; in many cases, such men still drink but more moderately (Fillmore & Midanik, 1984). In women, alcohol problems appear to peak in the 30s (compared to the 20s for men). Also, women are more likely than men to display considerably higher rates of remission across all decades of life (Fillmore, 1987b).

Even among clinical populations (treated alcoholics and problem drinkers), evidence appeared to dispute the conception of alcoholism as a progressive disorder. For example, in Norway, Skog and Duckert (1993) tracked the drinking behavior of 182 alcoholics (men and women) over a 4½-year period following inpatient treatment, and that of 135 problem drinkers (men and women) over a 2¼-year period following outpatient treatment. All clients were assessed by a standardized alcoholism assessment instrument and by a personal interview that focused on patterns of drinking during the previous year. In the outpatient group, blood samples were collected and analyzed for a liver enzyme (gamma-glutamyl transferase, or GGT) that is responsive to the presence of alcohol. This was done to determine whether self-reported light drinking was actually the result of consistent underreporting (i.e., minimizing alcohol intake). The data analyses included the calculation of one-step transition matrices that estimated the likelihood that a participant would move from one level of drinking to another between two successive follow-up assessments.

Skog and Duckert (1993) found that 1 year following treatment, only 11% of the inpatients and 5% of the outpatients were abstinent. However, treatment appeared to have a substantial positive impact on the drinking practices of both client groups. At each follow-up, self-reported alcohol intake was considerably lower than at admission to treatment. This was true for both groups of clients. Among the outpatient group, liver enzyme levels were consistent with self-report intake—making it unlikely that the results (at least for this group) were biased by underreporting.

Although there was a good deal of change in the drinking patterns of individuals from one assessment interval to the next, the investigators could find no strong or clear trends for the groups as a whole (Skog & Duckert, 1993). Some participants were increasing their drinking, whereas a nearly equal number was consuming less. When change did occur, it most likely was to a "neighboring" consumption category (e.g., from abstinence to moderation). According to the investigators, "Very large and dramatic jumps are, in effect, unlikely. Hence, the data suggest that processes of change are reasonably smooth" (Skog & Duckert, 1993, p. 183). Furthermore, there was no evidence of loss of control or heavy consumption following periods of abstinence or light drinking, and heavy drinkers tended to gradually decrease their intake rather than quit abruptly. None of these findings fit with the conception of a "progressive disease." Skog and Duckert (1993) concluded that among treated clients, "the observed pattern of change more resembles an indeterministic (or stochastic) process than a systematic natural history of a disease" (p. 178).

An Alternative Model: Maturing Out

In the 1980s, Peele (1985) advanced the concept known as *maturing out* (still used today) to explain how many alcoholics and addicts give up substance abuse without the benefit of treatment or self-help programs. The term was coined earlier by Winick (1962), who sought to explain the process by which many heroin addicts cease using the drug as they grow older. Today, the concept has been applied more broadly to include alcohol and other drugs.

This natural remission is believed to be related to developmental issues. Peele (1985) suggests that addiction is a maladaptive method of coping with the challenges and problems of young adulthood. Such challenges may include establishing intimate relationships, learning to manage one's emotions, finding rewarding work, and separating from one's family of origin. Abuse of alcohol or drugs is a way to evade or postpone dealing with these challenges. Peele contends that as addicts tire of the "night life" and the "fast lane" and become more confident in their ability to take on life challenges (i.e., responsibilities), they will gradually (in most cases) give up substance abuse.

In a series of empirical studies, the process of maturing out was examined among a group of heroin addicts who had been admitted to the California Civil Addict Program during the years 1962–1964 (see Anglin, Brecht, Woodward, & Bonett, 1986). In 1974–1975, the investigators conducted a follow-up assessment of the original sample using a longitudinal retrospective procedure. The studies revealed that maturing out was prevalent in this population, but it was conditional on a number of factors. For example, 75% of "older addicts" and 50% of "younger addicts" had ceased heroin use if they lacked antisocial characteristics and were not involved in crime/drug dealing (Anglin et al., 1986). However, among those still involved in crime/drug dealing to some degree, there was no relationship between maturing out and age. Furthermore, younger addicts assessed as high in "personal resources"—an aggregate measure combining educational status, post–high school vocational training, employment history, and parents' socioeconomic status—were found to cease heroin use at a somewhat earlier point in their addiction careers (Brecht, Anglin, Woodward, & Bonett, 1987). Finally, participation in methadone maintenance facilitated maturing out more in older addicts than in younger addicts, but legal supervision had no differential effect across age categories (Brecht & Anglin, 1990).

Evidence also shows that the alcohol consumption of young adults tends to follow the process of maturing out. Similar to heroin, the process seems to be conditional on a number of individual characteristics and social variables. Gotham, Sher, and Wood (1997) assessed 284 college students, most of whom were seniors. Three years later, after all of them had earned a bachelor's degree, they were assessed a second time. At this follow-up, the cohort's frequency of weekly intoxication had dropped substantially. Three variables were associated with decreased college drinking: having a full-time job, being male, and being less "open to experience." Individuals who scored relatively high on a measure of extraversion were most likely to have continued a pattern of frequent intoxication during the 3-year period. In another study, Miller-Tutzauer, Leonard, and Windle (1991) conducted a 3-year longitudinal study of 10,594 individuals, ages 18–28. The purpose of their investigation was to examine the impact of marriage on alcohol use. They found that individuals tended to moderate their alcohol use prior to actually becoming married and that drinking continued to decline into the first year of marriage. This decline in alcohol use appeared to stabilize by the end of the first year. Miller-Tutzauer and colleagues concluded that the transition to marriage is often associated with maturation in drinking behavior.

Why did the disease model proponents contend that the course of addiction is invariably progressive in the face of evidence indicating that natural remission increases with age? This discrepancy can probably be traced to the fact that the disease models emerged from recovering alcoholics' first-person accounts and from clinical anecdotes. All these reports were given by alcoholics who recovered through AA or presented themselves for treatment. Such individuals probably represent just a subgroup of all persons with addiction problems. Thus, although the concept of addiction as a progressive disease may fit some alcoholics and addicts, it does not apply to most with these problems.

Addiction as a Chronic Disease

For many years, questions about the "chronicity" of addiction have been among the most controversial issues in the field and a source of tension between the treatment and research communities (Marion & Coleman, 1991; Peele, 1985). The disease models maintain that addiction is a chronic disorder, meaning that it never disappears (e.g., "Once an alcoholic, always an alcoholic"). The disease can be readily treated with sustained abstinence and growth within AA or NA, but it is never "cured." For this reason, most individuals in AA or NA refer to themselves as "recovering" rather than "recovered." In this way, substance dependence is likened to other chronic diseases, such as cancer, diabetes, or heart disease.

Abstinence from all mood-altering substances, then, is the imposed goal of most treatment programs in the United States (it should be noted, however, that caffeine and nicotine are not usually prohibited). In contrast, the research literature going back into the 1970s contains a large number of clinical studies indicating that controlled drinking is a viable treatment strategy for many alcoholics, particularly those of younger ages (e.g., Heather & Robertson, 1983; Miller, 1982; Sobell & Sobell, 1976). Furthermore, many contemporary evidence-based clinical strategies for helping persons with addictions do not impose treatment goals of abstinence on clients. Instead, therapy is viewed to be a collaborative process in which the client's autonomy is respected and behavior change targets are identified by the client (Tooley & Moyers, 2012).

Denial

Historically, the denial exhibited by the addict received a great deal of attention in the traditional disease model. According to Massella (1990), it is the "primary symptom of chemical dependence" (p. 79). Denial is best characterized as an inability to perceive an unacceptable reality; the unacceptable reality is being an "alcoholic" or an "addict." Denial is not lying. It is actually a perceptual incapacity—the most primitive of the psychological defenses. Denial protects the ego from the threat of inadequacy. George (1990) recognized that it also "protects the option to continue to use, which for the addicted individual is the essence of life" (p. 36). Further discussion of denial and other defense mechanisms is reviewed in Chapter 5.

Certainly, denial is a common aspect of alcoholism and other addictions. However, instead of narrowly defining it as a symptom of a disease, it is useful to take a broader view and to consider how other forces, in combination, foster its use (see E. S. Carr, 2011). For instance, the general social stigma attached to addiction is responsible in part for the frequent emergence of the defense. There are few labels today worse than that of *alcoholic* or *addict*. With this moral condemnation, it is no wonder that individuals unconsciously react the way they do when initially offered help. Another contributing factor is the coercive methods that are sometimes used to force clients into treatment. The use of confrontational procedures (e.g., family interventions, employee assistance program efforts, and group confrontation) to break down the denial may, in many situations, have the unintended effect of actually strengthening it.

This is not to say that substance abuse should be ignored or "enabled." However, it should be kept in mind that at least in some cases, denial is a product of well-intentioned coercion by "concerned others" or treatment personnel. To describe denial as a disease symptom is to ignore its social origins and the universality of its use by almost all humans, addicted as well as nonaddicted.

CHAPTER SUMMARY

The enduring value of the disease models is that they remove alcohol and other drug addictions from the moral realm. They propose that addiction sufferers should be treated and helped rather than scorned and ridiculed. Although the moral model of addiction has by no means disappeared in the United States, today more resources are directed toward rehabilitation rather than just toward punishment. The emergence of the disease models is largely responsible for this shift in resource allocation. Increasingly, it is being recognized that harsh penal sentences do little to curb substance abuse in our society.

The contributions of molecular genetics and neuroscience in recent years have begun to elucidate the genetic parameters of addiction. These developments will likely solidify the treatment community's conception of addiction as a disease state. If technological advances lead to implementation of genetic screening as a diagnostic tool, the credibility of the disease view may increase among the general public. From a public policy perspective, the more addiction can be attributed to genetic factors (as opposed to willful misconduct), the greater the likelihood of public support for increased resources being directed to treatment.

Putting science aside, another strength of the *classic* disease model is its simplicity. Recall from Chapter 1 that a good theory is one that is parsimonious. This applies to the traditional disease model: It can be taught to clients in a relatively simple and straightforward manner. Clients, in turn, are often comfortable with the disease conception because it is familiar. Most clients have known someone with a disease (heart disease, diabetes, etc.), so it is not a foreign notion.

The disease models provide the individual who is new to recovery with a mechanism for coping with any guilt and shame stemming from past misdeeds. This framework teaches that problem behaviors are symptoms of the disease process. The alcoholic or addict is not to blame; the fault rests with the disease process. As one alcoholic with many years in recovery once shared, "Calling it [alcoholism] a disease allows us to put the guilt aside so that we can do the work that we need to do."

The unwavering commitment to abstinence as the goal of treatment and sobriety as a way of life is a principle promoted by the disease models and a source of their strength as well. Clearly, the large majority of clients who appear for treatment would benefit most by complete abstinence from psychoactive drugs (other than prescribed medications). Hundreds of thousands, if not millions, of recovering persons have rebuilt their lives as the result of achieving and maintaining a sober life. In this regard, disease models are distinguished from other theories on addiction. On the issue of abstinence, the disease models are clear and direct. Other models dodge the issue a bit, do not address it directly, or contend that "it depends" on the individual client.

The weaknesses of the disease models have been identified throughout this chapter; they are not repeated here in detail. Simply put, some of the historical concepts of the disease models are not well supported by science. The notions that have been particularly discredited are that addiction is a progressive disease and that it involves a literal loss of control. Clearly, the best-supported proposition is that alcoholism and other substance use disorders have varying degrees of genetic etiology. However, as argued earlier, the fact that a human trait, behavior, condition, syndrome, or disorder is, to some degree, rooted in genes does not necessarily require us to think of it as disease (see Lewis, 2017). Furthermore, it is clear that environmental factors contribute greatly to all forms of substance use, misuse, and dependence.

The major limitation of the disease conception in general is that it gives too little emphasis to the impact of psychosocial variables and particularly the role of learning as etiological bases. Moreover, the classic disease model has contributed little to skill-based relapse prevention strategies that rely on learning principles to enhance coping. Subsequent chapters in this volume explore some alternatives to the disease models. None of them is without significant limitations either, as we will see.

REVIEW QUESTIONS

1. Why are the disease models of addiction controversial in many quarters?

2. How does Stanton Peele distinguish between types of disease models?

3. What is the relationship between genes and the environment in influencing complex human traits such as addiction?

4. What is the difference between genotype and phenotype?

5. With respect to genetics, how is addiction fundamentally different from sickle cell anemia and cystic fibrosis?

6. What does the study of epigenetics explain about genetic expression and the role of the environment in determining addiction?

7. What is the significance of the mesolimbic dopamine pathway for understanding addiction?

8. What is meant by addiction as a "primary disease"?

9. What is meant by "loss of control"?

10. Does research support the loss-of-control concept?

11. In what ways do research findings dispute the concept of alcoholism as a "progressive disease"?

12. What is meant by addiction as a "chronic disease"?

13. How is denial different from lying? What are the problems with calling it a "symptom" of a disease?

14. What are the strengths and weaknesses of the disease models?

CHAPTER 3

Public Health
and Prevention Approaches

WHAT IS PUBLIC HEALTH?

The World Health Organization (1998) provides two definitions of public health. The one-sentence definition simply states that public health is "the science and art of promoting health, preventing disease, and prolonging life through the organized efforts of society" (p. 3). The elaborated definition distinguishes between traditional and more contemporary conceptions of public health:

> Public health is a social and political concept aimed at improving health, prolonging life and improving the quality of life among whole populations through health promotion, disease prevention and other forms of health intervention. A distinction has been made in the health promotion literature between public health and a new public health for the purposes of emphasizing significantly different approaches to the description and analysis of the determinants of health, and the methods of solving public health problems. This new public health is distinguished by its basis in a comprehensive understanding of the ways in which lifestyles and living conditions determine health status, and a recognition of the need to mobilize resources and make sound investments in policies, programmes and services which create, maintain and protect health by supporting healthy lifestyles and creating supportive environments for health. Such a distinction between the "old" and the "new" may not be necessary in the future as the mainstream concept of public health develops and expands. (p. 3)

Public health is often contrasted with medicine: Public health is concerned with promoting and protecting the health of populations, whereas medicine is primarily focused on the care of individual patients.

A Brief History of Public Health in America

The earliest attempts to address public health problems in America can be traced to the colonies of the 17th century (Duffy, 1992). Infectious diseases brought by western European settlers were the chief health problems of that period. Smallpox, malaria, diphtheria, yellow fever, diarrheas and dysenteries, scarlet fever, cholera, typhoid, and other diseases were endemic in the colonial period and contributed to enormous suffering. For instance, in Cotton Mather's diary, the famous New England minister noted that his wife, three children, and a maid died during a single measles outbreak in the winter of 1713–1714 (Duffy, 1992, p. 11). Colonists treated disabling conditions such as malaria and some forms of dysentery with resignation, but the more deadly diseases, such as smallpox, were feared because they appeared without apparent explanation and killed at random.

At that time, and until the 1880s, infectious disease was not well understood. The prevailing medical theories employed a poorly defined concept known as *miasma,* which was thought to be an invisible, toxic matter coming from the earth or from rotting tissue or human waste, or other sources that contaminated the atmosphere and led to widespread illness and death (Stone, Armstrong, Macrina, & Pankau, 1996). Thus, the early approaches to improve the public health were usually confined to the cities and took the form of municipal sanitary regulations that sought to reduce overcrowding in city buildings, control the dumping of garbage, improve the disposal of human waste, manage livestock better, and so on. These regulations were typically reactive in nature; that is, they were enacted in response to a local outbreak of disease. Their enforcement was often inconsistent and subsequently ignored after an illness waned (Duffy, 1992).

As the U.S. urban population grew in the 1800s, health conditions in the cities deteriorated, particularly in impoverished sections of urban areas. Duffy (1992) noted that affluent families typically moved out of older parts of U.S. cities at this time, and they became filled with the poor. The great influx of immigrants from Ireland and other countries in the 1840s and 1850s made this situation worse. Often, entire families would live in small one- or two-room apartments. In most slum housing, the only water source was an outside well or standpipe, if the city had a water system at all. Frequently, multiple families would share a single toilet facility. Disease spread rapidly under these living conditions.

Public health advocates, often members of civic groups and sometimes well-educated, progressive physicians, led reform efforts in a number of cities during the 1800s (Duffy, 1992). Collectively, these reforms came to be known as the *sanitary movement,* the forerunner of the modern public health movement that became institutionalized in the early part of the 20th century. Despite being based on the erroneous miasmatic disease concept, the sanitary reforms were mostly successful in reducing the incidence of infectious disease. In contrast, medicine played little part (Duffy, 1992). These developments clearly showed that the private medical treatment of individual sufferers was not an adequate community response. To prevent disease, there was a need to (1) focus on the environment, (2) alter the living conditions of citizens, and (3) educate citizens about how to protect themselves and their community. The origins of the tensions between medicine and public health, then, can be traced to the sanitary movement.

By the turn of the 20th century, scientists had identified a number of pathogenic organisms that caused common infectious diseases, including the germs causing tuberculosis, typhoid, and diphtheria (Stone et al., 1996). This new *germ theory* gradually supplanted miasmatic theory and revolutionized both public health and medicine. Better management and inspection of food and water supplies, preventive vaccines, quarantine of the sick, and health education campaigns were remarkably successful in reducing the morbidity and mortality of common infectious diseases. Thus, public health began to rely more on science and research as a means to improve health conditions. However, even as more attention was given to scientific methods, the experience with tuberculosis and infantile diarrheas, in particular, forced public health officials to recognize that environmental factors and living conditions, often associated with poverty, remained important causal factors in the development of disease (Duffy, 1992). Thus, the "new public health" official could not retreat into a narrow science based on germ theory. Political advocacy and activities directed toward improving living conditions remained an important public health function (which continues today).

The 20th century saw a number of important developments in public health. One was the institutionalization of public health work. The federal government established a number of agencies with missions to focus on specific public health problems (e.g., the Substance Abuse and Mental Health Services Administration [SAMHSA]). Most of these agencies are under the umbrella of the U.S. Department of Health and Human Services (DHHS). State, county, and municipal public health departments were created as well.

Another development was the professionalization of the public health field. Civic groups and some physicians spearheaded most of the reforms during the sanitary movement of the 1800s. The 20th century witnessed the advent of formal public health training typically provided by schools of public health. Initially, much of this training was geared toward the physician. Today, many students receive training in public health without a background in medicine.

The scope of public health also expanded greatly in the last century. Though much effort remains directed at infectious disease, many other health concerns are the focus of public health practice today. Chief among these problems are tobacco, alcohol, and other drug use. Some of the other major public health issues today include HIV/AIDS, obesity, chronic disease, injuries and violence, and bioterrorism.

It is important to recognize that significant advances were made in public health during the 20th century (Centers for Disease Control and Prevention [CDC], 1999). Since 1900, the average lifespan of Americans has increased by more than 30 years, and 25 years of this increase can be attributed to public health efforts (Bunker, Frazier, & Mosteller, 1994). Without ranking them in order of importance, the CDC (1999) has identified 10 great public health achievements of the 20th century (see Table 3.1).

Philosophical Foundations of Public Health

For some time, the public health enterprise in the United States has been involved in debate about the best approach to promote health and prevent disease in the population. The debate can be traced to the different social philosophies undergirding these approaches (Nijhuis & van der Maesen, 1994). The dominant approach of the 20th century was medical science. However, the view that public health practice is but one of many subdivisions of the field of medicine has had severe critics (e.g., McKinlay & Marceau, 2000). Proponents of a more progressive model have argued that to further strengthen the health of the population, a paradigm shift is needed in which medicine is subsumed under the more comprehensive structure of the public health system (Nijhuis & van der Maesen, 1994).

Figure 3.1 depicts the competing visions of the public health enterprise. McKinlay and Marceau (2000) contend that the conventional public health model is driven by a social philosophy of individualism, a dominant

TABLE 3.1. Ten Great Public Health Achievements in the United States, 1900–1999

1. Vaccination
2. Motor vehicle safety
3. Safer workplaces
4. Control of infectious disease
5. Decline in deaths from coronary heart disease and stroke
6. Safer and healthier foods
7. Healthier mothers and babies
8. Family planning
9. Fluoridation of drinking water
10. Recognition of tobacco use as a health hazard

Note. From Centers for Disease Control and Prevention (1999).

perspective in the United States today that emphasizes the traits, motives, and actions of distinct individuals as the primary determinants of health status. In this traditional approach, medical science is viewed as the means to best promote and preserve the health of the population. An alternative model arises from a collectivist social philosophy that is more holistic and ecological and points to multilevel intervention activities (Levin, 2017). In short, the holistic/ecological conception recognizes that health is a dynamic state influenced by determinants both within and outside the individual.

The conventional strategies employed in the United States for preventing and treating tobacco, alcohol, and other drug abuse have mostly followed the individualistic approach noted in Figure 3.1. That is, intervention strategies focus on risk factors usually "within the skin" of the individual and have largely ignored multilevel strategies that seek to address community and environmental risk factors. Much of this chapter is devoted to reviewing public health and prevention approaches that rely on innovative, multilevel interventions.

The Triad of Causation in Public Health

The public health experience with tuberculosis in the early part of the 20th century made clear that the disease was not caused merely by the presence of a germ, in this case, tubercle bacillus (Duffy, 1992). Gradually, public health officials came to recognize that more than one factor contributes to the occurrence of disease. For instance, it is now known that many persons exposed to tubercle bacillus do not develop tuberculosis and that poverty, overcrowding, malnutrition, and alcoholism are important causal factors in its occurrence (Friedman, 2004). Thus, germ theory is an inadequate basis for understanding the development of disease and other health problems.

Social Philosophy		Conception of Health		Determinants		Public Health Activities
Individualism	→	Absence of disease	→	Physiological and lifestyle influences	→	Conventional medical care; early screening/detection; disease prevention; focus on treating patients
Collectivism	→	Holistic/ecological view of health	→	Physiological, lifestyle, social, and environmental influences	→	Advocacy for change in public health policies; increasing health care access; community-level intervention; health promotion initiatives; focus on population health

FIGURE 3.1. Competing visions of public health in the United States.

In public health, the triad model of causation involving *host, agent,* and *environment* is often used to explain the development of disease and other health problems. The model provides a better understanding of the interactive nature of the multiple factors that produce disease and other health problems, such as alcohol dependence. Although the agent (i.e., alcohol) must be present for dependence to occur, its presence alone does not produce alcoholism in an individual (the host). Hence, the agent, in this case alcohol, is best considered a necessary factor, but not a sufficient factor, for a health problem, in this case alcohol dependence (or alcoholism), to occur. As depicted in Figure 3.2, the triad model proposes that the multiple characteristics of the host (in this case the alcoholic) determine susceptibility or resistance to the agent (alcohol). In general, host characteristics include such factors as genetic vulnerability, age, attitudes and expectancies, and habits (lifestyle variables), but with disorders that tend to be chronic, such as alcohol dependence, the range of determinants can be very broad and complex (Friedman, 2004). In addition, health problems, such as alcohol dependence, are instigated or suppressed by the environment. Again, a wide range of environmental variables may be involved in the development of the disorder, including availability of the drug, community and peer drinking norms, and family influences. Furthermore, subsets of agent,

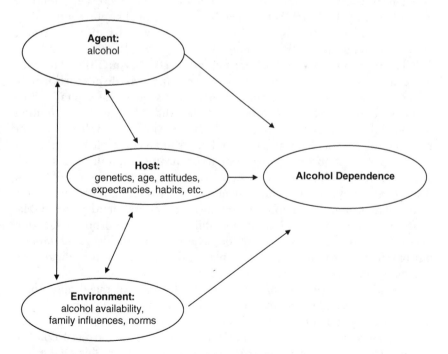

FIGURE 3.2. Agent–host–environment interaction model of alcohol dependence.

host, and environmental factors may interact to retard or promote disease and other health problems in specific populations. For example, Asian Americans appear to have lower rates of both alcohol dependence and drug dependence than other ethnic and racial groups in the United States (Hasin & Grant, 2015).

Health Disparities and Poverty

A central concern of public health is reducing the many health disparities that exist today in the United States and around the world. Health disparities refer to "differences in health outcomes that are closely linked with social, economic, and environmental disadvantage—are often driven by the social conditions in which individuals live, learn, work and play" (DHHS, 2011, p. 1). Although they are often associated with race and ethnicity, health disparities take place across many dimensions, including income/wealth, geographic location, age, gender, disability status, sexual orientation, and other population characteristics. Relative to whites and persons with higher incomes, African Americans, Hispanics, Native Americans, and lower-income groups often experience a wide variety of worse health outcomes, including colorectal cancer, asthma, binge drinking, diabetes, health-related quality of life, HIV infection, severe periodontitis, pregnancy and childbirth before age 20, preterm births, preventable hospitalizations, hypertension, tuberculosis, coronary heart disease, stroke, homicide, infant mortality, and motor vehicle-related death (CDC, 2013).

The root cause of health disparities is poverty (Levin, 2017). The public health consequences of poverty are many, and they disproportionately affect certain populations because they are the sequelae of capitalist economic systems based on the efficient, rather than the equal, distribution of material resources to individuals. In other words, capitalism was not designed to care for the health of populations in an equitable manner.

With respect to protecting population health, capitalism has social and structural weaknesses that operate as upstream determinants of health disparities. These determinants include, but are not limited to, income inequality, movement of jobs to low-income nations, inadequate public education, community and family instability related to corporate decision making, lack of access to healthy food, exposure to unhealthy and dangerous physical environments and workplaces, limited access to medical care, and many other conditions.

Health disparities not only increase health risks of racial and ethnic minority groups and the poor, but also limits the extent to which the health of the wider population can be improved so that unnecessary costs are reduced for society as a whole (LaVeist, Gaskin, & Richard, 2009). The urgency to address disparities is underscored by demographic changes in the U.S. population. Members of racial and ethnic minority groups are expected to make up over one-half of the U.S. population by 2043 (U.S. Census Bureau, 2012).

HEALTHY PEOPLE 2020: THE NATIONAL HEALTH PRIORITIES ON TOBACCO, ALCOHOL, AND DRUG USE

Healthy People 2020 is a public health initiative that has established a set of health objectives for the nation (DHHS, 2017). The initiative also monitors the progress made in achieving these objectives over the first decade of the new millennium. Its four broad goals are as follows:

1. Attain high-quality, longer lives free of preventable disease, disability, injury, and premature death.
2. Achieve health equity, eliminate disparities, and improve the health of all groups.
3. Create social and physical environments that promote good health for all.
4. Promote quality of life, healthy development, and healthy behaviors across all life stages (DHHS, 2017).

Healthy People 2020 (DHHS, 2017) developed more than 1,200 health objectives covering 42 topic areas. From these objectives, it selected 26 leading health indicators to identify the highest priority public health problems in need of action. A total of five leading health indicators address tobacco, alcohol, and other drug problems. Table 3.2 on the next page displays the baseline and 2020 target measure reductions for these indicators.

PUBLIC HEALTH SURVEILLANCE OF SUBSTANCE ABUSE

Public health surveillance is the ongoing assessment of the health of a community or population based on the collection, analysis, interpretation, and use of health data (CDC, 2017b). Surveillance work provides the factual information needed for public health decision making, program promotion, and public advocacy. The data generated from surveillance activities provide an empirical basis for establishing priorities and planning programs that might not be well understood by the public or may even be controversial because they often address sensitive topics (e.g., regulation of cigarette smoking in public areas and reducing HIV transmission). Furthermore, as Duffy (1992) has noted, throughout U.S. history the public's attention span to health issues has been short (p. 313). There is a continual need to maintain awareness of the importance of these issues among the public. The sustained, ongoing nature of surveillance programs serves the

TABLE 3.2. Healthy People 2020: National Objectives for Tobacco, Alcohol, and Other Drug Use

Topic area: Tobacco use

Tobacco use

1. Reduce tobacco use by adults.
2. Reduce tobacco use by adolescents.
3. Reduce the initiation of tobacco use among children, adolescents, and young adults.
4. Increase smoking cessation attempts by adult smokers.
5. Increase recent smoking cessation success by adult smokers.
6. Increase smoking cessation during pregnancy.
7. Increase tobacco use cessation attempts by adolescent smokers.

Health systems change

8. Increase comprehensive Medicaid insurance coverage of evidence-based treatment for nicotine dependency in states and the District of Columbia.
9. Increase tobacco screening in health care settings.
10. Increase tobacco cessation counseling in health care settings.

Social and environmental changes

11. Reduce the proportion of nonsmokers exposed to environmental tobacco smoke.
12. Increase the proportion of persons covered by indoor worksite policies that prohibit smoking.
13. Establish laws in states, District of Columbia, territories, and tribes on smoke-free indoor air that prohibit smoking in public places and worksites.
14. Increase the proportion of smoke-free homes.
15. Increase tobacco-free environments in schools, including all school facilities, property, vehicles, and school events.
16. Eliminate state laws that preempt stronger local tobacco control laws.
17. Increase the federal and state tax on tobacco products.
18. Reduce the proportion of adolescents and young adults, grades 6–12, who are exposed to tobacco advertising and promotion.
19. Reduce the illegal sales rate to minors through enforcement of laws prohibiting the sale of tobacco products to minors.
20. (Under development) Increase the number of states and the District of Columbia, territories, and tribes with comprehensive, evidence-based tobacco control programs.

Topic area: Substance abuse

Policy and prevention

1. Reduce the proportion of adolescents who report that they rode, during the previous 30 days, with a driver who had been drinking alcohol.
2. Increase the proportion of adolescents never using substances.
3. Increase the proportion of adolescents who disapprove of substance abuse.
4. Increase the proportion of adolescents who perceive great risk associated with substance abuse.
5. (Under development) Increase the number of drug, driving while impaired (DWI), and other specialty courts in the United States.
6. Increase the number of states with mandatory ignition interlock laws for first and repeat impaired driving offenders.

(continued)

TABLE 3.2. *(continued)*

Screening and treatment

7. Increase the number of admissions to substance abuse treatment for injection drug use.
8. Increase the proportion of persons who need alcohol and/or illicit drug treatment and received specialty treatment for abuse or dependence in the past year.
9. (Under development) Increase the proportion of persons who are referred for follow-up care for alcohol problems, drug problems after diagnosis, or treatment for one of these conditions in a hospital emergency department.
10. Increase the number of Level I and Level II trauma centers and primary care settings that implement evidence-based alcohol screening and brief intervention (SBI).

Epidemiology and surveillance

11. Reduce cirrhosis deaths.
12. Reduce drug-induced deaths.
13. Reduce past-month use of illicit substances.
14. Reduce the proportion of persons engaging in binge drinking of alcoholic beverages.
15. Reduce the proportion of adults who drank excessively in the previous 30 days.
16. Reduce average annual alcohol consumption.
17. Decrease the rate of alcohol-impaired driving (.08+ blood alcohol content [BAC])
18. Reduce steroid use among adolescents.
19. Reduce the past-year nonmedical use of prescription drugs.
20. Decrease the number of deaths attributable to alcohol.
21. Reduce the proportion of adolescents who use inhalants.

Note. From U.S. Department of Health and Human Services (2010).

important societal function of reminding the public about potential health threats and new emergencies.

Discussed next are three national surveillance systems of substance use operated by public health agencies of the U.S. federal government: the Youth Risk Behavior Surveillance Survey (YRBSS), which is a school-based survey of high school students; the National Survey on Drug Use and Health (NSDUH), which relies on a household survey; and the National Vital Statistics System (NVSS), which collects and disseminates the official vital statistics for the United States. Each relies on a different method to collect data from nationally representative samples of Americans.

Youth Risk Behavior Surveillance Survey

The CDC (2016) operates the YRBSS. The YRBSS collects self-report survey data on a biennial basis from a nationally representative sample of U.S. high school students (grades 9–12). The surveillance system monitors priority health-risk behaviors that have been documented to contribute substantially to the social problems, disabilities, and death of American youth and adults. The multiple behaviors that are assessed include tobacco, alcohol and other drug use, sexual behaviors, violence, safety behaviors, eating behavior, and exercise behavior. These behaviors also are associated with educational outcomes and dropping out of school.

The YRBSS was designed with multiple purposes in mind: (1) to determine the prevalence of health risk behaviors among high students; (2) to examine change in these behaviors over time; (3) to study the co-occurrence of health-risk behaviors; (4) to compare national, state, and local prevalence rates as well as those among subpopulations of adolescents (e.g., sex, age, and racial/ethnic groups); and (5) to monitor progress toward achieving national health objectives (DHHS, 2017). Table 3.3 shows the lifetime prevalence rates of each of eight drugs found in 2015 to illustrate the type of data collected by the YRBSS.

In addition to documenting the relatively high prevalence of substance use among American high school students, the surveillance data in Table 3.3 reveal several noteworthy patterns. First, with the exception of inhalants, drug use prevalence rates generally increase with grade level. Second, alcohol is the most commonly used drug, followed by electronic cigarettes and marijuana, then nonmedical use of prescription drugs. Third, inhalant use generally decreases with grade level. Findings such as these can be useful for establishing prevention priorities and designing programs of intervention.

National Survey on Drug Use and Health

Another example of a national surveillance system is the NSDUH (Center for Behavioral Health Statistics and Quality, 2015). Formerly known as the National Household Survey on Drug Abuse, this surveillance survey is

TABLE 3.3. Percentages of High School Students Using Each of Eight Drugs in Their Lifetime: United States, Youth Risk Behavior Survey, 2015

Grade	E-Cigarettes	Alcohol	Marijuana	Nonmedical use of prescription drugs	Inhalants	Cocaine	Synthetic marijuana	Hallucinogens
9	37.2	50.8	25.9	13.0	8.3	3.4	7.1	5.2
10	43.3	60.8	35.5	15.3	7.5	5.1	8.8	7.7
11	49.5	70.3	45.2	18.9	5.9	5.0	10.0	9.2
12	50.9	73.3	49.8	20.3	6.0	7.2	11.0	11.3

Note. Data from the Centers for Disease Control and Prevention (Kann et al., 2016). Nonmedical use of prescription drugs category includes: Oxycontin, Percocet, Vicodin, codeine, Adderall, Ritalin, or Xanax. Inhalants measure used the following prompt: "Sniffed glue, breathed the contents of aerosol cans, or inhaled any paints or sprays to get high." Cocaine category includes crack. Hallucinogens category includes LSD, acid, PCP, angel dust, mescaline, or mushrooms.

managed by SAMHSA. Conducted since 1971, the NSDUH is the primary source of data on the incidence and prevalence of tobacco, alcohol, and other drug use in the civilian, noninstitutionalized population 12 years of age and older in the United States. Data are collected in all 50 states and the District of Columbia.

Each year, about 67,500 face-to-face interviews are conducted in a representative sample of U.S. households (Center for Behavioral Health Statistics and Quality, 2015). Introductory letters precede the interviewer visits to the selected NSDUH households. Within these sampling units (which can be a household or another type of living unit), survey participants are randomly selected using an automated program on a handheld computer. Prior to conducting these interviews, the interviewers explain the purpose of the study, how the data will be used, and the confidentiality protections provided under federal law. The names of the respondents are not collected, and their addresses are stored separately from their survey responses.

The selected participant is asked to identify a private area in the home away from other household members for the purpose of conducting the 1-hour interview (Center for Behavioral Health Statistics and Quality, 2015). The interview relies on both computer-assisted personal interviewing (CAPI) and audio computer-assisted self-interviewing (ACASI). The interviewer begins the interview in CAPI mode by reading the questions from the screen and entering the participant's responses into the database. For sensitive questions, the interviewer shifts to ACASI, with the participant reading the questions silently on the screen and/or listening to them through available headphones. In ACASI mode, the participants enter their responses directly into the computer database. A $30 cash payment is given to each participant who completes a NSDUH survey.

One example of findings reported from the NSDUH appears in Figure 3.3 on the next page. As the pie chart shows, in 2015 there were approximately 2.3 million people (over 11 years old) meeting DSM-IV criteria (American Psychiatric Association, 2000) who received substance abuse treatment in the previous year. This treated population constituted just 11% of the 21.7 million U.S. residents who needed treatment (Lipari, Park-Lee, & Van Horn, 2016). Clearly, substance use disorders are undertreated problems in the United States.

National Vital Statistics System

Located within the CDC, the National Vital Statistics System (NVSS) is the oldest collaborative governmental data-sharing organization in the field of public health. The NVSS registers vital events such as births, deaths, marriages, divorces, and fetal deaths. The legal authority for the registration of these events is vested in the 50 states, two cities (Washington, DC, and New York City), and five U.S. territories. These entities share their data with the NVSS, which is then responsible for reporting national vital statistics.

21.7 Million U.S. Residents Meeting Criteria for Substance Use Disorder

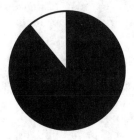

■ 89% did not receive treatment (19.3 million persons)

☐ 11% did receive treatment (2.3 million persons)

FIGURE 3.3. Proportion of U.S. residents with substance use disorder who received treatment in 2015.

The current opioid epidemic in the United States is perhaps the nation's foremost public health challenge (Burke, 2016). Based on NVSS data, Figure 3.4 displays the trends in opioid overdose deaths in the United States for the period 1999–2016. As can be seen, deaths resulting from heroin, natural and semisynthetic opioids, and synthetic opioids other than methadone have more than quadrupled since 1999 (Hedegaard, Warner, & Miniño, 2017). According to Rudd, Seth, David, and Scholl (2016), in 2014 there were 28,647 opioid-related deaths in the United States. This number comprised 61% of all drug overdose deaths that year. The deaths were the result of using heroin, natural/semisynthetic opioids, methadone, and synthetic opioids other than methadone, particularly fentanyl and tramadol. The overdose death rate associated with these latter two drugs increased 72.2% from 2014 to 2015. The CDC (2017c) reports that over 1,000 people each day are treated in U.S. hospital emergency departments for failing to use prescription opioids as directed. NVSS data also reveal that in 2015 the states with the 10 highest age-adjusted drug overdose deaths were West Virginia (41.5), New Hampshire (34.3), Kentucky (29.9), Ohio (29.9), Rhode Island (28.2), Pennsylvania (26.3), Massachusetts (25.7), New Mexico (25.3), Utah (23.4), and Tennessee (22.2) (CDC, 2017c).

An Example of a Public Health Investigation in One Community

On August 15, 2016, the Cabel–Huntington Health Department in Huntington, West Virginia, was notified that the local emergency medical

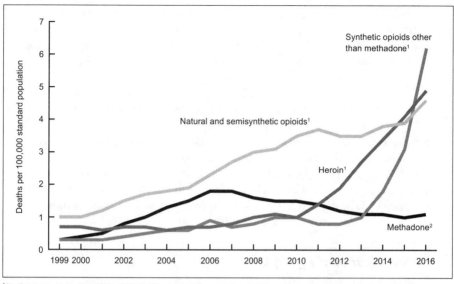

¹Significant increasing trend from 1999 to 2016 with different rates of change over time, $p < 0.05$.
²Significant increasing trend from 1999 to 2006, then decreasing trend from 2006 to 2016, $p < 0.05$.
NOTES: Deaths are classified using the *International Classification of Diseases, Tenth Revision*. Drug-poisoning (overdose) deaths are identified using underlying cause-of-death codes X40–X44, X60–X64, X85, and Y10–Y14. Drug overdose deaths involving selected drug categories are identified by specific multiple-cause-of-death codes: heroin, T40.1; natural and semisynthetic opioids, T40.2; methadone, T40.3; and synthetic opioids other than methadone, T40.4. Deaths involving more than one opioid category (e.g., a death involving both methadone and a natural or semisynthetic opioid) are counted in both categories. The percentage of drug overdose deaths that identified the specific drugs involved varied by year, with ranges of 75%–79% from 1999 to 2013, and 81%–85% from 2014 to 2016. Access data table for Figure 3.4 at: *www.cdc.gov/nchs/data/databriefs/db294_table.pdf#4* .
SOURCE: NCHS, National Vital Statistics System, Mortality.

FIGURE 3.4. Trends in opioid overdose deaths in the United States, 1999–2016.

system had received multiple telephone calls reporting opioid overdoses that had occurred that day between the hours of 3:00 and 8:00 P.M. (Massey et al., 2017). A public health investigation and response was immediately conducted by the West Virginia Bureau for Public Health and the Cabel–Huntington Health Department. In a short period of time, public health officials discovered that 20 opioid overdose cases had occurred in Cabell County in the prior 53 hours. In all cases, the overdose patients were treated in hospital emergency departments in the county. Emergency medical service personnel, other first responders, and hospital providers administered the opioid antidote naloxone to 16 of the patients. Underscoring the potency of the opioids that had been used, it was necessary to administer multiple naloxone doses to six patients to revive them. None of the patients were provided referrals to substance abuse treatment services upon discharge from the emergency departments, highlighting the lack of care continuity. A subsequent investigation analyzed patient specimens and found that the patients had used synthetic opioid fentanyl and novel analogs, such as carfentanil. The findings of these two investigations draw attention to the need for enhanced community-level partnerships between public health departments, public safety agencies, and health care systems to produce rapid, in-depth surveillance information to respond effectively to opioid overdose outbreaks and to connect these patients with follow-up care.

AGE OF ONSET AND THE GATEWAY HYPOTHESIS

From a public health perspective, the optimal way to reduce the human costs associated with substance use is to *prevent or delay* the onset of tobacco, alcohol, and other drug use. Although a number of unanswered questions remain about the best way to characterize the developmental sequence of substance use, in the last 30 years much has been learned about its initiation and the risk factors associated with its onset.

The Significance of Age of Onset

It is well established that the onset of cigarette smoking can be predicted by early conduct problems in school, poor academic performance, weak school bonds, peer smoking and perceived peer norms, lower socioeconomic status, poor refusal skills, and other variables (Bryant, Schulenberg, Bachman, O'Malley, & Johnston, 2000; Conrad, Flay, & Hill, 1992; Olds, Thombs, & Ray-Tomasek, 2005). In turn, adolescents who currently smoke have been found to be 3 times more likely than teen nonsmokers to drink alcohol, 8 times more likely to smoke marijuana, and 22 times more likely to use cocaine (CDC, 1994). Furthermore, teenage smoking has been linked to higher rates of other risk behaviors, including fighting and engaging in unprotected sex (CDC, 1994).

Research also has documented that the early onset of use (late childhood/early adolescence) of a particular drug increases the risk of experiencing problems with that same substance at a later point in life. For example, findings from the NSDUH (see Table 3.4) show that those Americans who initiated alcohol use before the age of 14 were three times more likely to have met criteria for alcohol abuse or alcohol dependence in the past year than those who started drinking at, or after, the age of 18, and five times more likely to meet these same criteria than those starting to drink at, or after, the age of 21 (SAMHSA, 2011). Using data from a separate national probability sample, Grant and Dawson (1997) found that the odds of alcohol abuse in adulthood decreased 8% with each increasing year of age at drinking onset, whereas the odds of alcohol dependence decreased 14% with each increasing year of age at drinking onset. More recent research has found that it is not early adolescent drinking that is so problematic, but instead early-onset *drunkenness* (Kuntsche et al., 2013). Age of first drunkenness also has been linked to elevated mortality rates for

TABLE 3.4. Rates of Alcohol Abuse or Dependence among American Adults by Age of Drinking Onset, 2010

Age at first use of alcohol	Percentage experiencing alcohol abuse or dependence in past year
14 or younger	15.1
15–17	9.1
18–20	4.4
21 or older	2.7

Note. From Substance Abuse and Mental Health Services Administration (2011).

persons who were first drunk before, at, or after the age of 15, as compared to persons who had never been drunk (Hu, Eaton, Anthony, Wu, & Cottler, 2017). From a public health perspective, these findings suggest that a goal of prevention strategies should be to delay or postpone the onset of alcohol use until at least the legal drinking age of 21.

The Gateway Hypothesis

Although early onset is clearly a risk factor for subsequent alcohol and drug abuse problems, there are more complex models that seek to explain the progression into use of so-called hard drugs, such as cocaine and heroin (see Klein & Riso, 1993). The most prominent (and probably controversial) model is the *gateway hypothesis* (Vanyukov et al., 2012). This hypothesis proposes that there is a predictable sequence to the process by which people become involved in drug use (Kandel & Faust, 1975; Kandel, Yamaguchi, & Chen, 1992). The sequence involves four stages in which the use of beer or wine is followed by hard liquor or cigarettes, which, in turn is followed by marijuana and then other illicit drugs (see Figure 3.5 on the next page). An important point to keep in mind is that, although the large majority of persons who reach Stages 3 and 4 have previously used gateway substances, most people at Stages 1 and 2 never advance to Stage 3 or 4.

A compelling piece of evidence supporting this developmental sequence is that, though not every drug user follows this specific sequence, only about 1% began their substance use with marijuana or another illicit drug. Thus, for young people, the legal drugs (i.e., alcohol and cigarettes) seem to function as a "gateway" to marijuana and possibly other illicit drug use. Furthermore, Kandel and colleagues (1992) have found that the progression to a subsequent stage is strongly predicted by both age of onset and frequency of use in the previous stage.

Without doubt, the most controversial aspect of the gateway hypothesis is whether the sequence and association of drug use identified in Figure 3.5

Stage 1		Stage 2		Stage 3		Stage 4
Beer or wine	→	Hard liquor or cigarettes	→	Marijuana	→	Other illicit drugs

FIGURE 3.5. The gateway hypothesis: A developmental sequence of drug involvement.

should be considered a *causal* model (Kandel, 2003; Vanyukov et al., 2012). In public policy debates about the legal control of cannabis, proponents of laws prohibiting marijuana use and distribution frequently assert that the gateway sequence involves causation; that is, marijuana use is a cause of "hard" drug use (e.g., methamphetamine, heroin, cocaine). Thus, those in favor of restrictive cannabis laws may argue that even though the use of marijuana by itself may sometimes not be highly addictive or dangerous, it often leads young people to other more serious drug use that is very harmful to the individual, his or her family, and society.

Opponents of strong legal controls on marijuana typically argue that the stage sequence in Figure 3.5 does not establish causality but, rather, represents a series of spurious correlations. In this view, it is contended that there is no plausible biological mechanism by which drug use at one stage would cause drug use at a subsequent stage. Therefore, the observed correlation between marijuana and hard drug use is the result of some third factor, such as an underlying proneness to deviance, which puts individuals at risk for use of both cannabis and hard drugs as well as a range of other unconventional behavior (Jessor, Donovan, & Costa, 1991). Furthermore, opponents of marijuana prohibitions maintain that the gateway hypothesis is simplistic and directs attention away from the actual root causes of hard drug use, which are believed to be such factors as limited economic opportunity and poverty, poor education, weak family bonds and inadequate parental supervision, neighborhood disorganization, and so on.

Two twin studies conducted to test the gateway hypothesis have arrived at somewhat different conclusions about the role of marijuana use as a possible cause of other drug abuse and dependence. In one study, Lynskey and colleagues (2003) assessed 311 monozygotic (MZ) and dizygotic (DZ) same-sex twin pairs discordant for early marijuana use (before age 17). The participants ranged in age from 24 to 36 (median = 30 years). The design of their investigation was based on the assumption that same-sex twins share the same environmental and family experiences and that the MZ pairs share the same genetic risk factors. Therefore, if the relationship between early marijuana use and other drug use later in life can be explained by shared environmental factors, then in those twin pairs who were discordant for early marijuana use, the twin who did not initiate early marijuana use should be at the same risk for developing later drug problems as the twin who did start using marijuana early. In addition, if shared genetic variables explained the relationship between early marijuana use and other drug use in later life, then the MZ twin pairs discordant for early marijuana should still have the same risk for developing later drug problems (Lynskey et al., 2003). Alternatively, if the relationship between early marijuana use and other drug use in later life is causal, or accounted for by nonshared environmental factors, it would be expected that higher rates of later drug problems would be observed in the twins who had initiated marijuana early in life.

Lynskey and colleagues (2003) found that the relationship between early marijuana use and other drug use later in life could not be adequately explained by either shared environmental factors or genetic factors, providing support for the gateway hypothesis. (The investigators controlled for a host of other known risk factors, such as parental conflict/separation, sexual abuse during childhood, conduct disorder, and social anxiety.) Compared to the twins who had not used marijuana by the age of 17, those who had done so were 2.1–5.2 times more likely to have experienced other drug use, alcohol dependence, and drug abuse/dependence. The investigators speculated that the gateway mechanism operates within a social context of peers to reduce the perceived barriers against other drug use and to increase access to them. They also cautioned that their findings do not provide definitive evidence that early marijuana use plays a causal role in producing other drug use. Rather, they suggested that their study lends strong support to the view that individuals who start smoking marijuana early in life are at greatly elevated risk for other subsequent drug abuse and drug dependence (Lynskey et al., 2003).

In a separate twin study, Agrawal, Neale, Prescott, and Kendler (2004) evaluated an expanded set of relational models (compared to those examined by Lynskey et al., 2003). Using data from a sample of 1,191 male and 934 female same-sex twin pairs, the investigators tested 13 genetically informed models that offered distinct explanations about the nature of the association between marijuana use and other illicit drug use. Agrawal and colleagues (2004) found that a correlated liabilities model provided the best fit to the data for marijuana use and its association with both other illicit drug use and abuse/dependence. Distinct from the gateway hypothesis, which maintains that marijuana use directly increases the subsequent risk of other drug use and abuse/dependence, the correlated liabilities model proposes that "cannabis use and other illicit drug use are influenced by genetic and environmental factors that are correlated across the drugs" (Agrawal et al., 2004, p. 219). That is, they found evidence that the co-occurrence of marijuana use and other illicit drug use arises from correlated genetic and environmental influences that exist for both classes of drugs—not a causal mechanism involving marijuana. This finding is supported by previous research that examined these relationships in a sample of men (Tsuang et al., 1998).

Agrawal and colleagues (2004), however, acknowledge that their study yielded some evidence to support a modified gateway model for *high-risk* marijuana users. In this model, individuals are at risk for other illicit drug use only after they reach a high threshold of risk for marijuana use. This finding appears to be consistent with the earlier epidemiological work of Kandel and colleagues (1992). Furthermore, the Agrawal and colleagues study did not account for the impact of age of onset of marijuana use, as did Lynskey and colleagues (2003). Thus, the existing evidence establishes an observable sequence and a relatively strong association between marijuana use and other illicit drug use, which may involve a marijuana risk gradient. However, at this time, it is probably premature to conclude that the co-occurrence arises from a causal mechanism.

TYPES OF PREVENTION PROGRAMS AND STRATEGIES

Today, the categorization of substance abuse prevention programs is most often based on the target population that the programs are designed to assist (National Institute on Drug Abuse [NIDA], 2003). In an attempt to clarify confusion about different types of prevention, the Institute of Medicine (1994) has proposed the following classification scheme: (1) *universal prevention*—programs designed for the general population, such as all students in a school; (2) *selective prevention*—programs targeting groups at risk or subsets of the general population, such as students performing poorly in school or children of drug abusers; and (3) *indicated prevention*—programs designed for people already using drugs, such as high-risk youth and their families. Effective prevention programs within each of these three categories address the protective factors and risk factors associated with substance use (NIDA, 2003).

At different stages of development, youth are exposed to different sets of protective factors and risk factors, and these influences may be altered by the presence of preventive interventions. For instance, it has been found that children and adolescents who have been exposed to positive youth development programs are less likely to use tobacco, alcohol, and other drugs (Catalano, Bergland, Ryan, Lonczak, & Hawkins, 1998; Flay & Allred, 2003). Moreover, it is important that negative behaviors in early childhood, such as aggression, be changed because they can lead to social and academic difficulties that further heighten risk for later drug abuse.

One important aim of all preventive interventions is to alter the balance between protective factors and risk factors, such that the former outweigh the latter in the life experience of children and adolescents (NIDA, 2003). Table 3.5 provides examples of common protective factors and risk factors that affect young people in five developmental spheres.

TABLE 3.5. Protective Factors and Risk Factors for Youth Substance Use

Protective factors	Developmental sphere	Risk factors
Positive self-concept	Individual	Negative self-concept
Parental monitoring	Family	Inadequate parental monitoring and supervision
Primary friendships with positive youth	Peers	Primary friendships with troubled youth
Academic success with strong school bonds	School	Academic difficulties with weak school bonds
Strong neighborhood attachment	Community	Weak neighborhood attachment

Evidence-Based Prevention Programs

Over the past two decades, the federal government has invested a considerable amount of money into the research and development of programs to prevent substance use and abuse. These efforts have been fruitful, and today a number of effective prevention approaches have been identified through rigorous testing and evaluation. SAMHSA (2017) maintains the National Registry of Evidence-Based Programs and Practices (NREPP) to assist in the dissemination of tested interventions. Three of the preventive interventions in the registry are discussed here to provide some perspective on the range of prevention strategies that have empirical support. The identification of these three programs should not be considered an endorsement of them.

LifeSkills® Training

Today, LifeSkills® Training (LST) is one of the most widely used, evidence-based prevention programs. LST is a universal, school-based program designed for both elementary and middle school students. The program has been successfully tested in white, suburban student populations as well as in ethnic and minority populations and in inner-city schools (National Health Promotion Associates, 2017).

The LST program does not spend a great deal of time reviewing information about the pharmacological actions of drugs or the medical and legal consequences of drug use. Instead, the program addresses protective and risk factors by attempting to build skills in three areas: drug resistance skills, personal self-management skills, and general social skills. For example, through coaching and practice, students learn (1) to deal with social pressures to use drugs, (2) how to reevaluate personal challenges in an optimistic manner, and (3) ways to overcome shyness.

LST can be taught once a week over an extended period of time, or it can be offered in an intensive miniseries format where it is taught every day or two to three times a week (National Health Promotion Associates, 2012). The elementary school LST curriculum is normally taught in 24 class sessions (30–45 minutes long) over a 3-year period in either grades 3–5 or grades 4–6. Ideally, the elementary curriculum is followed by booster sessions in middle school. The LST curriculum designed for middle school is normally taught in 30 class sessions (45 minutes long) over a 3-year period in either grades 6–8 or grades 7–9.

In the first test of LST, Botvin, Eng, and Williams (1980) examined short-term cigarette smoking outcomes in 281 8th- to 10th-grade students in suburban New York. The program appeared to produce a 75% decrease in the number of new cigarette smokers after an initial posttest and a 67% decrease in new smoking at 3-month follow-up (Botvin et al., 1980). During the 1980s and early 1990s, Botvin and colleagues continued to be successful in testing LST with longer-term follow-ups for reducing tobacco use (e.g., Botvin & Eng, 1982; Botvin, Renick, & Baker, 1983), for reducing alcohol and other drug use (Botvin, Baker, Botvin, Filazzolla, & Millman, 1984; Botvin, Baker, Dusenbury, Tortu, & Botvin, 1990), and in minority populations (Botvin et al., 1992).

LST began to draw serious attention in 1995 when Botvin and colleagues published their work in the prestigious *Journal of the American Medical Association*. Botvin and colleagues reported the long-term outcomes of a randomized trial involving 56 public schools that were assigned to LST or a control condition. School, telephone, and mail surveys were used to collect follow-up data for 6 years after baseline. The investigators detected significant reductions in both drug and polydrug use for the groups that received LST, with the strongest effects observed among those who participated in a program that was implemented with the greatest fidelity. The Botvin and colleagues investigation was one of the first studies to provide compelling evidence that a properly implemented, school-based prevention program could produce meaningful and sustained reductions in student tobacco, alcohol, and marijuana use.

More recent evaluations of LST have offered further verification that the program is effective for other populations and drug problems. For instance, Botvin, Griffin, Paul, and Macaulay (2003) conducted another randomized trial of LST in elementary school students (grades 3–6). In 20 schools, rates of knowledge, attitudes, normative expectations, and substance use and related variables were assessed among students who were assigned to either LST (nine schools; $N = 426$) or to a control group (11 schools; $N = 664$). Individual-level analyses revealed that after controlling for gender, race, and family structure, students in LST reported less cigarette smoking in the past year, higher antidrinking attitudes, increased substance use knowledge and skills-related knowledge, lower normative expectations for smoking and alcohol use, and higher self-esteem at a posttest assessment (Botvin et al., 2003). Furthermore, at the posttest assessment, school-level analyses showed that the annual prevalence rate was 61% lower for smoking and 25% lower for alcohol use in schools that received the LST than in control schools. These findings suggest that LST reduces substance use at the elementary school level.

Botvin, Griffin, Diaz, and Ifill-Williams (2001) examined the efficacy of LST in a predominantly minority student population (29 New York City schools; N = 3,621), and Griffin, Botvin, Nichols, and Doyle (2003) evaluated LST in a subsample of this group that had been identified as being at high risk for substance use initiation. In both the total sample (Botvin et al., 2001) and the high-risk sample (Griffin et al., 2003), students who received LST reported less cigarette smoking, alcohol consumption, drunkenness, inhalant use, and polydrug use compared with controls. LST also had a direct positive effect on several cognitive, attitudinal, and personality variables that have been theoretically linked to adolescent substance use (Botvin et al., 2001). These findings support the use of LST in schools that serve disadvantaged, urban, minority adolescents and that assist high-risk, adolescent populations (Botvin et al., 2001).

Guiding Good Choices®

Another example of a universal prevention program is Guiding Good Choices® (Catalano, Kosterman, Haggerty, Hawkins, & Spoth, 1998; Channing Bete Company, 2017). This program was designed for parents of preadolescents. As implied by the name of the program, the aim of the Guiding Good Choices curriculum is to reduce the risk for alcohol and other drug problems during adolescence by empowering parents of 8- to 14-year-olds. Specifically, Guiding Good Choices teaches parents how to enhance important protective factors and reduce risk factors during the later elementary and middle school years. An important feature of the program is that it was designed for adult learners with varying learning styles and levels of education.

The conceptual foundation of Guiding Good Choices is the social development model (Catalano & Hawkins, 1996). A unifying construct of this framework is *bonding*, which is viewed as consisting of both attachment and commitment. In the context of a family, a strong parent–child bond is expected to lead to the child's acceptance of the beliefs and standards of the parent. When a bond generates beliefs that are prosocial and healthy, it serves as a protective factor. Of course, children can bond with antisocial parents, peers, or other harmful persons as well. The social development model and its Guiding Good Choices application stress the importance of bonding to prosocial family, school, and peers as a protection against the development of conduct problems, school misbehavior, and drug abuse (Catalano, Kosterman, et al., 1998).

The Guiding Good Choices program was originally developed in 1987 for use in the Seattle Social Development Project, a longitudinal research study funded by the NIDA (Catalano, Kosterman, et al., 1998). According to Catalano, Kosterman, and colleagues (1998), more than 120,000 families have been trained in the program. The Guiding Good Choices program is a 3-day parent-training course, composed of five 2-hour sessions. For use in the workplace, the program has been offered as a series of 10 1-hour sessions. In most cases, two trained leaders from the community conduct the workshops. The content of Guiding Good Choices focuses on three core beliefs:

1. Parents can play an important role in the reduction of risk factors for other drug and alcohol use by their children.
2. Parents can take an active role in the enhancement of protection for their children by offering them opportunities for involvement within the family, teaching them skills to be successful, recognizing and rewarding their involvement, and communicating clear family norms on alcohol and other drug use.
3. Regular family meetings provide a mechanism for family involvement and serve as a tool to transfer content and skills learned in the workshop into the home environment. (Catalano, Kosterman, et al., 1998, pp. 135–136)

The initial evaluations of Guiding Good Choices were focused mostly on dissemination issues, for example, answering such questions as whether parents would participate in the program and use recommended family management practices. In attempting to reach parents, these are important issues to consider in designing a prevention program. Dissemination obstacles can range from logistical problems, such as lack of transportation or child care, to the manner in which the program is marketed to parents (Catalano, Kosterman, et al., 1998).

In Oregon, Heuser (1990) evaluated the statewide dissemination of Guiding Good Choices in 32 counties and within four state agencies. Television, radio, and newspaper announcements; posters and brochures; and announcements at public agencies, schools, and churches were used to recruit parents. It was found that the largest proportion of participants learned of the Guiding Good Choices workshops through their child's school (45%) or from a friend or family member (34%). Overall, attendance dropped about 33% during the course of the workshops. Again, participant ratings of the workshops were quite favorable, and between 49 and 61% of the parents reported that they had organized and held a family meeting in the past week, as instructed in each session (Heuser, 1990).

In the Seattle metropolitan area, Hawkins, Catalano, and Kent (1991) had broadcast a 1-hour television special on the local NBC affiliate (at 9:00 P.M. on a Tuesday evening) that vividly documented the risk factors and consequences of adolescent drug abuse and presented strategies that parents could use to prevent these problems. About 98,000 households were estimated to have viewed the program. In addition, public service announcements were broadcast to alert parents to the availability of 87 local Guiding Good Choices workshops.

Hawkins and colleagues (1991) found that about 2,500 participants attended the voluntary Guiding Good Choices workshops in the Seattle area. About 90% of the parents were identified as European American, and a majority had children in the targeted ages (grades 4–7). Over half of the participants had seen the television special (53%) and had learned about the workshops either through this special (29%) and/or through their child's school (72%). At the final session, about 69% of the original attendees remained in the program. Overall, the participants provided very favorable program ratings, and at posttest, there was evidence of increases in knowledge about good family management and utilization of program parenting strategies (Hawkins et al., 1991).

Guiding Good Choices has also been tested among families with sixth and seventh graders in rural Iowa (Catalano, Kosterman, et al., 1998). Through nine different schools, parents were invited to participate. The families were nearly all white and mostly working class. At the initial assessment, data were collected from 209 families. At the final assessment, 175 of these families (84%) provided posttest data. The relatively high participation rate was probably motivated by the use of financial incentives (approximately $10 per hour per family member for completing assessments). However, the incentives were not given for program participation itself. About 88% of participating mothers and 69% of participating fathers attended at least three of the five sessions (mean attendance rate for mothers = 3.9 sessions; fathers = 3.1 sessions). In addition to responding to questionnaires, participating families also were videotaped in two structured interaction tasks. One task involved responding to general questions about their family life, such as chores, roles, and parental monitoring. The other task was focused on family problems and attempts at problem solving.

Families were randomly assigned to either the Guiding Good Choices intervention condition or a wait-list control condition (to receive the Guiding Good Choices program after the trial). Families were administered posttest assessments 2–9 weeks following completion of the program. Trained community members conducted the workshops. The investigators collected data on the fidelity of the delivery of the workshops. Across workshops, it was found that 74–82% of the complete Guiding Good Choices curriculum was delivered by the community members (Catalano, Kosterman, et al., 1998).

The analysis of parent outcomes revealed significant improvement in parenting behavior, child management, and the affective quality of parent–child relations for both mothers and fathers in the intervention group (Catalano, Kosterman, et al., 1998). Specifically, mothers who had participated in Guiding Good Choices were significantly more likely to report that they (1) provided rewards to their child for prosocial behavior, (2) communicated rules about substance use, (3) appropriately punished their child for misbehavior, (4) restricted alcohol use by their child, (5) expected their child to refuse a beer if offered by a friend, (6) expressed less conflict toward their spouse, and (7) attempted to involve themselves more with their child. Fathers in the Guiding Good Choices program were significantly more likely to report that they (1) communicated rules about substance use and (2) attempted to involve themselves more with their child.

The effects of the Guiding Good Choices program on adolescent substance use have been positive as well. In a study reporting the adolescent outcomes of the Iowa trial, Spoth, Redmond, and Shin (2001) found that in families in which the parents had received the Guiding Good Choices program, 3½ years later their 10th-grade children were 19% less likely to report ever being drunk, 37% less likely to report ever smoking marijuana, and 41% less likely to have used alcohol in the past month—compared to 10th graders in a no-treatment control condition. These long-term outcomes are particularly impressive given that Guiding Good Choices is a brief, five-session intervention for parents. Also, it is possible that the differences between adolescents in the intervention and control groups could have continued to increase over time (Spoth et al., 2001).

The research on the Guiding Good Choices program suggests that one viable universal prevention strategy is parent education and training delivered via community-based workshops. It appears that with appropriate promotion and marketing, parents can be successfully recruited to participate and that the content of a program such as Guiding Good Choices is found to be acceptable to most parents. Furthermore, the program appears to strengthen parental family management practices that are critical for enhancing protective factors and reducing risk factors for adolescent substance use.

Project Towards No Drug Abuse

Project Towards No Drug Abuse (Project TND) is an example of an intervention that can be classified as both a selective and an indicated prevention program (Sussman, Dent, & Stacy, 2002). The program is designed for the heterogeneous population of high school youth, ages 14–19, who may or may not have prior experience with substance use and violence. In three experimental trials, Project TND has been tested in both traditional and alternative high schools in Southern California. At 1-year (Sussman et al., 2002) and 2-year (Sussman, Sun, McCuller, & Dent, 2003) follow-up assessments, reductions in cigarette smoking, alcohol use, marijuana use, hard drug use, and victimization have been detected in these trials. (The investigators defined a "hard" drug as any one of the following: cocaine/crack, hallucinogens, stimulants, inhalants, depressants, PCP, steroids, heroin, etc.)

The conceptual framework of Project TND is the motivation–skills–decision-making model (Sussman, 1996). This model proposes that teenage problem behavior such as drug use arises from deficits in three classes of variables. First, motivational deficits that instigate teen drug use include (1) believing that drug use is not wrong, (2) misunderstanding the effects of drugs, and (3) possessing a desire to use them. Second, skill deficits decrease the likelihood of bonding with lower-risk peer groups. These include poorly developed social conversation skills and weak self-control. Third, deficits in rational decision making facilitate choices to use drugs.

The current Project TND curriculum consists of a set of twelve 40-minute interactive sessions for the high school classroom (Sussman et al., 2002). The goals of these sessions are to teach active listening skills, challenge stereotypes that drug use is the norm among teens, debunk various myths about drug use, identify the consequences of substance dependence, teach ways to deal with stress and the importance of health as a means of achieving life goals, teach skills for bolstering self-control and assertiveness, teach how to avoid unproductive ways of thinking, encourage the adoption of more conservative views on drug use, and encourage personal commitments to avoid drug use. Rather than using a lecture format in class, the teaching of these topics relies heavily on prescribed interactive activities, including role plays, mock talk shows, and games (Sussman, Rohrbach, Patel, & Holiday, 2003).

The first randomized trial of Project TND involved 21 continuation (or alternative) high schools assigned to one of three conditions: a nine-session classroom curriculum combined with a school-led extracurricular activities component, the nine-session curriculum by itself, and a "standard care" control (Sussman, Dent, Stacy, & Craig, 1998). In California, continuation high schools serve students who are unable to remain in the traditional high school setting because of conduct problems related to poor attendance, academic underachievement, drug use, and so on. At 1-year follow-up (Sussman et al., 1998), it was found that compared to those in the control schools, the students in both of the intervention conditions had a 25% lower rate of hard drug use and a 21% lower rate of weapon carrying. Among males in the intervention conditions, there was a 23% reduction in being a victim of violence. Furthermore, among students who were using alcohol at baseline, there was a 7% decrease in alcohol use. Project TND did not appear to have an impact on either cigarette or marijuana use (Sussman et al., 1998). The school-led extracurricular activities component did not appear to offer any protective benefit to students above and beyond that provided by the classroom curricula at the 1-year follow-up.

A long-term evaluation also was conducted of the nine-session Project TND trial (Sun, Skara, Sun, Dent, & Sussman, 2006). At 5-year follow-up, no intervention effects were detected for 30-day use of cigarettes, alcohol, or marijuana. However, there was approximately a 50% decrease in the 30-day rate of hard drug use among the students who received the classroom-only intervention and about an 80% reduction in the 30-day rate of hard drug use among those students who had received the classroom plus extracurricular activities components. The investigators speculate that hard drug use may be more amenable to intervention because compared to tobacco, alcohol, and marijuana, use of these substances is viewed as more immediately dangerous (Sun et al., 2006).

A second Project TND trial tested the program in three regular high schools in California (Dent, Sussman, & Stacy, 2001). Within each school, classrooms were assigned to either the nine-session TND curriculum or a no-treatment control condition. The results paralleled those found in the first trial. At 1-year follow-up, hard drug use was reduced by 25%, and alcohol use was reduced by 12% in the baseline users. Among males, weapon carrying was reduced by 19%, and being a victim of violence was reduced by 17%. Cigarette and marijuana use did not appear to be reduced by the TND curriculum.

In the third Project TND trial, the curriculum was expanded to 12 sessions (Sussman et al., 2002; Sussman, Sun, et al., 2003). The new sessions were added to better address tobacco and marijuana use as well as violence prevention. A total of 18 alternative high schools were assigned to one of three conditions: the 12-session TND classroom curriculum, a self-instructed TND curriculum, or control. The findings of this trial revealed that the teacher-led TND curriculum reduced substance use and violence at both a 1-year (Sussman et al., 2002) and a 2-year (Sussman, Sun, et al., 2003) follow-up assessment (the self-instruction version did not reduce substance use or violence relative to the control condition). At 1-year follow-up, a 27% reduction in cigarette use was observed, followed by other reductions of 26% for hard drug use, 22% for marijuana use, and 9% for alcohol use among baseline users (Sussman et al., 2002). Furthermore, a 6% decrease in being a victim of violence was observed among males, and a 37% decrease in weapon carrying was detected in baseline non-weapon-carrying students. At 2-year follow-up, the reductions in substance use associated with having been exposed to the teacher-led program appeared to have increased further: cigarette use, 50%; hard drug use, 80%; alcohol use, 13%. Marijuana use was reduced by 88% in the subsample of male students who had never used the drug at baseline (Sussman, Sun, et al., 2003). Although Project TND needs further testing in other populations, these findings indicate that school-based curricula can be developed and used to prevent substance use and violence in high school students. In addition, the results suggest that classroom interactivity is a critical feature of effective substance abuse curricula (Sussman, Rohrbach, et al., 2003).

Research to Practice: The Challenges of Dissemination and Implementation

Unfortunately, the transfer of research findings to practice is a relatively slow process. To assess the extent of this problem in the United States, Ennett and colleagues (2003) studied the prevention practices of middle school program providers in 1999. The 1,795 providers were selected from a national sample of public and private middle schools. The investigators administered surveys to these personnel after determining that they were the individuals most knowledgeable about the substance abuse program in their middle school. The assessment compared the substance use prevention practices in place in the schools against standards previous research determined to be necessary for effective curriculum content and delivery.

The findings of this study highlighted the limited extent to which prevention research findings had been disseminated or transferred to the nation's schools (Ennett et al., 2003). For instance, in 1999, only 35% of the middle school providers reported that they had implemented an evidence-based prevention program at their school. A majority of the providers were found to teach effective content (62%), but only a small proportion used effective delivery (17%), and even a smaller percentage relied on both effective content and delivery (14%). The providers most likely to have implemented both effective content and delivery were those who had adopted evidence-based programs, such as LST. In addition, the use of effective content and delivery methods was found to be positively related to (1) being recently trained in substance use prevention, (2) being comfortable with using interactive teaching methods in the classroom, (3) possessing a graduate degree, and (4) being female. Use of effective content and methods was not related to a specific set of school capabilities, number of years the provider had been teaching substance use prevention, provider age, school status (public vs. private), school enrollment, geographic location of the school, or other variables (Ennett et al., 2003). Clearly, a great deal of works needs to be done to strengthen the prevention capacity of schools.

The Diffusion of Innovation

One way to understand the speed at which communities and schools adopt evidence-based drug prevention programming is to apply the diffusion of innovation model. According to Rogers (1995), "an innovation is an idea, practice, or object that is perceived as new by an individual or other unit of adoption" (p. 11). Study of the diffusion of innovation has revealed that new ideas and practices are often adopted slowly, even when they appear to have advantages over traditional views and practices. As indicated previously, this is frequently the case with evidence-based prevention programming in many communities and schools.

The speed at which an innovation is adopted is thought to be influenced by five general factors: (1) the perceived attributes of the innovation; (2) the type of innovation decision; (3) the communication channels; (4) the nature of the social system, including the views of opinion leaders and community norms; and (5) promotion efforts by change agents. These also are discussed in Chapter 12.

The specific perceived attributes that foster diffusion are the innovation's *relative advantages* over the customary practice, its *compatibility* with existing values, past experiences, and needs of potential adopters, its *complexity* to use, its *trialability* or the degree to which the innovation can be experimented with on a limited basis, and its *observability* or the degree to which the effects of the innovation are visible to others (Rogers, 1995). Adoption decisions that depend on an individual making a decision generally speed up diffusion of innovation, whereas adoption decisions that require a large number of stakeholders in a community, school, or organization to decide slows down diffusion. Furthermore, when diffusion depends on interpersonal communication channels, it will generally occur more quickly than when it depends on mass media. In social systems in which the views of opinion leaders and the norms of the community support change, innovation is more likely to occur. Finally, the intensity of change agents' efforts to promote the adoption of an innovation may make it more likely to occur. Figure 3.6 depicts these factors as they apply to the decision to adopt a new drug prevention program in a community.

The Politics of Diffusion: The History of DARE and the keepin' it REAL Curriculum

In 1983, the Chief of the Los Angeles Police Department, Daryl Gates, and the Los Angeles Unified School District cofounded a drug abuse prevention program known as the Drug Abuse Resistance Education or Project DARE (DARE, 2017). The goal of the demand reduction program was to teach elementary school students decision-making skills so that they would not use drugs and not join gangs. A central feature of DARE was that it would use uniformed police officers to instruct students on the dangers of drug and alcohol use. School districts across America adopted DARE rapidly, in part because of the promotion efforts of its national office, but also because the prevention of drug use among youth had become a national priority and a subject of political debate. Twenty years after its founding, the U.S. General Accounting Office (2003b) estimated that 80% of the nation's school districts had adopted DARE, making it, by far, the most widely used drug prevention program in the United States.

The rapid diffusion of DARE caught the attention of university researchers in the late 1980s and early 1990s. By the mid-1990s, DARE's

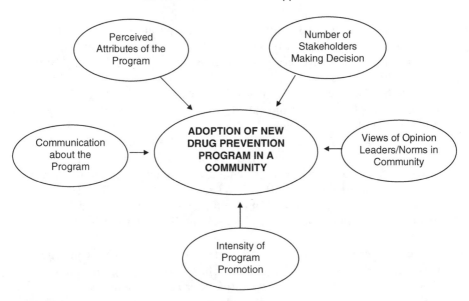

FIGURE 3.6. Factors determining adoption of new drug prevention programs.

growing popularity, despite lack of empirical support, drew the concern of a number of investigators and social critics interested in the diffusion of evidence-based drug prevention programs (e.g., Clayton, Leukefeld, Harrington, & Cattarello, 1996; Elliot, 1995). They noticed that the speed of program dissemination did not seem to be based on evidence of program efficacy, but rather on the success of law enforcement and other groups in program promotion and marketing. Then, a series of university-based studies in the 1990s found that the program was ineffective in deterring drug and alcohol abuse in youth, and some studies found that exposure to DARE actually increased youth use of some drugs (e.g., Clayton, Cattarello, & Walden, 1991; Clayton et al., 1996; Dukes, Stein, & Ullman, 1997; Ringwalt, Ennett, & Holt, 1991; Rosenbaum & Hanson, 1998).

For a number of years, DARE officials ignored the emerging and growing science suggesting that the program was ineffective. However, in 2001, with the help of a research grant from the Robert Wood Johnson Foundation titled "Take Charge of Your Life," DARE America partnered with a university to develop and evaluate a new middle school drug prevention program based in part on DARE principles. Unfortunately, the longitudinal trial found that students who were exposed to the revised program actually reported increased alcohol and cigarette use, and overall the program had no effect on marijuana use (Sloboda et al., 2009). Subgroup analyses revealed that the increases in alcohol and cigarette use occurred among baseline nonusers and primarily among white students.

As a result of Sloboda and colleagues' disappointing findings, DARE America decided to take a different path. The organization partnered with Pennsylvania State University researchers who had developed a culturally sensitive program known as keepin' it REAL (Hecht, Colby, & Miller-Day, 2010). Their collaboration resulted in a new DARE-based version of keepin' it REAL (Nordrum, 2014). SAMSHA's National Registry for Evidence-based Programs and Practices (NREPP; *https://www.samhsa. gov/nrepp*) had already recognized keepin' it REAL as an evidence-based program. At first, DARE employed keepin' it REAL in middle schools. However, by 2013, DARE America had developed and begun to implement a version for elementary school entitled keepin' it REAL DARE Elementary (DARE, 2017). According to Caputi and McLellan (2017) and Nordum (2014), today about 75% of American school districts are using keepin' it REAL.

In the keepin' it REAL program, DARE police officers continue to deliver the curriculum (DARE, 2017). The 10-lesson program relies on a "from kid through kid to kids" narrative approach. Each interactive lesson begins with a story about real-life persons and events. Role-play situations are integrated into the lessons to provide students with opportunities to develop skills necessary for avoiding substance use. The program is based on four resistance strategies: refuse, explain, avoid, and leave. The learning objectives of keepin' it REAL include the following: exercise self-control; identify the risks and consequences of making choices; make safe and responsible decisions; communicate confidently and effectively; and become safe and responsible citizens. Each lesson ends with a closing story (DARE, 2017).

Recently, Caputi and McLellan (2017) conducted a systematic review of the research literature on the keepin' it REAL program. These investigators found no published studies on the DARE versions of keepin' it REAL. Thus, they expanded their review to include studies that examined the effectiveness of the keepin' it REAL program when administered outside of the DARE. network and found 11 studies.

Caputi and McLellan (2017) found mixed results in support of keepin' it REAL's effectiveness. The investigators' concerns were the following: (1) keepin' it REAL had been tested in a narrow population and thus may not be effective in DARE's massive U.S. network, (2) in elementary school populations, keepin' it REAL may be ineffective, and (3) DARE's specific versions of keepin' it REAL that have been implemented since 2012 or 2013 have not been tested for efficacy. Caputi and McLellan recommended that DARE versions of keepin' it REAL undergo independent, randomized trials to determine their effectiveness. Thus, questions continue to linger about the effectiveness of the most widely used substance abuse prevention program in the United States.

The Role of the School Superintendent

In most communities, the public school superintendent is an important opinion leader on school-based drug prevention practices. As the senior school district official, superintendents are expected to provide leadership on issues affecting students' academic performance, health, and safety. These officials also are significant change agents who can wield considerable influence on a school district's approach to drug abuse prevention, if they choose to do so.

Thus, in a study one of the authors of this book (D.L.T.) conducted with a colleague, we examined the specific role of the public school superintendent in the decision to keep or replace DARE (Thombs & Ray-Tomasek, 2001). The specific aim of the study was to explain superintendents' intentions toward future reliance on the DARE program. In June 2000, we mailed an anonymous survey to all 611 superintendents in the state of Ohio (the response rate was 71%). At that time, we found that 85–87% of the state's public school districts used DARE. A large majority of the superintendents (88%) reported that they intended to continue using the program in the future. Most of the superintendents held either incorrect knowledge about DARE's effectiveness in deterring substance use (29%) or acknowledged that they were uninformed about DARE outcome research (34%).

Results from a multivariate analysis indicated that the intention to use DARE in the future was positively associated with the superintendents' beliefs about community support for the program and negatively associated with perceptions of their ability to replace drug prevention curricula in their district. Perhaps most troubling was the finding that accurate knowledge of the research on DARE outcomes had no relationship to intentions toward DARE, suggesting that these school officials do not use research findings as a guide for making decisions about prevention programming. Overall, we concluded that superintendents' positive intentions toward continued use of DARE were formed to avert conflict with adults in the school district and community (Thombs & RayTomasek, 2001). This study provides some insight into the challenges of adopting evidence-based programs.

COMMUNITY COALITION BUILDING

During the past 20 years, coalition building has become a common grassroots response to public health problems in communities throughout the United States (Kreuter, Lezin, & Young, 2000; Wolff, 2001a). There are many reasons for the rise of the community coalition. Recent interest comes from the increasing recognition that problems such as substance abuse do not result only from characteristics within the individual but are instigated and maintained by conditions in the community as well (Kreuter et al., 2000; Wolff, 2001a). Interest in coalitions also comes from (1) the shift of responsibility for health and social problems from the federal government to state and local levels; (2) the societal expectation that these problems will be adequately addressed with fewer resources; (3) the widespread belief that health and human service systems are too bureaucratic to adequately address community needs; and (4) the hope that volunteer work in coalitions will restore civic engagement in the United States (Wolff, 2001a).

Though not well documented, public health officials and other community practitioners typically report that the process of coalition building is not well understood and that the many coalition success stories are probably matched by a comparable number of failures (Wolff, 2001b). However, according to Wolff (2001a), it also is possible to identify a number of functional features of effective community coalitions (see Table 3.6).

The research base on community coalitions is limited at this time. The systematic studies that have been conducted raise questions about their potential to have a positive impact on public health problems, such as substance abuse (e.g., Green & Kreuter, 2002; Hallfors, Cho, Livert, & Kadushin, 2002). One problem may be the insistence of funding agencies that community initiatives adopt "best practices," as identified by past research conducted in different locations and/or with different populations. Unfortunately, these so-called best practices may not be well suited for a specific community or culture. Conversely, community initiatives can make the mistake of ignoring research altogether in favor of an unproven, "homegrown" intervention (Green & Kreuter, 2002, p. 305). These problems reveal the complexities of public health interventions that rely on community collaboration.

In one comprehensive review of the research literature, Kreuter and colleagues (2000) found that only six of 68 published studies reported that a coalition or consortium produced a positive health status or health system change. Based on the descriptions found in these 68 studies, the investigators concluded that there were three possible, overlapping explanations for the lack of positive coalition outcomes:

1. Collaborative mechanisms are inefficient and/or insufficient for carrying out planning and implementation tasks.
2. Expectations of health status/health systems change outcomes are unrealistic.
3. Health status/health systems change may occur but may go undetected because it is difficult to demonstrate a cause-and-effect relationship. (p. 52)

These conclusions should not be considered the definitive and final word on community coalition building. However, they should be sobering to those

TABLE 3.6. Seven Functional Features of Effective Community Coalitions

1. *Holistic and comprehensive.* Breadth allows a community to address those issues that it believes are a priority.

2. *Flexible and responsive.* Adaptability allows a coalition to respond to emerging needs and sudden threats.

3. *Build a sense of community.* The coalition serves as a recognized forum for problem solving in a community.

4. *Build and enhance citizen engagement in community life.* The coalition promotes civic engagement and connectedness.

5. *Provide a vehicle for community empowerment.* The coalition creates the capacity to impact a problem.

6. *Allow diversity to be valued and celebrated as a foundation for the wholeness of the community.* The coalition can assist with finding common ground on issues that generate conflict.

7. *Serve as an incubator for innovative solutions to large problems facing not only their community, but also the nation as a whole.* The coalition can challenge government and other established institutions to think differently about a problem.

Note. Data from Wolff (2001a).

who advocate for coalitions as a means of changing community conditions that promote substance abuse.

RESULTS FROM COMMUNITY INTERVENTION TRIALS

Increasing Cessation among Adult Smokers

Since the 1990s, a number of community interventions have attempted to increase smoking cessation in populations of adult smokers. A variety of intervention strategies have been used to increase quit attempts. The designs and outcomes of several of these interventions are described below.

The COMMIT Trial

Although the prevalence of cigarette smoking among Americans steadily dropped in the 1980s (CDC, 1987), to reduce morbidity and mortality associated with tobacco use there was a need to identify ways to assist adult smokers to quit. Thus, in 1986, the National Cancer Institute funded the Community Intervention Trial for Smoking Cessation, known more simply as the COMMIT Trial (COMMIT Research Group, 1995a, 1995b). The large randomized trial involved 10 matched pairs of communities in the United States and one pair in Canada (within each pair, one community was randomly assigned to the intervention). The research design of the trial relied on rigorous, state-of-the-art methods to test the following hypothesis: "a defined intervention, delivered through multiple community sectors and organizations over a 4-year period and using limited external resources, would result in higher quit rates among heavy cigarette smokers in the intervention communities than in the comparison communities" (COMMIT Research Group, 1995a, p. 184). The trial was based on a collaborative conceptual framework that sought to bring together diverse organizations, institutions, and individuals for the purpose of conducting smoking cessation activities in the community. This framework was based on the premise that a comprehensive community-based strategy would decrease the likelihood that adult smokers could avoid exposure to cessation messages and opportunities for quitting smoking.

The COMMIT Trial was carried out in communities with populations ranging from 49,421 to 251,208 residents (COMMIT Research Group, 1995a). Prior to implementation, a community board, composed of key community representatives, was formed in each community. These boards had responsibility for overseeing the implementation of COMMIT in their communities. The intervention activities were implemented via four channels: (1) public education delivered by media and at community events, (2) health care providers, (3) workplaces and other organizations, and (4) smoking cessation resources. The intervention protocol required that 58 activities had to be implemented in each of the intervention communities. Systematic monitoring indicated that across the 11 intervention communities, the mean attainment rates for implementing intervention activities were 90–93%. Optional intervention activities also were encouraged to allow for variability in community needs.

In each community, about 550 light-to-moderate smokers (1–24 cigarettes per day) and 550 heavy smokers (25 or more cigarettes per day) were randomly selected at baseline and tracked over the 4-year trial (COMMIT Research Group, 1995a). All these smokers were 25–64 years of age. The data collected from the two cohorts of 10,328 light-to-moderate smokers and 10,019 heavy smokers were analyzed separately in the study.

At the end of the COMMIT trial, there was no difference between the intervention and comparison communities on a measure of current smoking status in either the light-to-moderate smoking cohort or the heavy smoking cohort. The observed "quit smoking" rate appeared to be modestly increased by the intervention (1.8%) in the light-to-moderate smoking cohort, but there was no observed increase on this same measure in the heavy smoking cohort. Consistent with these findings, it was found that in the light-to-moderate smoking cohort, the 4-year intervention appeared to slightly reduce the "daily number of cigarettes smoked" (mean reduction of 2.7 cigarettes per day in the intervention condition). There was no significant change in daily number of cigarettes smoked in the heavy smoking cohort. Overall, the COMMIT intervention appeared to have a small, positive impact on cigarette smoking in light-to-moderate smokers but no significant effect on heavy smokers (COMMIT Research Group, 1995a).

Profiling the "Hard-Core" Smoker

Research conducted after the COMMIT Trial sheds some light on the failure of the community-based intervention to reduce cigarette use in heavy smokers. Emery, Gilpin, Ake, Farkas, and Pierce (2000) defined "hard-core" smokers as those reporting that they (1) smoke at least 15 cigarettes per day, (2) have no recent quit attempts, and (3) have no intention to quit smoking at any time. In a random sample of California households, these investigators found that an estimated 1.3% of the state's population, 26 years of age or older, met the criteria for being classified as a hard-core smoker (Emery et al., 2000). This group of smokers made up 5.2% of the smoking population (26 years of age or older). Hard-core smokers were typically retired, white men living alone, with 12 years or less of education and annual income below $50,000. In addition, these smokers were distinguished from other smokers by being less likely to believe that (1) negative health consequences were associated with their smoking, (2) tobacco is an addictive drug, and (3) secondhand smoke harms other people. Compared to other smokers, the hard-core smokers also were more likely to have begun experimenting with smoking at a younger age and to report that they were younger when they became regular smokers (Emery et al., 2000). This relatively unique profile suggests that it may be unrealistic to expect some individuals to ever quit smoking.

Neighbors for a Smoke Free North Side

Another example of a community intervention seeking to increase smoking cessation among adult smokers was the Neighbors for a Smoke Free North Side Project (Fisher et al., 1998). The intervention sites were located in three predominantly low-income neighborhoods in St. Louis. Three similar neighborhoods in Kansas City were selected as the comparison group. The intervention stressed neighborhood-based governance and resident involvement in the design of strategies to reduce smoking. Using neighborhood volunteers and paid staff members, wellness councils were established to carry out the program for a 24-month period. The program relied on smoking cessation classes, billboard advertisements, door-to-door promotion campaigns, and a "gospel fest." In 1990 and 1992, results from random-digit dial telephone surveys indicated that smoking prevalence in St. Louis declined 7% compared to only 1% in Kansas City—a difference that was statistically significant.

The investigators speculated that the Smoke Free North Side intervention was more successful than COMMIT because the former program was developed in the targeted St. Louis neighborhoods and thus may have had greater "community ownership" (Fisher et al., 1998). In contrast, COMMIT was centrally developed at the national level and then delivered to communities with only a limited number of tailoring options.

Decreasing Youth Access to Tobacco

Other community interventions have sought to restrict youth access to tobacco products. For instance, Rigotti and colleagues (1997) compared three communities in Massachusetts that increased enforcement of youth tobacco laws with three matched comparison communities. In the intervention communities, health departments started quarterly compliance checks with underage tobacco purchase attempts. At baseline, 68% of vendors sold to minors. The difference between the intervention and control communities was not statistically significant at baseline. At a 2-year follow-up, only 18% of the vendors in the intervention communities, compared with 55% in the comparison communities, sold tobacco to minors. Yet, three annual surveys of more than 17,600 respondents revealed only a small decrease in the perceived ability of underage adolescents to purchase tobacco and no decline in tobacco use itself.

The Tobacco Policy Options for Prevention Project was a 32-month intervention that attempted to restrict tobacco use among youth through a community mobilization effort (Forster et al., 1998). This initiative centered its energy on changing local ordinances, altering retailer and other adult practices regarding the provision of tobacco to youth, and increasing the enforcement of laws that prohibit sales to underage youth. A total of 14 Minnesota communities were randomly assigned to intervention and control conditions. In June 1993 and June 1996, youth under the control of investigators attempted to purchase tobacco at all tobacco outlets in the communities.

During the trial (1993–1996), school surveys of more than 6,000 students indicated that adolescent smoking had increased in both sets of cities, but less in the intervention communities (Forster et al., 1998). It appeared that the intervention had little effect on perceptions of tobacco availability through social sources such as peers or parents, but it reduced perceived availability through commercial sources. Furthermore, in the intervention communities, purchase attempts declined significantly during the trial. In all communities in the trial, there was a large decrease in youth purchase attempts that resulted in sales, and it was not significantly greater in the intervention cities. The investigators attributed the overall reduction in tobacco purchase success in both the intervention and the control communities to changes in state laws that restricted youth access to tobacco and to the increased awareness created by news reports of these changes in law that took place during the course of the trial (Forster et al., 1998).

A similar intervention program designed to bolster tobacco enforcement took place in Erie County, New York (Cummings et al., 1998). Six pairs of communities were matched on number of tobacco outlets, population size, and other demographic variables. Directed by police, underage purchase compliance checks were conducted in 366 tobacco outlets at baseline and 319 outlets at follow-up. In the intervention communities, all retailers were sent a letter about tobacco laws and sales to minors that also warned that compliance checks were planned for the area. Distribution of the letter was followed by a dramatic increase in purchase compliance in both enforcement and nonenforcement communities. Interestingly, compliance rates between the two groups of communities did not vary, however. It seems that most vendors in both areas learned about the enforcement program and perceived enforcement as more vigilant in the entire region.

Gemson and colleagues (1998) conducted a similar trial in central Harlem (New York City). In a randomized trial of 15 tobacco vendors, retail outlets selling tobacco were randomly assigned to three conditions: enforcement, education, and control. In October 1993 and April 1994, surveys of underage tobacco purchase compliance were conducted in the community. During both surveys, violators from the outlets in the enforcement condition were only fined (in accordance with the state law). At 6-month follow-up, underage sales had declined 56% among enforcement outlets, 34% among education outlets, and 16% among control stores (Gemson et al., 1998).

Decreasing Youth Access to Alcohol

Another community intervention was designed to decrease the availability of alcohol to youth. At the University of Minnesota, Wagenaar, Murray, Gehan, and colleagues (2000) developed and tested a community intervention known as Communities Mobilizing for Change on Alcohol. This community-organizing project aimed to reduce the number of outlets selling alcohol to underage youth and restrict the availability of alcohol to youth through noncommercial sources, such as peers and parents. A total of 15 communities were randomly assigned to intervention and comparison conditions. A leadership strategy team worked to strengthen numerous policies, procedures, and practices in the intervention communities. Community action was pursued through public and private organizations, including city councils, school and enforcement agencies, alcohol merchants, business associations, and the media.

Several assessments were made to evaluate the project. Approximately 4,500 12th graders were surveyed in 1992 and 1995. In addition, a telephone survey of 3,095 18- to 20-year-olds was conducted in 1992 and repeated in 1995. Also, during the same years, alcohol purchase compliance checks, using study confederates who appeared underage, were conducted at more than 25 off-sale outlets.

Relative to the communities in the comparison condition, those in the intervention condition showed a 17% greater rate of checking age identification of youthful-looking purchasers and a 24% lower rate of sales to potential underage purchasers at bars and restaurants. Furthermore, in the intervention communities, there was a 25% decrease in the proportion of older teens providing alcohol to younger teens, and a 7% decrease in underage respondents who reported drinking in the previous 30-day period. There also was a statistically significant decrease in DUI (driving under the influence) arrests among 18- to 20-year-olds (Wagenaar, Murray, & Toomey, 2000).

Community-Based Prevention for Youth

The Midwestern Prevention Project

Several community interventions have been tested for their ability to delay the onset of substance use among adolescents with no history of use and to decrease use in adolescents who have previous experience with one or more drugs. The Midwestern Prevention Project (MPP) attempted to deter cigarette, alcohol, and marijuana use among 10- to 14-year-olds in two U.S. cities: Kansas City, Missouri, and Indianapolis, Indiana. A quasi-experimental design in Kansas City (Pentz et al., 1989) and a randomized experimental design in Indianapolis (Chou et al., 1998) evaluated the program. From September 1984 to January 1986, the Kansas City students received a 10-session training program that included skills for resisting substance use, homework exercises relying on interviews of others, and role plays with parents and family. Most students interviewed parents and family members about family rules on substance use, effective techniques for avoiding use, and how to deal with media and community influences. Among other activities, teen participants also made statements of public commitments to avoid tobacco, alcohol, and other drug use; practiced role playing of resistance skills; and discussed homework results.

Among the 42 schools in the MPP trial, four were randomly assigned to the intervention condition and four to the control condition (Pentz et al., 1989). The remaining 34 schools were assigned based on their willingness to participate—20 were willing, 14 were not. School willingness may have been associated with perceptions that substance abuse was or was not a high-priority concern in the school. The 20 willing schools received the intervention, increasing the total number of intervention schools to 24 (18 schools served as controls).

At 1-year follow-up, students in the intervention condition reported lower rates for all three drugs compared to those in the control condition: 17% versus 24% for cigarette use, 11% versus 16% for alcohol use, and 7% versus 16% for marijuana use. Although cigarette, alcohol, and marijuana use had increased in both groups of schools, 2 years after the program the increases for these three substances were significantly lower in the intervention group. This finding provides evidence that the MPP effects were sustained, at least for 2 years following the intervention (Pentz et al., 1989).

Chou and colleagues (1998) implemented and evaluated the MPP in Indianapolis by tracking 1,904 students in intervention schools and 1,508 students in control schools. The schools were randomly assigned to these conditions, and after baseline, student follow-up assessments were conducted at 6 months, 1½ years, 2½ years, and 3½ years. After statistically adjusting for ethnicity, gender, socioeconomic status, father's occupation, and school type and grade, the researchers discovered that among those adolescents who had a baseline history of tobacco, alcohol, or other drug use, alcohol use had been decreased at the 6-month and 1½-year follow-ups and for tobacco use at 6-month follow-up only. Results for marijuana use were not consistent over time.

Project Northland

Located in Minnesota, Project Northland was designed to reduce alcohol use among preteens and younger adolescents (Perry et al., 1996). The intervention was community-based but had a significant school component. A 3-year behavioral curriculum was provided to sixth, seventh, and eighth graders that emphasized peer leadership, parental involvement, and community task force activities. The program taught students to resist negative peer influence and sought to instill conservative norms about the use of alcohol. In addition, students learned methods with which to bring about community social, political, and institutional change in alcohol-related programs and policies. Students interviewed parents, local government officials, law enforcement personnel, retail alcohol merchants, schoolteachers, and administrators to learn about their views and activities relative to teenage drinking. Students also conducted "town meetings" and developed recommendations for community action to deter adolescent drinking.

Project Northland also organized community task forces to press for passage of local ordinances to prevent sales of alcohol to minors and intoxicated patrons of drinking establishments (Perry et al., 1996). The task forces consisted of government officials, law enforcement personnel, school representatives, health professionals, youth workers, parents, concerned citizens, and teenagers. In addition, students who pledged to be alcohol and drug free were eligible for discounts at local businesses.

At baseline, 2,351 students were surveyed in Project Northland (Perry et al., 1996). The investigators were able to obtain 2-year follow-up rates greater than 80% in both the intervention and control groups. At baseline, a higher percentage of students in the intervention group were alcohol users. However, at follow-up, the proportions of students who had used alcohol in the past week and past month were lower in the intervention group than in the control group. The intervention effects of Project Northland appeared to be greatest (and statistically significant) among students with no history of alcohol use at baseline. The intervention did not reduce cigarette smoking or marijuana use in the participating youth (Perry et al., 1996).

Reducing Impaired Driving and Alcohol-Related Injuries and Deaths in the General Population

Community Prevention Trial Program

Two community interventions have attempted to reduce alcohol-related injuries and deaths in the general population. The Community Prevention Trial Program was a 5-year project designed to decrease the number of alcohol-related injuries and death in three experimental communities (Holder, 1997; Holder et al., 2000). The model for this intervention relied on five reinforcing components to change individual behavior by changing the environmental, social, and structural contexts of drinking in the community. The first component of the intervention model was community mobilization. Local residents were organized to press for public policy change. These efforts increased general awareness and concern about alcohol-related trauma. In each community, the media, mobilization, and intervention activities had specific objectives tailored to their needs.

The second component of the intervention model was responsible beverage service. This component attempted to reduce sales to intoxicated patrons in drinking establishments and to strengthen local enforcement of alcohol control laws by collaborating with restaurants, bars, and hotel associations; beverage wholesalers; and the Alcohol Beverage Control Commission.

The third component of the intervention was a drinking and driving component to improve traffic safety. This component sought to increase the number of DWI (driving while intoxicated) arrests in the community through officer training, use of passive alcohol sensors (at DWI checkpoints), and media-publicized sobriety checkpoints.

The fourth intervention component was a media advocacy initiative. These efforts attempted to focus news attention on underage drinking, enforcement of underage sales laws, and training of personnel to prevent alcohol sales to minors. The fifth intervention component sought to reduce alcohol outlet density through local zoning regulations.

The Community Prevention Trial Program relied on a quasi-experimental design to evaluate the effects of each intervention component in intervention and comparison communities as well as the overall project effects on alcohol-related injuries (Holder et al., 2000). During the trial, local regulation of alcohol outlets and public sites for drinking were altered in all three experimental communities. Furthermore, compliance checks at 150 outlets revealed a significant decrease in successful alcohol purchases by youth.

Holder and colleagues (2000) found that the DWI intervention component produced increased news coverage about drinking and driving, heightened police enforcement, and increased their use of roadside breath-testing equipment. Data collected via telephone surveys indicated a significant increase in the perceived likelihood of a DWI arrest and a decrease in the self-reported frequency of driving and drinking. Data collected at roadside surveys corroborated the reduction in driving after drinking found in the telephone survey. Most important, alcohol-related crashes, as measured by single-vehicle night crashes, fell by 10–11% in the intervention communities, and alcohol-related trauma visits to emergency departments declined by 43% in the intervention communities.

Massachusetts Saving Lives Program

The Massachusetts Saving Lives Program was a comprehensive community intervention designed to reduce drinking and driving and alcohol-involved traffic deaths (Hingson, McGovern, Howland, & Hereen, 1996). The intervention began in 1988 and ended in 1993. A competitive proposal process was used to select six program communities for the trial. The six intervention communities were compared with five matched communities that also submitted applications but were not funded. The remaining communities of Massachusetts served as a comparison group as well. Outcome data were collected for the period 5 years before and after the intervention.

From the mayor's office in each intervention community, a full-time coordinator organized a task force of private citizens, organizations, and public officials. Each year, the intervention communities received approximately $1 per inhabitant in program funds. One-half of these funds supported the program coordinator. The balance provided for increased law enforcement, other program activities, and educational materials. The intervention also encouraged citizens to volunteer their time to program activity. In each intervention community, active task force participation ranged from 20 to 100 individuals, and about 50 organizations participated in each of these cities (Hingson et al., 1996).

In the Massachusetts Saving Lives Program, the intervention communities were responsible for developing most of the program activities. Communities adopted such objectives as reducing alcohol-impaired driving, speeding, "running" red lights, failing to yield to pedestrians in crosswalks, and failing to use seat belts. To address the problems of drinking and driving and speeding, intervention communities implemented media campaigns, sobriety checkpoints on roadways, speed-watch telephone hotlines, alcohol-free prom nights, beer keg registration, police surveillance of alcohol outlets, and a number of other activities. To address the problems of pedestrian safety and seat belt use, intervention communities conducted media campaigns and police checkpoints, posted crosswalk signs warning motorists of fines for failure to yield, increased the number of crosswalk guards at schools, and other activities (Hingson et al., 1996). The effects of the Massachusetts Saving Lives Program were positive. For example, among drivers under the age 20, the proportion reporting driving after drinking in random-digit-dialing telephone surveys decreased from 19% in the first year of the trial to 9% in subsequent years. In the comparison cities, there was little change on this measure. A 7% increase in seat belt use was observed in the intervention cities, a significantly greater increase than found in the comparison cities. Fatal motor vehicle crashes declined from 178 during the 5 preintervention years to 120 during the 5 intervention years, representing a 25% greater reduction than existed in the remainder of the state. Moreover, fatal crashes involving alcohol decreased by 42%, and the number of fatally injured drivers with positive blood alcohol levels was reduced by 47% compared to the rest of the state. The evaluation found that all six of the intervention cities had greater decreases in fatal and alcohol-related fatal crashes than did the comparison cities or the rest of the state (Hingson et al., 1996).

Lessons Learned about Community Interventions

Four conclusions can be drawn from this review of comprehensive community interventions. First, most of the trials reviewed here produced reductions in substance abuse and related problems (e.g., drinking and driving) and/or increased protective actions in the community (e.g., refusing alcohol sales to minors). These findings indicate that community interventions can be designed to effectively address substance abuse problems. Second, though community interventions have the potential to produce far-reaching effects, including an impact on high-risk, "hard-to-reach" groups, the *size* of the effects generated from these interventions is often relatively small. For instance, the MPP reduced adolescent alcohol use by an estimated 5% (Pentz et al., 1989). Thus, it becomes a matter of judgment as to whether the costs of an intervention are justified when the effect size is not large. Third, the design of the interventions reviewed here suggests that positive outcomes depend on combining community mobilization and local policy change with public education and awareness activities (Hingson & Howland, 2002). Sole reliance on substance abuse education and awareness activities does not seem to be adequate community prevention strategy. Fourth, interventions that can somehow foster and promote community collaboration, input, and ownership seem to be more likely to succeed than those interventions that are imported from outside the community.

THE PARTICIPATORY RESEARCH APPROACH

In the field of public health, there has long been a tension between researchers, who believe it is necessary to investigate research questions, and practitioners and citizens, who favor action, community development, and possibly social change. These tensions have led to appeals to researchers to better serve the needs of community members by treating them more as research "users" than merely as research "subjects." On this point, Brownson, Baker, and Kreuter (2001) commented: "It is recognized increasingly that effective research in communities should be conducted *with* and *in* communities rather *on* communities" (p. vii). Thus, researchers have been challenged to be more attentive to the application of research findings, their dissemination, and the formulation of best-practice guidelines for practitioners. It is in this context that the concept of "participatory research" has become a dominant theme in public health practice in recent years (Green & Mercer, 2001).

Participatory research is not a specific research method but, rather, a mindset and an approach that attempts to engage all potential users of the research in the community (and possibly elsewhere, e.g., state health department) in the generation of the research questions and the implementation of the research itself (Green et al., 1995). The core beliefs of the participatory research approach are that public health research can be (1) sensitive to unique circumstances in a specific locale, (2) under local control, (3) trusted by communities and involve collective decision making, and (4) conducted without compromising the quality of the evaluation (Brownson et al., 2001; Mercer, MacDonald, & Green, 2004).

A range of participatory research approaches exist, such that any specific community's participation in public health research will vary by project (Green & Mercer, 2001). Maximum community participation would involve collaborating with stakeholders to identify research questions, select research methods, and assist in data analysis and interpretation and the application of findings. Minimum community participation is limited to formative work at the beginning of a research project and to interpretation and application at the end of an investigation. Proponents argue that integrating stakeholder values into the design of participatory research projects does not compromise the scientific integrity of the study and its evaluation.

Although U.S. government funding for participatory research has been limited thus far, the approach has shown promise (Frankish et al., 1997; Langton, 1995; Mercer et al., 2004; Minkler & Wallerstein, 2003). This optimism is based on the democratic and inclusive values that are implicit in the approach. Nevertheless, at this point, significant questions remain about (1) the extent to which communities are interested in, and capable of, participating in public health research and (2) the potential of this research process to produce knowledge that has generalizibility and usefulness beyond the specific community or communities in which it was applied (Green et al., 1995).

THE COMMUNITY MOBILIZATION APPROACH

Wagenaar, Gehan, Jones-Webb, Toomey, and Forster (1999) have outlined a *process* for mobilizing communities to take action to change local institutional polices on substance abuse issues. The seven stages identified in Table 3.7 are not sequential sets of activities, however. Rather, during a mobilization effort, there typically is ongoing work in other stages but perhaps at a lower level of intensity, when the focus turns to a new stage. Action and vigor characterize community organizing. Wagenaar and colleagues describe the functions of the organizers at each stage as "advising, teaching, modeling, persuading, selling, agitating, facilitating, coaching, confidence-building, guiding, mobilizing, inspiring, educating, and leading" (p. 317).

Both the community mobilization model and the participatory research model recognize the need for collaborative work and community input. However, the community mobilization model is the more strategic and targeted approach; the investigator determines the specific aims of the research, and these goals may not be the highest health priorities in the community. In contrast, the participatory research model is more egalitarian and allows communities to set the priorities and decide the direction of the research to best meet their needs. Although this latter emphasis may present communities with special opportunities, and thus at first appear to be an obvious advantage of the participatory research model, it should be kept in mind that substance abuse problems may become secondary or even low priorities in comprehensive initiatives seeking to enhance public and community health. For example, Green (1992), a proponent of participatory research, has suggested that alcohol abuse would seldom if ever be identified by a community as its number-one health problem. The community

TABLE 3.7. A Community Organizing Process for Changing Local Institutional Policy

1. *Making a comprehensive assessment of community interests, needs, and resources.* What is the range of perceptions on various tobacco, alcohol, and other drug problems? Who wields power on these issues in the community? Who are likely supporters and opponents of local policy changes? What arguments should be anticipated from opponents of a policy change? Where do the self-interests of various stakeholders collide with potential policy changes?

2. *Establishing a core group of support.* Who supports local policy change? Who is connected to a network of potential supporters? How do we find supporters from diverse public and private sectors of the community?

3. *Developing an action plan.* Which local policy or policies do we work to change? How do we develop a consensus on identifying a policy for change? Do we focus on one policy at a time or on multiple policies? Are we willing to develop an action plan that may be perceived to be controversial in some circles in the community?

4. *Expanding the base of support for the action plan.* What activities should the core group implement to build broad support for the action plan? (letters, e-mails, mass e-mailings, Twitter, Facebook, texting, phone calls, one-to-one negotiation, public speaking, working with news media, etc.)

5. *Implementing the action plan.* What specific strategies do we need to secure changes in local policy? When do we propose policy change to various public and private groups?

6. *Maintaining the effort and institutionalizing it.* How do we continue this work without grant support? Where can we find other sources of funding?

7. *Evaluating and disseminating the results of the community mobilization effort.* What are the outcomes of our work? Who are the stakeholders that need to have knowledge of these outcomes?

Note. See Wagenaar, Gehan, Jones-Webb, Toomey, and Forster (1999).

mobilization model might be more appropriate for public health problems that require the community to be *coaxed* to address them.

CHAPTER SUMMARY

Historically, the federal government of the United States spent most of its drug control dollars on interdiction and law enforcement, with substantially smaller amounts of funds directed to prevention and treatment (Haaga & Reuter, 1995; U.S. Office of National Drug Control Policy, 2016). This longstanding "war-on-drugs" policy begun during the Nixon Administration may be changing as recognition grows among both conservatives and liberals that this approach has not achieved the goals that the nation had hoped for when it was implemented in the early 1970s (Smith, 2009). The continual appearance of new and recurring drug problems including the drug trade and related violence in Mexico, the large-scale smuggling of fentanyl into the United States from China, the return of large-scale opium production in Afghanistan (United Nations Office on Drugs and Crime, 2017), the domestic epidemic of narcotic pain medication overdoses, and many other developments, have prompted many reactive, micro-shifts in the U.S. national drug control strategy over the years (U.S. Office of National Drug Control Policy, 2016). However, the primary focus of U.S. policy has remained law enforcement.

Almost two decades ago, Des Jarlais (2000) laid out criteria for drug control policy change based on a public health model. First, such a policy would have to rely on science and recognize that psychoactive substance use is nearly a universal human experience. Second, heavy emphasis would be placed on the prevention of substance use, especially the primary prevention of cigarette smoking. Third, there would be a shift in public policy so that treatment would become the primary method for addressing problems of illicit drug abuse. Fourth, communities would adopt harm-reduction strategies (see Chapter 11) to help active users protect themselves from modifiable risks and to possibly motivate them to move toward abstinence. Fifth, the development of a drug control policy would explicitly consider the potential benefits of some forms of psychoactive drug use in some situations (Des Jarlais, 2000).

Judged by Des Jarlais (2000) criteria, the federal government's national strategies in recent years do not represent a bold step away from law enforcement and toward a public health and safety model. The Obama administration's proposed fiscal year 2017 budget for national drug control devoted only 5.0% to prevention (U.S. Office of National Drug Control Policy, 2016). Most funds were devoted to law enforcement and interdiction. The national drug control strategy of the Trump administration is unknown. However, it will be surprising if substantial new federal investments are made in prevention and treatment, given the nation's indifference to the opioid epidemic and relentless debate about health care reform. Thus, it remains to be seen whether meaningful changes in U.S. drug control policy will actually be implemented in a meaningful way.

Why is it unlikely that public health concepts will entirely supplant policies concentrated on law enforcement? Among the impediments are a basic human fear of pleasure and the enduring belief that it must be regulated (Linden, 2011). Throughout human history, the widespread ambivalence about the experience of pleasure has been the fuel for drug regulation and prohibition. Another obstacle to a public health approach is simply the fear of change. Many citizens underestimate the hazards of some current forms of legal drug use, such as cigarette smoking, and possibly overestimate the dangers of some types of drug use that are currently illegal, such as marijuana use as an adjunct to cancer chemotherapy. Misplaced moral judgments also serve as hindrances to adopting a public health model. The tendency to condemn the drug user is ingrained in American culture and in conventional belief systems. Finally, the widespread adoption of public health approaches could threaten the economic status quo of U.S. industries (e.g., tobacco, alcohol, and pharmaceutical companies that overproduce opioid medications) that benefit from either the manufacture of legal drugs or the incarceration of illicit drug users.

REVIEW QUESTIONS

1. What is the focus of public health, and how is it different from medicine?

2. What were the great public health achievements of the 20th century?

3. What are the competing visions of public health in the United States?

4. How can the triad model of causation be applied to substance abuse and dependence?

5. What are examples of national surveillance systems on substance use and abuse?

6. From a prevention perspective, why is age of onset an important issue?

7. Does existing scientific evidence support the view that marijuana use is a gateway to other illegal drug use?

8. Have prevention programs been shown to reduce substance use in youth?

9. What factors influence the diffusion of prevention programs?

10. Why is DARE the most widely used substance abuse prevention program in the United States?

11. Does the research literature support the use of community coalitions to address substance use problems in the community?

12. Overall, what lessons have been learned from community interventions seeking to reduce substance use and misuse?

13. What is the participatory research approach, and how is it different from the community mobilization approach?

14. What are the prospects in the United States for a drug control policy based on public health concepts?

CHAPTER 4

Understanding the Co-Occurrence of Substance Use and Psychiatric Conditions

Historically, the classification of mental disorders by the psychiatric profession was driven by a desire to identify discrete, independent illnesses (Faraone, Tsuang, & Tsuang, 1999). Although comorbidity was recognized, early versions of the American Psychiatric Association's *Diagnostic and Statistical Manual of Mental Disorders* (DSM) encouraged diagnostic hierarchies that focused attention on a "primary" disorder while assigning less clinical significance to the "secondary" disorder, and frequently substance abuse or dependence was considered the secondary disorder. However, as a result of epidemiological research (reviewed later) as well as clinical experience, the emphasis on hierarchical approaches to diagnosis and treatment gradually waned (Mueser, Drake, & Wallach, 2003).

Today the co-occurrence of substance use disorders with other psychiatric conditions is recognized as a pervasive feature of the mental health problems experienced in the general population (Grant et al., 2015, 2016) and in clinical samples (Krawczyk et al., 2017). In part, the comorbidity of substance abuse and severe mental illness, specifically, can be traced to the deinstitutionalization movement that began in the United States in the 1960s and continued through the 1980s (American Hospital Association, 1995). Prior to the 1960s, persons with severe mental illness (typically schizophrenia) were confined indefinitely in state psychiatric facilities. Now they are treated in community-based programs and thus are often left unprotected from the dangers of street life, including alcohol and illicit drug use. As Drake and Wallach (1999) observed two decades ago, "Like homelessness itself, a comorbid substance use disorder is an unintended consequence of a deinstitutionalization policy that paid more attention to closing hospitals than to providing affordable housing that is also safe from the predators of urban street culture" (p. 589).

Today, the co-occurrence of substance abuse and *severe* mental illness has become an obvious public health problem in the United States because of pervasive homelessness and the use of jails to treat people with these disorders (Dart, 2016; Greenberg & Rosenheck, 2008; 2010; Parker et al., 2018). According to the 2015 results from the National Survey on Drug Use and Health (Center for Behavioral Health Statistics and Quality, 2016a), 8.1 million adult Americans, or about 2.5% of the U.S. population, report experiencing a comorbid condition involving mental illness and substance use disorder. Among those persons with a substance use disorder, 41.2% met criteria for any mental illness. In contrast, among persons with mental illness, 18.6% met criteria for substance use disorder. In the United States, 52% of persons with co-occurring disorders (or approximately 4 million Americans) had not received treatment for either condition in the previous 12-month period (Center for Behavioral Health Statistics and Quality, 2016b). Only 6.8% of persons with a comorbid condition received treatment for both their substance abuse and mental health problems.

This chapter first reviews the epidemiology of comorbid disorders to establish the broadest picture of the problem in the United States. Comorbidity should be recognized as a heterogeneous problem in the general population—it clearly takes many forms. Consistent with conventional clinical practice, in this chapter the term *dual diagnosis* is reserved for the subset of co-occurrences that involve a substance use disorder and a severe mental illness, such as schizophrenia or bipolar disorder (Kikkert, Goudriaan, de Waal, Peen, & Dekker, 2018). After the epidemiology section, we review explanatory models of comorbidity and integrated treatment.

THE EPIDEMIOLOGY OF COMORBIDITY IN THE UNITED STATES

The National Epidemiologic Survey on Alcohol and Related Conditions-III (NESARC-III) is the fourth national survey conducted by the National Institute on Alcohol Abuse and Alcoholism (Grant et al., 2015, 2016). NESARC-III is the most comprehensive surveillance study ever conducted on alcohol and drug use and their associated comorbidities. The target population was the civilian noninstitutionalized population residing in the United States. The study relied on a nationally representative face-to-face retrospective survey of American adults, ages 18 or older. Data were collected in randomly selected households in 2012 and 2013. African

Americans, Hispanics, and Asians were oversampled to ensure reliable estimates for these groups. The study's sample size was 36,309. Participants were offered two $45 incentives to complete data collection.

The NESARC-III relied on DSM-5 criteria (American Psychiatric Association, 2013). The study's semistructured diagnostic interview assessed the following: alcohol consumption and experiences; treatment utilization; family history; tobacco and nicotine use; medication, nonalcohol drug use, and related experiences; mood disorders; social situations; traumatic experiences; medical conditions; eating behavior; and other conditions. Saliva samples were also collected for DNA analysis. The overall survey response rate was 60.1% (Grant et al., 2015, 2016).

NESARC-III provides prevalence estimates of substance use disorders in the U.S. population for 2012–2013 (McCabe, West, Jutkiewicz, & Boyd, 2017). As shown in Table 4.1, 13.9% of the U.S. population met DSM-5 criteria for alcohol use disorder in the past year, followed by cannabis disorder with a prevalence rate of 2.5%. Past-year prevalence rates for other substance use disorders were less than 1.0%. Table 4.1 also provides prevalence ratios for each of the 10 drug classes. The prevalence ratios identify the extent to which a substance use disorder co-occurred with other substance use disorders. Alcohol use disorder was the drug class least likely to co-occur with another substance use disorder; that is, only 15.0% of the alcohol diagnoses were accompanied by another substance use disorder.

TABLE 4.1. Prevalence of Coexisting DSM-5 Substance Use Disorders in the U.S. Population: Past-Year Findings from the NESARC-III

10 SUDs	Past-year prevalence in U.S. population (%)	Percentage of SUD cases in the drug class that co-occur with other SUDs[a]
Alcohol	13.9	15.0
Cannabis	2.5	63.5
Prescription opioid	0.9	56.8
Prescription sedative	−0.4	73.7
Cocaine	−0.3	86.0
Prescription stimulant	−0.3	73.1
Other drug	0.2	82.3
Heroin	0.1	77.1
Hallucinogen	<0.1	91.0
Inhalant	<0.1	97.5

Note. N = 36,309. SUD, substance use disorder. Data from McCabe et al. (2017).
[a]As percentages approach 100%, nearly all of the substance use disorders in that drug class co-occurred with one or more substance use disorders from the other nine classes.

By comparison, 63.5% of the cannabis use disorder diagnoses were accompanied by another substance use disorder. Inhalant use disorder was the drug class most likely to co-occur with other substance use disorders, that is, 97.5% of the time. These data show a high degree of co-occurrence in nonalcohol drug use in the U.S. population (McCabe et al., 2017).

NESARC-III data also have been used to examine associations between psychiatric disorder and multiple substance use disorder (McCabe et al., 2017). As shown in Table 4.2, 8.7% of persons with a personality disorder also had multiple substance use disorders in the past year, followed by persons with posttraumatic stress disorder in which 8.0% had multiple substance use disorders. Anxiety disorder was less likely to be associated with multiple substance use disorder.

Findings from NESARC-III reveal that persons with alcohol use disorder or drug use disorder are at heightened risk for also having coexisting DSM-5 psychiatric conditions. The adjusted odds ratios in Table 4.3 represent the probability of individuals with an alcohol use disorder or a drug use disorder having a coexisting condition, compared to those individuals without the disorder. The odds ratios are adjusted statistically to account for potentially confounding effects of demographic characteristics and other psychiatric comorbidity. Thus, the adjusted odds ratios in Table 4.3 represent conservative estimates of the associations between alcohol/drug use disorder and the coexisting DSM-5 conditions.

As illustrated in Table 4.3, persons with alcohol use disorder were 3.3 times more likely than those without the disorder to have a drug use disorder. In contrast, persons with drug use disorder were 3.2 times more likely than those without the disorder to have an alcohol use disorder. Though not surprising, these analyses confirm that alcohol use disorder and drug use disorder often co-occur in individuals. Furthermore, alcohol

TABLE 4.2. Prevalence of Multiple Substance Use Disorders by Type of Psychiatric Disorder in the U.S. Population: Past-Year Findings from the NESARC-III

DSM-5 psychiatric disorder	Past-year prevalence of multiple SUDs in U.S. population (%)
Personality disorder	8.7
Posttraumatic stress disorder	8.0
Multiple psychiatric disorders	6.6
Eating disorder	6.0
Mood disorder	5.0
Anxiety disorder	4.6

Note. N = 36,309. SUD, substance use disorder. Data from McCabe et al. (2017).

use disorder and drug use disorder are associated with other coexisting psychiatric conditions. For instance, persons with alcohol use disorder are 40% more likely to have a bipolar I diagnosis than persons without alcohol use disorder, whereas persons with drug use disorder are 50% more likely to have a bipolar I diagnosis than persons without it.

The adjusted odds ratios in Table 4.3 also indicate that alcohol and drug use disorders coexist less frequently with anxiety disorders. In contrast, alcohol/drug use disorders and personality disorders are frequently associated with one another. Persons with alcohol use disorder are 60% more likely to have a diagnosis of antisocial personality disorder and 90% are more likely to have a diagnosis of borderline personality, compared to persons without an alcohol use disorder. With regard to persons with drug use disorders, heightened risk exists for antisocial (40%), borderline (80%), and schizotypal (50%) personality disorders.

TABLE 4.3. Past 12-Month Comorbidity in the U.S. Adult Population: Adjusted Odds Ratios from the NESARC-III

Coexisting DSM-5 condition	Adjusted odds ratios (95% confidence interval)	
	Alcohol use disorder	Drug use disorder
Alcohol use disorder	—	3.2 (2.81–3.66)*
Any drug use disorder	3.3 (2.88–3.76)*	—
Nicotine use disorder	2.5 (2.24–2.69)*	3.2 (2.78–3.68)*
Any mood disorder	1.3 (1.18–1.47)*	1.9 (1.58–2.77)*
Major depressive disorder	1.2 (1.08–1.36)*	1.3 (1.09–1.64)*
Bipolar I disorder	1.4 (1.08–1.78)*	1.5 (1.06–2.05)*
Bipolar II disorder	1.3 (0.70–2.39)	1.3 (0.63–2.69)
Persistent depression	0.9 (0.72–1.15)	1.5 (1.09–2.02)*
Any anxiety disorder	1.1 (0.97–1.27)	1.2 (0.99–1.50)
Panic disorder	1.1 (0.89–1.42)	1.0 (0.73–1.44)
Agoraphobia	1.1 (0.81–1.44)	1.0 (0.63–1.43)
Social anxiety disorder	0.8 (0.63–0.98)*	1.1 (0.84–1.49)
Specific phobia	1.2 (1.03–1.43)*	0.9 (0.73–1.20)
Generalized anxiety disorder	1.0 (0.86–1.22)	1.2 (0.89–1.55)
Posttraumatic stress disorder	1.0 (0.86–1.22)	1.6 (1.27–2.10)*
Personality disorder	—	—
Antisocial	1.6 (1.28–1.94)*	1.4 (1.11–1.75)*
Borderline	1.9 (1.66–2.23)*	1.8 (1.41–2.24)*
Schizotypal	1.1 (0.95–1.28)	1.5 (1.18–1.87)*

Note. N = 36,309. Data from B.F. Grant et al. (2015, 2016). Drug use disorder excludes alcohol. Adjusted odds ratios represent the probability of individuals with a DSM-5 alcohol use disorder or a drug use disorder having the coexisting condition, compared to those individuals without the disorder. The odds ratios are adjusted for a number of potential confounders, including age, race/ethnicity, sex, education, family income, marital status, urbanicity, geographic region, and additional psychiatric comorbidity. Asterisks indicate a statistically significant adjusted odds ratio ($p < .05$).

Comorbidity among Persons Who Seek Treatment

An earlier 2001–2002 NESARC survey relying on DSM-IV criteria found that relatively small percentages of persons with substance use, mood, and anxiety disorders sought treatment for these conditions (Grant et al., 2006). In the previous 12-month period, only 5.8% of those diagnosed with alcohol abuse or alcohol dependence sought treatment, compared to 13.1% meeting criteria for any drug abuse or drug dependence diagnosis. Among those with mood disorders, 26.0% sought treatment for these conditions. Among those with anxiety disorders, 12.1% sought treatment.

An important set of findings from the 2001–2002 NESARC reveals that many persons who seek treatment for a mood or anxiety disorder also have some type of substance use disorder (Grant et al., 2006). Table 4.4 shows that 15.4% (panic disorder without agoraphobia) to 31.0% (hypomania) of persons seeking treatment for specific mood or anxiety disorders in the past year had coexisting substance use problems during the same time period. These findings are of considerable clinical significance because if a substance use disorder is not recognized in the treatment of mood and anxiety disorder, the prognosis for both disorders may be poor.

NESARC survey data indicate that the co-occurrence of alcohol/drug problems with mental health problems represents a common psychiatric syndrome in the U.S. population. Thus, comorbidity should be an expectation rather than viewed as the exception (SAMHSA, 2002). Persons with substance dependence disorders (alcohol and other drugs) are much more likely to have a coexisting mood, anxiety, or personality disorder than persons without substance dependence diagnoses. These mental health problems appear to be independent of alcohol/drug intoxication and

TABLE 4.4. Prevalence of Substance Use Disorders among Respondents Seeking Treatment for Mood or Anxiety Disorders in the Past 12 Months: Findings from the NESARC, 2001–2002

Condition for which treatment sought	Percentage with any SUD
Any mood disorder	20.8
Major depression	20.3
Dysthymia	18.5
Mania	22.5
Hypomania	31.0
Any anxiety disorder	16.5
Panic disorder with agoraphobia	21.9
Panic disorder without agoraphobia	15.4
Social phobia	21.3
Specific phobia	16.0
Generalized anxiety disorder	15.9

Note. N = 43,093. SUD, substance use disorder. Data from B. F. Grant et al. (2006).

withdrawal. Furthermore, many persons who seek treatment for mood or anxiety disorders have a substance use disorder as well, which highlights the need for careful, systematic client assessment and integrated treatment of both disorders. As noted by SAMHSA (2002) in a report to the U.S. Congress: "Improving the Nation's public health demands prompt attention to the problem of co-occurring disorders" (see Executive Summary). Unfortunately, little progress has been made in the past 15 years.

Levels of Comorbidity across Patterns of Substance Use Disorder

Kandel, Huang, and Davies (2001) examined the extent to which individuals with one or more drug use disorders had coexisting major depression or any anxiety disorder (i.e., a mood disorder of some type). The investigators found that a *single* substance use disorder of any type had similar degrees of association with the mood disorders. However, the co-occurrence of a licit substance use disorder (nicotine or alcohol) and an illicit drug use disorder was associated with nearly a doubling of the odds of a coexisting mood disorder. The odds of having a coexisting mood disorder did not appear to be elevated by the co-occurrence of nicotine use and alcohol use disorders, however. Kandel and colleagues concluded that persons seeking treatment for substance use disorders that involve both a licit and an illicit drug will likely be those most in need of mental health services. In other words, a multiple substance use disorder of this type may be a marker for other psychiatric problems.

Cannabis Use and Psychiatric Comorbidity in Adults

Among the federally defined illegal substances, cannabis is the most widely used drug in the United States, with an estimated 22.2 million past-month users in 2015 (Center for Behavioral Health Statistics and Quality, 2016a). This number represents about 8.3% of the 2015 U.S. population. The drug also is the source of a great deal of controversy and public debate because many users and groups that advocate for reform of marijuana laws contend that the drug causes little harm (see *www.norml.org*). A Quinnipiac University national poll found that in February 2017, 59% of U.S. voters believed that marijuana should be legalized; 93% thought physicians should be able to prescribe marijuana; and 71% indicated that federal laws prohibiting marijuana use should not be enforced in states that legalized medical or recreational use of marijuana (Quinnipiac University Poll, 2017). As a result of these changing norms, a number of American states have legalized recreational cannabis use in recent years, and it appears more may do so in the future (Chilkoti, 2017).

Blanco and colleagues (2016) used NESARC data to examine the prospective relationship between cannabis use and risk of developing a psychiatric disorder at a subsequent 3-year assessment. Cannabis use at baseline was not associated with mood disorders or anxiety disorders at follow-up. However, baseline cannabis use was significantly associated with a number of substance use disorders 3 years later. For instance, as illustrated by the adjusted odds ratios in Table 4.5 on the next page, persons were 2.3 times more likely to meet criteria for alcohol dependence at follow-up if they had used cannabis at baseline, compared to those who had no baseline cannabis use. Similar patterns of association existed for all of the other substance use disorders identified in Table 4.5. Thus, in this nationally representative sample of U.S. adults, cannabis use was associated with substantially increased risk of developing alcohol and other drug disorders within a 3-year period. Although these associations should not be interpreted as evidence that cannabis use *causes* subsequent alcohol/drug disorders, it does appear that marijuana use is a marker for subsequent alcohol and other drug problems—but not for mood or anxiety disorders.

Cannabis Use and Psychiatric Comorbidity among Adolescents

Many studies on cannabis use and its relation to psychiatric conditions among adolescents have suffered from flaws in study design. Some studies have relied on cross-sectional designs, whereas other longitudinal studies did not repeatedly assess cannabis use at multiple time-points throughout adolescence. Moreover, until recently, longitudinal studies did not examine cannabis usage and psychotic symptoms *within individuals*, thereby allowing for an examination of two important questions: (1) Do psychotic symptoms increase during periods of regular cannabis use (a concurrent effect)? and (2) Does regular, multiyear use of cannabis produce an incremental and sustained increase in subclinical psychotic symptoms even after periods of abstinence from cannabis (a cumulative/sustained effect)?

Employing a within-individuals design, Bechtold, Hipwell, Lewis, Loeber, and Pardini (2016) recruited a sample of 1,009 boys in the first and seventh grades from the Pittsburgh public schools. Data were initially collected in 1987–1988. Boys in the first-grade cohort were interviewed every 6 months for 4 years, followed by nine annual assessments and follow-ups when participants were usually ages 26 and 29. Boys in the seventh-grade cohort were assessed every 6 months for 30 months, then annually for 10 years, and again when they were an average age of 36. Data from the two cohorts were combined by aligning assessments by participant age at the time of the interview. The assessments record self-reported frequency of cannabis use, subclinical psychotic symptoms, and a number of

TABLE 4.5. Past 12-Month Cannabis Use at Baseline and Substance Use Disorders at 3-Year Follow-Up: Adjusted Odds Ratios from the NESARC

DSM-IV substance use disorder	Adjusted odds ratios (95% confidence interval)
Any substance use disorder	2.8 (2.4–3.4)*
Any alcohol use disorder	2.5 (2.1–3.0)*
Abuse	1.8 (1.4–2.3)*
Dependence	2.3 (1.9–2.9)*
Any cannabis disorder	12.4 (8.9–17.2)*
Abuse	12.3 (8.9–17.0)*
Dependence	9.0 (3.9–20.8)*
Any other drug use disorder	3.1 (2.1–4.6)*
Abuse	3.0 (1.9–4.7)*
Dependence	3.0 (1.7–5.3)*
Nicotine dependence	1.5 (1.2–1.8)*

Note. N = 34,653. Data from Blanco et al. (2016). Adjusted odds ratios represent the probability of individuals with baseline cannabis use (in past 12 months) having a substance use disorder 3 years later, compared to those individuals with no baseline cannabis use. The odds ratios are adjusted for a broad range of potential confounders that assess individual characteristics at different stages of life. Asterisks indicate a statistically significant adjusted odds ratio ($p < .05$).

potential confounding variables (Bechtold et al., 2016). Subclinical symptoms included feelings of paranoia, hallucinations, bizarre thinking, and behavior other people think strange. Endorsement of these measures by teenagers has been found in previous research to be associated with the development of psychoses later in life (Kaymaz et al., 2012).

Bechtold and colleagues (2016) found that for each year adolescent boys engaged in regular marijuana use, their subsequent level of subclinical psychotic symptoms increased 21%; their expected odds of experiencing subsequent subclinical paranoia rose 133%; and their expected odds of reporting hallucinations jumped 92%. The effect of previous, regular cannabis use on later subclinical psychotic symptoms persisted even after boys abstained from cannabis for 12 months. Bechtold and colleagues tested for and found no evidence that subclinical psychotic symptoms caused cannabis use, that is, reverse causation. The researchers concluded that regular cannabis use during adolescence significantly increases the likelihood of persistent subclinical psychotic symptoms, that is, even after stopping use of the drug (Bechtold et al., 2016).

EXPLANATORY MODELS

The epidemiological data reviewed thus far indicate that substance use disorders co-occur with other psychiatric disorders at rates far exceeding that explained by chance or coincidence. Unfortunately, these data do little to elucidate the nature of these comorbid conditions. Much work has been devoted to establishing the onset order of the co-occurring disorders (e.g., does alcohol dependence typically predate the onset of major depression?). Though important, questions about order of onset fail to address the most fundamental issues at a nosological level. When comorbidity is observed, does it truly represent the presence of two distinct disorders or instead an uninformed appraisal that does not recognize a third *independent disorder* that encompasses the broader symptomatology of the comorbid condition? Eaton (2015) contends that DSM-5 nosology is inadequate because mental disorders are not true independent conditions. Instead, *transdiagnostic factors* produce co-occurring mental disorders and explain why comorbidity in the psychiatric patient population is the rule rather than the exception (Kim & Eaton, 2015). In the co-occurrence of substance use and other psychiatric problems, these issues of classification are among the most pressing questions for both clinical practitioners and researchers.

Table 4.6 identifies 10 models that attempt to clarify the association between substance use and other psychological problems (Neale & Kendler, 1995). The question each model attempts to address also appears in the table. Chance, sampling bias, and population stratification are models that assert that comorbid conditions are nothing more than artifacts (i.e., the co-occurrence is not significant or meaningful). Clearly, the epidemiological data reviewed here indicate that this is not the case. However, these models are useful for helping us to clarify our understanding of the nature of comorbidity and thus have been included in Table 4.6 on the next page.

The model labeled *alternative forms* maintains that the co-occurrence of substance use and other psychological problems arises from a single risk factor with a single threshold of severity (Agrawal et al., 2004). Others have referred to this as a *general latent factor model* (Sunderland, Slade, & Krueger, 2015). Regardless, the model proposes that a risk factor increases the likelihood of both substance use and psychiatric disorder. The common risk factors most discussed in the research literature are genetic vulnerability, antisocial personality disorder, disordered mesolimbic activity in the brain, and poverty (Mueser, Noordsy, Drake, & Fox, 2003). One landmark study in molecular genetics found that a variation in the muscarinic acetylcholine receptor M2 is a risk factor for the associated clinical characteristics of both alcohol dependence and major depression (Wang et al., 2004). More recently, studies have identified several genetic risk factors of the central nervous system that have been linked to comorbid bipolar disorder/alcohol dependence (Chang et al., 2015; Dalvie, Fabbri, Ramesar, Serretti, & Stein, 2016; Lydall et al., 2011; Sharp et al., 2014). Investigators believe that a shared molecular pathophysiology may underlie these two disorders. Findings such as these give rise to speculation that, in the future,

TABLE 4.6. Models of Comorbidity

Name	Question posed by the model
Chance	Is the co-occurrence of the disorders due simply to chance?
Sampling bias	Do we overestimate the prevalence of comorbid conditions in the general population because our observations are derived from a clinical population that has been referred for treatment?
Population stratification	Do we overestimate the prevalence of comorbid conditions in the general population because we fail to account for subgroup differences, such as socioeconomic status or other stratification variables?
Alternate forms	Is there one underlying risk factor that gives rise to both disorders?
Random multiformity	Does the comorbid condition represent an atypical form of one of the disorders with symptoms that overlap with those of the second disorder?
Extreme multiformity	Does the atypical form arise only after risk factors for either or both of the disorders reach extreme levels?
Three independent disorders	Does the comorbid condition represent a third disorder that is distinct from the other two disorders?
Correlated liabilities	Do the two disorders have a high probability of co-occurring because they arise from a set of shared risk factors?
Causation	Is one disorder a risk factor for the subsequent onset of the other disorder?
Reciprocal causation	Regardless of which disorder appears first, do the two disorders exacerbate one another with the passage of time?

other shared and specific genetic risk factors may be found to underlie a variety of comorbid conditions.

Random multiformity and *extreme multiformity* are models that assume that one disorder can take heterogeneous or atypical forms (Klein & Riso, 1993). In such situations, symptoms will appear that are typically associated with other disorders. Thus, multiformity does not represent true comorbidity but, instead, "indicates that the boundaries of a disorder have been drawn in the wrong place" (Klein & Riso, 1993, p. 44). Extreme multiformity is a variant model that assumes the atypical form will appear only when the severity of the risk factors for either or both of the disorders is at elevated thresholds. For instance, the co-occurrence of cannabis dependence and social phobia (an anxiety disorder) might not be likely to occur unless the frequency of marijuana smoking reaches some high threshold or there exists an extensive family history of anxiety disorder. These models challenge conventional diagnostic criteria, which do not rely on specific subcriteria for establishing diagnostic boundaries and symptom thresholds.

The model known as *three independent disorders* assumes that the comorbid condition is actually a distinct disorder itself. Neale and Kendler (1995) describe this model as "somewhat implausible" (p. 941). It is the only model that asserts that the co-occurrence arises from a process that is completely separate from those that instigate the development of the other two disorders.

The *correlated liabilities* model proposes that comorbid conditions arise because prevalent forms of co-occurrence tend to share common sets of risk factors (Neale & Kendler, 1995). Although any two disorders will have common and unique risk factors, the overlapping of them will contribute to a rate of co-occurrence that is higher than that expected by chance. For example, the co-occurrence of substance dependence and depression in adolescence may arise from a variety of forms of neglect and abuse experienced during childhood.

The straightforward *causation* model asserts that one disorder operates as a risk factor for the subsequent onset of a second disorder. For instance, alcohol dependence causes major depression. Causation models assert that one disorder predates the other in time of onset. Two types of causation models have been proposed to specify the order of onset of substance use and other psychiatric disorders (Mueser et al., 2003). The secondary substance abuse model proposes that psychopathology precedes and causes substance abuse. In contrast, the secondary psychiatric disorder model maintains that substance abuse precedes and causes psychopathology.

Finally, the *reciprocal causation* model proposes that, over time, substance use and psychopathology will exacerbate one another. Arising from clinical observations, this model is less concerned with the order of onset of the disorders and is more focused on integrated treatment options (Mueser et al., 2003). In addition, the reciprocal causation model tends to emphasize the role of multiple risk factors in the immediate social environment of the dual-diagnosis patient, including negative peer influences, employment problems, and limited recreational opportunities.

Problem Behavior Theory: A Social-Psychological Framework for Explaining Comorbidity

One alternative framework for understanding the co-occurrence of substance abuse and other mental health problems is problem behavior theory (Jessor & Jessor, 1977; Jessor et al., 1991). The result of longitudinal research on the development of adolescents and young adults, this longstanding social-psychological model maintains that human behavior is the result of person–environment interaction. The theory consists of three interdependent systems of variables: (1) the behavior system, which encompasses a conventional behavior syndrome or a problem behavior syndrome (substance abuse, low academic achievement, aggression, etc.); (2) the personality system, which particularly includes such variables as achievement motivation, affiliation–alienation, self-esteem, and mental health; and (3) the perceived environmental system, which includes "perceived controls and instigations from significant others in the life space, particularly parents and friends" (Jessor et al., 1991, p. 29).

In problem behavior theory, the variables from each system represent either instigations or controls that, in combination, generate "proneness" or the probability of resultant problem behavior. Although proneness can exist in one, two, or all three of the systems, overall *psychosocial proneness* is the central concept of the theory and is used to predict and explain variation in problem behavior. Psychological proneness can be considered the "outcome of the balance of instigation toward and controls against engaging in problem behavior" (Jessor et al., 1991, p. 19). In essence, the psychological concepts of *instigations* and *controls* can be thought of as analogous to the epidemiological notions of *risk* and *protective* factors.

A major proposition of this theory is that problem behaviors are highly interrelated (Jessor & Jessor, 1977). That is, *multiple* problem behaviors (often more than two) tend to co-occur within individuals. The data collected by Jessor and colleagues (1991) suggest that it is relatively unusual for individuals to have just one problem behavior. Instead, these problems tend to co-occur in prone individuals. For instance, Jessor and colleagues have noted that individuals who smoke cigarettes are much more likely to engage in a range of risk behavior, including sexual risk taking, drinking and driving, and other deviant behavior.

The tendency of multiple problem behaviors to cluster within individuals is described as *problem behavior syndrome*. The syndrome concept implies that a common factor (psychosocial proneness) underlies the development of different types of problem behaviors. The structural equation models created by Jessor and colleagues (1991) provide strong evidence to support the syndrome concept of both problem behavior and conventional (nonproblem) behavior. More than one half of the variance in both problem behavior involvement and conventional behavior involvement can be explained by the psychosocial measures assessed in their longitudinal investigation (Jessor et al., 1991). An important point is that "problem behavior" does not necessarily imply antisocial behavior. Rather, the term is reserved for a broad range of behaviors that undermine conventional (or normal) human psychosocial development.

Problem behavior theory does not encompass psychiatric/medical conceptions of mental illness but, instead, relies on traditional measures used in the field of social psychology. Nevertheless, the theory rests on a strong empirical foundation. Thus, the propositions of problem behavior theory have great significance for helping us to understand the co-occurrence of substance use disorder and mental health problems. In particular, the rather narrow psychiatric perspective focusing on two coexisting DSM disorders may not be an adequate or rich enough model for capturing the many psychosocial problems and life challenges of so-called dual-diagnosis patients (Drake, Wallach, Alverson, & Mueser, 2002). Our understanding of coexisting substance use and mental disorders may be enhanced by further interdisciplinary inquiry.

The Role of Discounting Delayed Consequences

Findings from an expanding body of research in the areas of behavioral economics and neuroscience suggest that persons with substance use disorders tend to *discount* both the value of delayed reinforcement and the severity of reinforcement losses encountered at a later time, compared to persons without these disorders (Amlung, Vedelago, Acker, Balodis, & MacKillop, 2017; Bickel & Marsch, 2001; Higgins, Heil, & Lussier, 2004; Owens, Amlung, Beach, Sweet, & MacKillop, 2017). In other words, substance abusers appear to prefer immediate reinforcement, even if it is of smaller magnitude, over delayed reinforcement of greater magnitude, and they prefer that punishment be delayed, even if it means that its magnitude will increase. This preference represents a proneness toward impulsive decision making.

An intriguing possibility is that increased rates of discounting may be associated with comorbidity. Substance abusers with co-occurring attention-deficit/hyperactivity disorder (Miguel et al., 2016) and pathological gambling (Krmpotich et al., 2015) have been found to discount delayed consequences more than substance abusers without these comorbid conditions. Furthermore, persons suffering from psychosis report that despite being aware of the long-term physical and mental consequences of substance abuse, they use drugs to obtain immediate pleasure and to find relief from dysphoria and the unpleasant side-effects of antipsychotic medication (Charles & Weaver, 2010). Thus, it is possible that in the population of mentally ill persons, comorbidity may be most likely to occur in those who have poor impulse control and are less sensitive to the longer-term contingencies associated with alcohol and drug use. More research is needed in this area.

Treatment of Adolescents with Comorbid Conditions

In the past decade, there has been significant growth in the research literature focused on the treatment of substance abuse in the adolescent population. Tanner-Smith, Wilson, and Lipsey (2013) conducted a comprehensive review of adolescent treatment studies and concluded that a majority of the studies reported positive treatment outcomes for teenagers. Treatments based on cognitive–behavioral therapy, motivational interviewing, and family/systems approaches were found to most consistently produce beneficial effects. Each of these three approaches has generated an overall level of empirical support that is regarded as acceptable for adoption by treatment programs (Becker & Curry, 2008). In addition, positive adolescent treatment outcomes have been observed in 12-step program participation (Kelly & Urbanski, 2012), but research on the use of this approach among teenagers is restricted (Donovan, Ingalsbe, Benbow, & Daley, 2013).

Although progress has been made in identifying effective interventions for adolescent substance abuse, the magnitude of treatment gains in this population can be moderated by the presence of comorbid conditions. Yet, adolescent substance abuse treatment that also addresses co-occurring psychiatric disorders is often underutilized or unavailable (Brewer, Godley, & Hulvershorn, 2017). This is unfortunate because in adolescent substance use disorder, the presence of co-occurring psychiatric conditions is more likely to exist than not (Godley et al., 2014; Hulvershorn, Quinn, & Scott, 2015). Among adolescents with substance use disorder, the most prevalent co-occurring psychiatric condition may be conduct disorder. However, attention-deficit/hyperactivity disorder, depression, anxiety, and traumatic distress are also common. These conditions have been found to moderate the effects of substance abuse treatment for adolescents (Godley et al., 2014; Hulvershorn et al., 2015). Adolescents with conduct disorder in particular are less likely to be engaged by treatment and more likely to leave it prematurely. Nevertheless, evidence indicates that treatment participation can produce significant improvements in the emotional and behavioral problems of adolescents with substance use disorders (Godley et al., 2014; Hulvershorn et al., 2015).

The National Registry of Evidence-based Programs and Practices, maintained by SAMHSA (2017), identifies 10 evidence-based approaches for treating adolescents experiencing substance abuse and any type of co-occurring psychiatric disorder. These include the adolescent community reinforcement approach, Chestnut Health Systems–Bloomington Adolescent Outpatient and Intensive Outpatient Treatment Model, family behavior therapy, family support network (comprising 12 sessions of motivational enhancement therapy/cognitive–behavioral therapy, a family component, and case management), multidimensional family therapy (discussed in Chapter 8), multisystemic therapy (also discussed in Chapter 8), Parenting with Love and Limits, Phoenix House Academy, The Seven Challenges, and Seeking Safety. However, the efficacy of these approaches for treating specific combinations of comorbid conditions is largely unknown. For example, effective treatment for adolescent substance use disorder that co-occurs with conduct disorder may require different strategies than when it co-occurs with depression or another type of psychiatric condition (Hulvershorn et al., 2015).

In the treatment community, questions have been raised about the usefulness of 12-step participation by people with psychiatric disorders and by those who are adolescents (Chi, Sterling, Campbell, & Weisner, 2013). The concerns are that the former group may not be accepted by AA and NA members who do not have a comorbid psychiatric condition and that the latter group, that is, adolescents, are developmentally incapable of working with the spiritual model of 12-step programs. To examine these issues, Chi and colleagues (2013) followed a sample of 419 adolescents, ages 13–18, who entered outpatient substance use treatment. Their participation in 12-step programs and its relationship to treatment outcomes were tracked over a 7-year period. Those teenagers who were diagnosed with a co-occurring psychiatric condition at treatment admission were found to have more intensive substance abuse, compared to those without a co-occurring condition at admission. Over the 7-year period, the comorbid adolescents participated in 12-step groups at the same or greater levels than those without a psychiatric diagnosis—which challenges the notion that psychiatric morbidities interfere with 12-step participation. Chi and colleagues found that those with a co-occurring psychiatric diagnosis had similar or better substance use outcomes at the 7-year follow-up, compared to those without such a diagnosis. Furthermore, in both the comorbid and noncomorbid groups, 12-step participation was associated with abstinence from drugs and alcohol. The investigators concluded that the comorbidity status of the adolescents was unrelated to substance abuse treatment outcomes and that the comorbid teenagers appeared to have benefited as much from 12-step participation as those without a co-occurring psychiatric disorder.

Treatment of Adults with Dual Diagnoses

The term *dual diagnosis* is often used to refer to the subset of possible comorbidities that involve a substance use disorder and a severe mental illness—usually schizophrenia or bipolar disorder. Persons with dual diagnoses pose special challenges to mutual-help organizations, such as AA and NA, and the treatment systems that offer them assistance. They may experience opposition from 12-step members who question their use of psychotropic medications (for treating the comorbid condition). They may be perceived to be disruptive or noncompliant with meeting or treatment rules. Others may be uncomfortable with persons with dual diagnoses because of their involvement in the criminal justice system or their risk for harming themselves (Drake et al., 2016; Greenberg & Rosenheck, 2008; Rush et al., 2008). Persons with dual diagnoses may frequently drop out of treatment or become involved in the "revolving door" of brief inpatient treatment admissions to resolve crises. Also, care of these patients also stretches the fiscal resources of the treatment system. One early study of dual-diagnosis patients found that their treatment costs were almost 60% higher than those for psychiatric patients without a substance use disorder (Dickey & Azeni, 1996). Although sound population-level prevalence rate estimates are not available, dual diagnosis patients may make up 25 to 28% of the total U.S. homeless population (Fletcher & Reback, 2017; Tsai, Kasprow, & Rosenheck, 2013).

In a review of the literature on substance use disorders and severe mental illness (schizophrenia or bipolar disorder), Mueser and colleagues (1998) suggested that these associations may be explained by more than one model. They proposed that the features of these comorbid conditions may be of two types: an antisocial personality disorder (ASPD) model and a supersensitivity model. The ASPD model conceptualizes the co-occurrence of substance use disorder and severe mental illness as a problem of developmental psychopathology. That is, ASPD—and its childhood precursor, conduct disorder—is viewed to be the common factor that increases risk for the subsequent development of both substance use disorder and serious mental illness in young adulthood. In contrast, the supersensitivity model posits that persons with a coexisting substance use disorder and severe mental illness are extremely vulnerable to stress. Psychotherapeutic medications usually decrease this vulnerability. However, alcohol and street drug use, even in relatively small quantities, may greatly exacerbate the psychiatric symptomatology. In essence, persons with dual diagnoses

TABLE 4.7. Two Models Explaining the Co-Occurrence of Substance Use Disorder and Severe Mental Illness

Feature	ASPD model	Supersensitivity model
Age of onset of substance use disorder	Earlier	Later
Quantity of substance use	Higher	Lower
Physical dependence on a drug	More likely	Less likely
Family history of substance abuse	More likely	Less likely
Age of onset of severe mental illness	Earlier	Later
Premorbid social functioning	Marginal	Good
Social functioning	Poor	Good
Psychiatric symptoms	More severe	Less severe
Aggression	More likely	Less likely
Prognosis	Guarded	Good

Note. From Mueser, Drake, and Wallach (1998). Copyright 1998 by Elsevier. Adapted by permission.

are "supersensitive" to the negative consequences of alcohol and drug use, even at low doses or infrequent use. Table 4.7 identifies the features of these two proposed models.

INTEGRATED TREATMENT FOR DUAL DIAGNOSIS

Not too long ago, discussions about treating persons with co-occurring substance use disorder and severe mental illness tended to focus on the most appropriate *sequence* of independently delivered treatment regimens (see NIAAA, 1994, pp. 51–53). Persons experiencing these problems were treated either at the same time in separate substance abuse and mental health treatment programs (i.e., parallel treatments), or in one program first, discharged, and then treated in the second program (i.e., sequential treatment). The advantages and disadvantages of these two approaches were weighed and evaluated in the context of traditional treatment delivery systems. Over the last 15 years or so, innovations have led to the development of the *integrated treatment model* (Drake & Mueser, 2001; Drake, Mueser, & Brunette, 2007). Though still evolving, the core feature of this model is the application of coordinated, concurrent treatment of two or more disorders in programs designed specifically for those patients with comorbid substance abuse and severe mental illness (Drake et al., 2007; Mercer, Mueser, & Drake, 1998; Pringle, Grasso, & Lederer, 2017).

During the 1990s, dissatisfaction with the traditional treatment modalities gave rise to a set of guiding principles for the provision of integrated treatment (Drake, Mercer-McFadden, Mueser, McHugo, & Bond, 1998). For persons who struggle with substance use and who also suffer from severe mental illness, such as schizophrenia, treatment should be provided by one integrated program that is designed to address both disorders. It is not adequate to sequentially treat one disorder and then the other at a later time. One feature, then, of integrated treatment is the employment of clinical staff members who are trained to treat both substance abuse and severe mental disorder. Another feature of integrated treatment is that many of the traditional practices used in addiction treatment programs need to be modified to properly assist those with severe mental illness. For instance, in integrated treatment, the emphasis is placed on establishing a relationship with patients and helping them to cope, whereas in traditional addiction treatment, confrontation often is used to break down denial (Mueser & Gingerich, 2013). Furthermore, to engage patients, integrated treatment endorses a harm reduction approach that may not insist on immediate abstinence from alcohol and illicit drugs. Consistent with this approach, there is recognition that treatment will probably be long term—at least for most patients. Thus, counseling is stage-based and motivational—not confrontational. In addition, to adequately attend to crises, integrated treatment needs to be provided in facilities that can offer around-the-clock access to treatment staff. In such an environment, 12-step programs must be available, but participation should be voluntary. Finally, in integrated treatment programs, the patient's severe mental illness is recognized as a biological disorder that usually needs to be treated with psychotherapeutic medication. Medication is not thought to compromise the treatment goals set for the substance use disorder. Table 4.8 summarizes these principles.

Effectiveness of Integrated Treatment

In two reviews of studies on integrated treatment, Drake and colleagues (1998) and Brunette, Mueser, and Drake (2004) concluded that the methodological limitations of the research conducted to date preclude any firm conclusions about the effectiveness of the approach. With these caveats in mind, the available evidence suggests that simply adding dual-diagnosis groups to traditional services is not effective. Also, integrated treatment, when delivered via *intensive* inpatient, residential, or day treatment, does not appear effective. The dropout rate in these programs is high, presumably because of the insistence on abstinence. Low-intensity programs may

---

TABLE 4.8. Guiding Principles of the Integrated Treatment Model

1. Treatment is provided by one integrated program designed to address both substance use disorder and severe mental illness.

2. The substance use disorder and the severe mental illness are treated by one team of dually trained clinicians.

3. The treatment for substance use disorder deviates from traditional "detox" and "rehab" practices and is tailored to the needs of those with severe mental illness.

4. Emphasis is placed on reducing anxiety—not breaking through denial about substance abuse.

5. Attempts are made to build trust and engage the patient in treatment— confrontation is avoided.

6. Priority is placed on reducing the harm associated with substance abuse— insistence on immediate abstinence may be counterproductive.

7. There is a recognition that treatment will probably be long term—rapid detoxification and short-term treatment followed by discharge is not realistic.

8. Counseling is stage based and motivational—not confrontational and time limited.

9. Around-the-clock access to treatment staff—not limited to daytime office hours— is essential.

10. Participation in 12-step programs is available and encouraged—but not mandatory.

11. Use of psychotherapeutic medications is based on the patient's psychiatric and medical needs—the goals of substance abuse treatment are not seen as compromising reliance on these medications.

---

be more effective. The authors found some reason to be optimistic about the prospects of newer comprehensive, integrated treatment approaches that rely on long-term, stage-based, motivational counseling. The somewhat better outcomes may be attributed to employing assertive outreach and possibly not insisting on immediate abstinence from alcohol and other illicit drugs.

Results from other studies bolster the view that long-term, comprehensive treatment is important for "engaging" patients with dual diagnoses (i.e., keeping them in treatment). For instance, one comparison of long-term and short-term residential programs found that at follow-up, patients with dual diagnoses in the former type of program were more likely to stay in treatment, more likely to maintain abstinence, and less likely to experience homelessness (Brunette, Drake, Woods, & Hartnett., 2001). There were no statistically significant differences between the two groups on measures of psychiatric hospitalization, incarceration, or number of moves. The investigators concluded that patients with dual diagnoses need safe, stable, sober living environments to learn skills for maintaining abstinence and that the acquisition of these skills is less likely to occur in intensive, short-term programs that may be too challenging. Another study of long-term outcomes of integrated treatment followed 126 dual-diagnosis patients for up to 3 years (Judd, Thomas, Schwartz, Outcalt, & Hough, 2003). The study found that integrated treatment produced statistically significant improvements in quality of life, substance use, and psychiatric symptoms. Moreover, these improvements were associated with decreases in health care and criminal justice costs (Judd et al., 2003).

Unfortunately, significant policy and organizational impediments are associated with the adoption, implementation, and maintenance of dual-diagnosis treatment programs (Clark, Power, Le Fauve, & Lopez, 2008; Mercer et al., 1998). One of the problems is an inadequate workforce prepared to deliver integrated treatment services (Flynn & Brown, 2008; McGovern, Xie, Segal, Siembab, & Drake, 2006). Although many states have implemented services for dual-diagnosis clients, high-quality treatment programs are the exception, not the rule (Clark et al., 2008; Flynn & Brown, 2008; Hawkins, 2009). Public investment in these programs may depend on research that can demonstrate cost-effectiveness.

CHAPTER SUMMARY

Comorbidity remains one of the most poorly understood areas in addictions and substance use treatment fields (Bennett, Bradshaw, & Catalano, 2017; Hasan et al., 2015). Although surveillance studies have begun to document the patterns of association between substance use disorders and mental disorders and have established that these associations are not due to chance, much remains to be understood about the etiology and treatment of the many types of comorbid conditions involving substance abuse and mental health disorders (Kushner, 2014). Treatment study reviews on persons with co-occurring mood/anxiety and substance use disorders conclude that there is a lack of evidence for most treatment recommendations (Tiet & Mausbach, 2007; Watkins, Hunter, Burnam, Pincus, & Nicholson, 2005). In addition, in a systematic review of 32 randomized controlled trials that tested interventions for dual-diagnosis patients, investigators found no evidence to support any particular type of psychosocial treatment for: (1) keeping persons in treatment, (2) reducing substance use, or (3) improving psychological functioning (Hunt, Siegfried, Morley, Sitharthan, & Cleary, 2013). Interdisciplinary research efforts may yield new insights because the questions about comorbidity range from problems in molecular genetics to those in the social environment and the public policy arena.

Clearly, there is a need to develop a service infrastructure to increase the capacity to provide accessible, integrated treatment and stable housing. At this time, the treatment system for persons with comorbid conditions is commonly described as *fragmented* and is fraught with barriers that prevent ready access to care (e.g., Padwa, Guerrero, Braslow, & Fenwick, 2015; Priester et al., 2016). Further research on integrated approaches to treating persons with dual diagnoses (i.e., substance abuse and severe mental illness) is needed. The integrated treatment model holds promise for helping this population of clients. As noted by Drake and colleagues (2016), the life course of persons suffering from both schizophrenia and substance use disorder "is variable but often quite positive" (p. 202).

REVIEW QUESTIONS

1. How is the deinstitutionalization movement implicated in the problem of dual diagnoses?

2. How prevalent are co-occurring mental disorders and substance use disorders in the general U.S. population?

3. How are the terms *comorbid conditions* and *dual diagnoses* used in different ways?

4. How common is it for persons with alcohol disorders and drug use disorders to seek treatment?

5. How much progress has been made in the United States in the past 15 years addressing the problem of co-occurring disorders?

6. To what extent is cannabis dependence associated with lifetime risk of alcohol dependence and mental disorder?

7. What are the associations between adolescent cannabis use and subsequent subclinical psychotic symptoms found in the study conducted by Bechtold and colleagues?

8. At a nosological level, why are DSM-5 criteria inadequate for understanding co-occurring disorders?

9. Which model of comorbidity indicates that the comorbid condition represents a disorder that is distinct from the other two?

10. In problem behavior theory, why is it predicted that multiple problem behaviors cluster in individuals?

11. What is the nature of the association between discounting delayed consequences and comorbidity?

12. What does the evidence indicate about the effectiveness of substance abuse treatment for adolescents?

13. Does 12-step participation help adolescents who have co-occurring disorders?

14. What are the challenges of treating adults with dual diagnoses?

15. What are the characteristics of integrated treatment for persons with dual diagnoses?

16. How effective is integrated treatment?

CHAPTER 5

Psychoanalytic Formulations

Alex is a 35-year-old primary care physician mandated to treatment as a result of a driving under the influence conviction. The son of two physicians, he describes his parents as demanding, cold, and distant. Although he had always been an excellent student and successful high school athlete, Alex feels that his parents were never satisfied with his achievements. He discussed several painful memories of his parents ridiculing his attempts to be a better son. Alex is also ashamed of how he occasionally bullied other students in school. He reports that he once violently threw a girl much younger than he was to the ground. Alex describes his clinical practice as highly stressful, and he questions whether he is in the right career. He wonders if he went into medicine, like his parents, because he was trying to please them.

In the first phase of treatment, Alex denies that he has a drinking problem. He clearly wants to please his therapist, but he does not want to stop drinking. Over time, Alex comes to see his two demons in life as his drinking and his relationship with his therapist. In essence, he develops the same type of relationship with his therapist that he had with his parents. In a subsequent phase of treatment, Alex accuses his therapist of trying to force him to stop drinking. This leads to many promises to the therapist that he will reduce his drinking, but all of these efforts are unsuccessful. After biweekly therapy sessions for 15 months, Alex realizes that his motivation to binge-drink is to get the therapist to take care of him—something his parents had not done for him when he was a child. In psychoanalysis, alcoholism and other addictions are seen as symptoms of underlying and unresolved conflicts.

PSYCHOANALYSIS: A TYPE OF PSYCHOTHERAPY

Dr. Sigmund Freud (1856–1939) was an Austrian neurologist who made the first systematic attempt to explain the origins of mental disorders. His theory, known as *psychoanalysis*, and his ideas have had a lasting impact on our culture. For example, Freud originated the notion of defense mechanisms (e.g., denial, rationalization), brought attention to the significance of anxiety in the human experience, and was the first to give an extensive description of the unconscious mind. He pointed to the importance of early childhood experience, and he was the first to insist that human sexual behavior is an appropriate subject for scientific scrutiny.

Freud derived psychoanalytic concepts from his clinical practice. His patients were predominantly white female residents of Vienna, Austria, from the 1890s to the 1930s. Psychoanalytic models continue to influence clinical practitioners in the substance abuse field today, particularly among psychotherapists who provide long-term, insight-oriented treatment in private practice settings (Rothschild & Gellman, 2009). These concepts also have historical significance because they provide perspective on the evolution of the addiction concept and the treatment of substance abuse.

The terms *psychoanalysis* and *psychotherapy* are not synonymous, though they are sometimes mistakenly thought to be. *Psychotherapy* is a more general term describing professional services aimed at helping individuals or groups overcome emotional, behavioral, or relationship problems. Over 30 years ago, George and Cristiani (1995) estimated that there were more than 240 methods of counseling and psychotherapy. This number is now over 500 (see Prochaska & Norcross, 2018). Psychoanalysis, also known as psychodynamic therapy, is one of these approaches.

Traditional psychoanalysis involves an *analyst* and an *analysand* (i.e., the client). Typically, the analysand lies comfortably on a couch while the analyst sits behind him or her, out of view. Often, the analyst takes notes while the analysand describes whatever comes into his or her mind. Interestingly, Freud discouraged analysts from taking notes; he cautioned that doing so would distract their attention (Gay, 1988).

Interpretation

Psychoanalysis relies heavily on the analyst's interpretation of the analysand's concerns. To this end, the analyst encourages the analysand to say absolutely everything that comes to mind. By contrast, the analyst remains as silent as possible, hoping that this silence will stimulate the analysand's uninhibited verbal activity. Gay (1988) describes the process in this way:

> In the strange enterprise that is psychoanalysis, half the battle and half alliance, the analysand will cooperate as much as his neurosis lets him.

The analyst for his part is, one hopes, not hampered by his own neurosis; in any event, he is required to deploy a highly specialized sort of tact, some of it acquired in his training analysis, the rest drawn from his experience with analytic patients. It calls for restraint, for silence at most of the analysand's productions and comments on a few. Much of the time patients will experience their analyst's interpretations as precious gifts that he doles out with far too stingy a hand. (p. 298)

Free Association

According to Freud, the fundamental principle of psychoanalysis is that *free association* should be encouraged. The analysand should be free to reveal the most sensitive things that come to mind, so that the analyst can interpret them. For this reason, the analyst positions him- or herself behind the analysand. The analyst's reactions to shocking disclosures could cause the analysand to be distracted and inhibit the free flow of associations.

Dream Interpretation

Another feature of psychoanalysis is dream interpretation. Its purpose is to uncover unconscious material, which the analysand typically represses. The task of the analyst is to study the symbols presented in the dreams and to interpret their disguised meanings. Psychoanalysts believe that dreams have two types of content: manifest and latent. The manifest content is the dream as it appears to the dreamer, whereas *latent* content is what is disguised to the dreamer. The latent content consists of the analysand's actual motives that are seeking expression but that are very painful or personally unacceptable (Coleman et al., 1980).

Resistance

In *The Interpretation of Dreams,* Freud (1900/1953) defined resistance as simply "whatever interrupts the progress of analytic work" (p. 555). According to Gay (1988), Freud warned: "Resistance accompanies the treatment at every step; every single association, every act of the patient's must reckon with this resistance, represents a compromise between the forces aiming at cure and those opposing it" (p. 299). For the psychoanalyst, resistance arises because the analysand becomes threatened by the uncovering of unconscious material. At such times, the analysand may attempt to change the subject, dismiss its importance, become silent, forget dreams, hold back essential information, be consistently late for appointments, become hostile, or employ other defensive mechanisms. Gay describes resistance as a "peculiarly irrational" but universal human tendency. The contradictory nature of resistance is underscored by the pointlessness of voluntarily seeking help (and paying for it) and then fighting against it.

Resistance can be viewed as a significant problem in counseling individuals with alcohol and other drug problems. Addiction practitioners who value the concept will see it in their clients and adopt helping strategies in accordance with it. Although traditional psychoanalytic thinking maintains that resistance arises from personality dynamics, Taleff (1997) and others have recognized that it has sources outside the person as well, such as counselor practices, inadequate treatment models, family and group dynamics, and the features of treatment programs. To a great extent, the challenge in helping persons with substance abuse problems is properly assessing and attending to these issues (Taleff, 1997).

Transference

In the process of psychoanalysis, the relationship between analyst and analysand becomes emotionally charged. In this situation, the analysand frequently applies to the analyst particular feelings, thoughts, attributes, and motives that he or she had in a past relationship with a parent or other significant person (a teacher, coach, clergyman, etc.). As a result, the analysand may respond to the analyst as he or she did to that particular person in the past. If the past relationship was characterized by hostility or indifference, the analysand may feel the same way about the analyst. The tasks of the analyst, then, are to help the analysand (1) "work through" these feelings, (2) recognize that the analyst is not the parent or significant other figure, and (3) stop living within the confines of past relationships.

PERSONALITY STRUCTURE

In the psychoanalytic perspective, human behavior is thought to result from the interaction of three major subsystems within the personality: the *id, ego,* and *superego.* Although each of these structures possesses unique functions and operating principles, they interact so closely with one another that it is often impossible to separate their distinct effects on behavior. In most cases, behavior is the result of the dynamic interaction among the id, ego, and superego. Each subsystem does not typically function in the absence of the other two (Hall et al., 1998).

The *id* is the original source of the personality and consists largely of instinctual drives. Psychoanalytic theorists have a specific understanding of the term *instinct.* It is defined as "an inborn psychological representation of an inner somatic source of excitation" (Hall et al., 1998, p. 39). The psychological representation is more commonly referred to as a *wish, internal urge,* or *craving.* The bodily excitations that give rise to wishes or urges are called *needs*. Thus, the sensation of hunger represents the physiological need of the body for nutrients. Psychologically, this need is expressed as a wish or craving for food. In addiction, drugs become sources of bodily excitation, which in turn give rise to cravings for that chemical. The chemical craving serves to motivate the addict to seek out the drug of choice. Psychoanalysts note that addicts' instinctual drives make them hypersensitive to environmental stimuli (e.g., offers from friends to "get high," the smell of a burning match, advertisements for alcohol). These stimuli elicit cravings and make them vulnerable to "slips" and relapses.

The id is present from birth. It is the basic life force from which the ego and superego begin to differentiate themselves. It supplies the psychic energy necessary for operation of the ego and superego. *Psychic energy* is defined as mental activity, such as thinking and remembering. Freud believed that the id is a bridge that connects the energy of the body to that of the personality. Interestingly, Freud noted that this psychic energy is not bound by logic and reality. It allows us to do such impossible things as to be in two places at once or to move backward in time.

Some of the instinctual drives of the id are constructive (e.g., sex). However, others are destructive (e.g., aggression, destruction, and death). Because the id cannot tolerate increases in psychic energy (they are experienced as uncomfortable states of tension), it is identified as the component of personality that is completely selfish. The id is only concerned with immediate gratification (i.e., discharge of tension). It has no consideration for reality demands or moral concerns.

The id is said to operate via the *pleasure principle*. That is, high tension levels (e.g., sexual urges or drug cravings) prompt the id to act to reduce the tension immediately and return the individual to a comfortably constant level of low energy. Thus, the id's aim is to avoid pain (e.g., the discomfort of abstinence) and to increase pleasure (e.g., drug-induced euphoria). The operation of the pleasure principle makes frustration and deprivation difficult to tolerate. Obviously, both frustration and deprivation are common in early recovery, and they make the addict susceptible to relapse.

The *ego* emerges from the id in order to satisfy the needs of the individual that require transactions with the external world (i.e., reality). Survival requires the individual to seek food, water, shelter, sex, and other basic needs. The ego assists in this effort by distinguishing between subjective needs of the mind (an id function) and the resources available in the external world.

Ultimately, the ego must answer to the demands of the id. However, it does so in such a way as to ensure the survival and health of the individual, which requires the use of reason, planning, delay of immediate gratification, and other rational resources in dealing with the external world. In "normal" individuals, the ego is able, to some degree, to control the primitive impulses of the id. As a result, the ego is said to operate via the *reality principle*. The aim of the ego is to suspend the pleasure principle temporarily, until a time at which an appropriate place and object can be found for the release of tension. In this way, the ego is the component of personality that mediates between the demands of the id and the realities of the external world.

The third subsystem of the personality is the *superego,* which is the moral component of the personality. It emerges from the learning of moral values and social taboos. The superego is essentially that which is referred to as the *conscience*; it is concerned with "right" and "wrong." The superego develops during childhood and adolescence in response to reward and punishment. It has three main functions: to suppress impulses of the id, particularly sexual and aggressive urges; to press the ego to abandon realistic goals in exchange for moralistic ones; and to impel the individual to strive for perfection.

Although the three subsystems of personality operate as a whole, each represents distinct influences on human behavior (see Figure 5.1 on the next page). The id is the biological force that influences human behavior. The ego represents the psychological origins of behavior, whereas the superego reflects the impact of social and moral forces. Both the id and superego can be thought of as the irrational or nonrational components of personality; the id strives for pleasure at all costs, whereas the superego always works to prevent it.

ANXIETY, DEFENSE MECHANISMS, AND THE UNCONSCIOUS

Anxiety plays a prominent role in psychoanalytic theory. The purpose of anxiety is to warn the individual that there is impending danger (i.e., pain). It is also a signal to the ego to take some preventive measure to reduce the threat.

Often the ego can cope with anxiety by rational measures. For example, a nervous student with an upcoming exam can spend extra time studying. A stressed-out employee can exercise, meditate, or turn to other constructive diversions. A parent can begin to save money now for a child's college education in 15 years. A recovering alcoholic who has cravings can call his or her AA sponsor. Such actions require reason, the ability to plan, and the delay of immediate gratification for long-term gain.

However, the ego is often overcome by anxiety it cannot control. In such situations, rational measures fail, and the ego resorts to irrational protective mechanisms, which are often referred to as *defense mechanisms.* These defense mechanisms, such as denial and rationalization, alleviate the anxiety. However, they do so by distorting reality instead of dealing directly with the problem. This distortion creates a discrepancy or gap between actual reality and the individual's perception of it. As a consequence, the

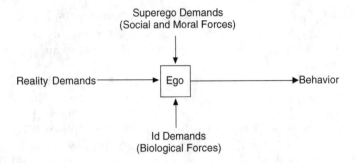

FIGURE 5.1. Influence of the id, ego, and superego and of reality demands on human behavior.

ego's ability to cope with reality demands becomes increasingly diminished. Such is the case with alcoholics, who, upon being confronted with their problematic drinking, rely on denial and rationalization. These defenses, in turn, allow the abusive drinking to continue and to become increasingly dysfunctional.

Typical ego defense mechanisms among the chemically dependent include:

1. *Compensation:* making up for the deprivation of abstinence by overindulging in another pleasure. (Example: A recovering drug addict becomes compulsive about gambling, work, eating, etc.)
2. *Denial:* inability to perceive an unacceptable reality. (Example: An employee denies he is suffering from alcoholism when confronted about the bottle he keeps hidden in his desk.)
3. *Displacement:* directing pent-up feelings of hostility toward objects less dangerous than those that initially aroused the anger. (Example: An addict in treatment comes home from a group counseling session and screams at his wife. In group, he had received feedback from the facilitator indicating that he was not actively participating.)
4. *Fantasy:* gaining gratification from past experiences by reliving the euphoria and fun. (Example: While in rehabilitation, a group of addicts experience cravings as they reminisce about the "good ol' times.")
5. *Isolation:* withdrawing into a passive state in order to avoid further hurt. (Example: A depressed alcoholic in early recovery refuses to share her problems.)
6. *Projection:* assuming that others think badly of one, even though they have never communicated this negative regard in any way.

(Example: An addict unexpectedly blurts out to a counselor, "I know you think I'm worthless.")

7. *Rationalization:* attempting to justify one's mistakes or misdeeds by presenting rationales and explanations for the misconduct. (Example: An addict reports that he missed a 12-step meeting because he had to take a very important telephone call from his attorney.)

8. *Regression:* retreating to an earlier developmental level involving less mature responses. (Example: In a therapeutic community, an adult resident "blows up" and makes a huge scene when she learns that iced tea is not available for lunch that day.)

9. *Undoing:* atoning for or making up for an unacceptable act. (Example: An alcoholic goes to a bar after work and gets "smashed." He doesn't get home until 4:00 A.M. His wife is furious. The next day he brings her flowers and cooks dinner.)

The defense mechanisms and other processes operate on an unconscious level. The unconscious, according to Freud, represents the largest part of the human mind. The individual is generally unaware of the content and process of this part of mind. The conscious mind, by contrast, is a function of the ego that has often been likened to the "tip of an iceberg" (see Figure 5.2 on the next page).

The unconscious mind holds forbidden desires, painful memories, and unacceptable experiences that have been "repressed" or pushed out of consciousness. Although individuals are unaware of unconscious material, it possesses energy and seeks expression. Thus, at times, unconscious material successfully penetrates the conscious mind. Typical examples of this are so-called Freudian slips (e.g., using the word *sex* when the word *stress* would have been appropriate). Unconscious material also surfaces during fantasies, dreams, and hypnosis. In each case, ego controls are lowered, allowing the unconscious to appear. Psychoanalysts believe that as long as unconscious material is repressed and not integrated into the ego (presumably through psychoanalysis), maladaptive behavior (e.g., addictions) will be maintained.

INSIGHTS INTO COMPULSIVE SUBSTANCE USE

Early psychoanalytic formulations insisted that substance dependence stems from unconscious death wishes and self-destructive tendencies of the id. It was believed that among alcoholics and drug addicts, the id is oriented toward death instincts rather than toward constructive (e.g., sexual) instincts. Thus, many early psychoanalysts cynically viewed compulsive substance abuse as a form of "slow suicide" (Khantzian, 1980). The

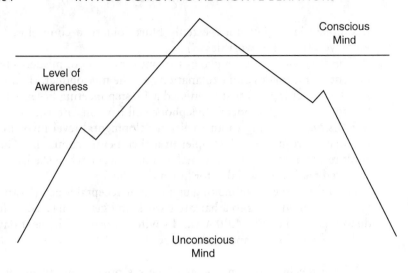

FIGURE 5.2. The "iceberg" view of the conscious versus the unconscious mind.

treatment focus was on the tendencies of the id. This traditional school of thought, known as *drive reduction,* holds that substance abuse is merely a manifest symptom of a repressed idea (or memory) that comes to consciousness (Director, 2002; Rothschild, 2010). The repressed idea is unrecognizable; that is, it appears as substance abuse because it is distorted by psychological defenses (Leeds & Morgenstern, 1996). In essence, substance abuse can be thought of as a compromise resulting from the conflict between a repressed idea and the defense against it (Leeds & Morgenstern, 1996).

A second school of thought within the psychoanalytic tradition is sometimes referred to as *ego psychology.* More contemporary psychoanalytic treatment of addiction seems to draw heavily on this conceptualization of addiction (Murphy & Khantzian, 1995). Here, substance abuse is seen as a symptom of a deficient ego. According to Murphy and Khantzian (1995), "it is the vulnerable and disregulated self which is the central problem in addiction" (p. 162). Individuals with addiction problems are seen as lacking the capacity to adequately care for themselves; they expose themselves unnecessarily to a variety of risks: health, safety, financial, legal, and so on. The consequences of risky or dangerous behavior can be ignored because drug intoxication provides a sense of well-being, security, and pleasure (Murphy & Khantzian, 1995). In this psychoanalytic approach, the goal of treatment is to build ego strength by helping the person develop the capabilities to cope with the demands of the external world. Thus, in challenging contemporary neurobehavioral explanations, Khantzian (2015) has argued that addiction is *not* about seeking either pleasure or self-destructiveness. Instead, he emphasizes that addiction is fundamentally a problem of *self-regulation*.

Despite the differences described previously, psychoanalytic formulations of addiction share a set of assumptions. Leeds and Morgenstern (1996) present the following assumptions:

1. The act of drug use is a symptom of some type of underlying psychological disorder.
2. The psychological problems of the addict precede and cause the substance abuse: There is little recognition that psychological problems are the consequence of substance abuse.
3. Addiction is seen as a uniform disorder: Relatively little consideration is given to disorder subtypes, different drugs of abuse, the course or severity of the addiction problem, and the like.
4. The presence of addiction indicates severe psychopathology. (p. 76)

Contemporary psychoanalysts tend to view addiction as a symptom of a deficient ego, that is, problems in coping. Essentially, they believe that substance abuse is only the obvious and outward manifestation of deeper personality problems. The goal of treatment in such cases is to build ego strength, so that the demands of the id can be better managed.

Two Necessary Conditions

According to Wurmser (1974), two general factors are always present in the development of compulsive substance use. The first is described as the *addictive search*. This internal urge is a psychological hunger or craving for an entire group of activities; the urge precedes the onset of chemical dependency but accompanies it and follows it, even after abstinence has been established. The activities may include compulsive gambling, overeating, indiscriminate sexual activity, irresistible violence, compulsive shoplifting, endless television viewing, and/or running away. All these activities can be used to provide external relief from overpowering internal drives.

The second necessary factor is referred to as the *adventitious entrance* of chemicals (Wurmser, 1974). This is the random introduction (in terms of accessibility and seductiveness) of alcohol or drugs into a person's life. They are typically introduced by peers or perhaps by drug dealers in the case of illicit drugs. Without access to and experimentation with these substances, addiction is obviously not possible.

Together, these two predisposing factors (i.e., the addictive search and the adventitious entrance) set the stage for the development of chemical dependency. Both must be present for the disorder to appear. According to Wurmser (1974), some people are driven by an addictive search, but they have not been exposed to the world of drug or alcohol abuse. In such cases, "there is no compulsive drug use without this trigger factor; but there is still an overriding emotional compulsiveness directed toward other activities and objects" (Wurmser, 1974, p. 829). This may also be the case for many chemically dependent persons in recovery. That is, they have removed themselves from the drinking/drugging scene and are abstinent, but they may continue old compulsions or develop new ones. They may be said to be continuing an addictive search even though they are abstinent.

These two predisposing factors could be used to explain why some people who gain access to the world of drug or alcohol abuse never become dependent on such substances (Khantzian, 2012). Despite the availability of various drugs, they may not possess the psychological hunger that is necessary to initiate or maintain compulsive drug or alcohol abuse. In other words, they may not need external relief from internal cravings or urges. Of course, an alternative "disease" explanation is simply that such individuals lack the *genetic* vulnerability to alcoholism and other drug addictions.

Abuse as Affect Defense

Contemporary psychoanalytic thinking maintains that substance abuse itself is a defense mechanism (Khantzian, 1980; Wurmser, 1980). Addicts are thought to abuse alcohol or drugs to protect themselves from overwhelming anxiety, depression, boredom, guilt, shame, and other negative emotions. One contemporary psychoanalyst contends that episodes of chronic drug use are fueled by needs for feelings of omnipotence (Director, 2002). Seeking omnipotence is considered a defensive reaction. Wurmser (1974) has stated that compulsive drug use is "an attempt at self-treatment" (p. 829). That is, it represents an attempt at self-medication, a way to relieve psychic pain. For the most part, contemporary psychoanalysts do not view negative affective states (e.g., anxiety and depression) as consequences of substance abuse but, rather, as its causes. According to Khantzian:

> I have become convinced, as has Wurmser, that becoming and remaining addicted to drugs is in most instances associated with severe and significant psychopathology. Necessarily, some of the deserved pathology evident in addicts is the result of drug use and its attendant interpersonal involvements. However, it is my opinion that drug-dependent individuals are predisposed to use and become dependent upon their substances mainly as a result of severe ego impairments and disturbances in the sense of self. (1980, p. 29)

Wurmser's (1978) analysis of this problem goes further. He believes that the greater the legal penalties and social stigma against a drug, the more likely its user is to have severe psychopathology. The lack of internal controls to resist engaging in conduct that society condemns is seen as pathology. Thus, Wurmser concludes that "a compulsive alcohol or nicotine abuser shows far less preexisting psychopathology than a compulsive (or even casual) user of heroin, LSD, or cocaine" (p. 9).

Wurmser (1978) refers to the link between severe psychopathology and addiction as the *hidden problem*. He contends that drug control bureaucrats, law enforcement officials, many physicians (including psychiatrists), and drug users themselves are in denial about this relationship. According to Wurmser, this collective unwillingness to acknowledge the emotional conflict underlying addiction has led to the development of misguided drug control policy and ineffective approaches to prevention and treatment. He believes that legal controls do little to address the demand for drugs and that much treatment is superficial because it focuses on the use or nonuse of substances rather than on underlying personality and emotional issues.

Does Research Support the "Self-Medication" Hypothesis?

For more than 25 years, the psychoanalytic belief that individuals are predisposed to substance addictions by the experience of negative affective states was viewed with skepticism by many in the addictions research field. Their skepticism was based largely on comprehensive summaries of research conducted in the 1980s. For example, Cox (1985) found that there was little evidence to support the view that psychological distress (e.g., anxiety, depression, and low self-esteem) leads to addiction. Rather, Cox and others concluded that studies of young people showed that future substance abusers possessed three preexisting *character* traits: independence, nonconformity, and impulsivity (Cox, 1985). Thus, rather than being instigated by negative affect or mood states, it was these character traits that were thought to be the important risk factors for subsequent substance use disorders. Furthermore, it was concluded that negative affective states were more likely to be the consequences of years of substance abuse, not the precursors, as psychoanalysts claimed.

Recent research has reopened this debate. In a methodologically rigorous prospective study, Conway, Swendsen, Husky, He, and Merikangas (2016) found evidence that many mental disorders, including disorders of affect and mood, are indeed associated with an increased risk of subsequent alcohol and other drug abuse. In a nationally representative sample of 10,123 American adolescents residing in the continental United States, Conway and his colleagues found that among adolescents who had never consumed alcohol, 38% had at least one DSM-IV mental disorder. Among adolescents who were not regular users of alcohol, 48% had a prior mental health disorder. Among those who would develop alcohol abuse or dependence, 67% had a prior mental health disorder. With regard to illicit drug use, 41% of the adolescents with no prior use had at least one DSM-IV mental disorder. Among adolescents who would initiate illicit drug use,

54% had a prior mental health disorder. Among those who would develop drug abuse or dependence, 67% had at least one prior DSM-IV disorder. These patterns indicate that mental health problems often precede the onset of alcohol and drug use disorders.

Conway and colleagues (2016) also report that among adolescents with anxiety disorders, alcohol abuse onset occurred later in 17% of the sample, with drug abuse appearing later in 20% of the sample. Among those with behavior disorders (ADHD, conduct, and oppositional defiant behaviors), alcohol abuse onset followed the behavior disorder in 16% of the sample, with drug abuse onset following the behavior disorder in 24% of the sample. The investigators could not determine why adolescents with prior mental health disorders later developed alcohol and/or drug problems. However, they speculated that alcohol may be used to seek relief from anxiety, whereas illicit drug use may arise from behavioral disorders characterized by impulsivity, defiance, and poor interpersonal relationships. Thus, at this point in time the self-medication hypothesis cannot be ruled out as a possible etiological explanation of alcohol and drug dependence. Chapter 4 provides more contemporary perspectives on the nature of comorbid substance abuse and mood disorders.

Specific Drugs to Correct Different Affects

Psychoanalysts are generally disinclined to accept the notion that an addict's drug of choice is determined by economic, environmental, or sociocultural factors. Instead, they maintain that addicts become dependent on the drug that will correct or counteract the specific negative emotional state from which they want relief. For example, Wurmser (1980) puts it this way:

> The choice of drugs shows some fairly typical correlations with otherwise unmanageable affects (moods): narcotics and hypnotics are deployed against rage, shame, and jealousy, and particularly the anxiety related to these feelings; stimulants against depression and weakness; psychedelics against boredom and disillusionment; alcohol against guilt, loneliness, and related anxiety. (p. 72)

Khantzian, Halliday, and McAuliffe (1990) claimed that differing types of emotional pain lead to dependence on different types of drugs. For example, they proposed that opiate or narcotic addicts are typically the victims of traumatic abuse and violence. As a result, they eventually become perpetrators of violence themselves. Their history causes them to suffer with acute and chronic feelings of hostility and anger, for which opiates provide relief. In contrast, individuals who are anxious and inhibited use sedative–hypnotics, including alcohol, to overcome deep-seated defenses and fears about interpersonal intimacy. Cocaine addicts were thought to select cocaine for its energizing qualities. These persons are now seen as seeking relief from depression, boredom, or emptiness. Cocaine is thought to be appealing because it bolsters feelings of self-esteem and assertiveness (Khantzian et al., 1990).

As noted previously, empirical data often appear to refute psychoanalytic concepts. This seems to be the case for "specific drugs to correct different affects." For example, it has long been recognized that alcoholism often co-occurs with antisocial personality disorder and depression (Holdcraft, Iacono, & McGue, 1998), which is somewhat inconsistent with the psychoanalytic profile of the alcoholic as guilt-ridden, lonely, and anxious. In teenagers, epidemiological data have shown that marijuana abuse is correlated with delinquency and depression (Greenblatt, 1998). These associations do not neatly fit in the psychoanalytic model either.

STAGES OF RECOVERY FROM ADDICTION

According to the psychoanalytic perspective, there are three stages to complete recovery, as shown in Table 5.1 on the next page (Zimberg, 1978). Stage I is characterized by the self-statement "I can't drink or drug." In this stage, external control (e.g., detoxification and use of Antabuse) is important. In essence, clients need protection from their own impulses. The second stage is characterized by the self-statement "I won't drink or drug." Here, the control becomes internalized. Many AA/NA members remain at this level indefinitely. The third stage is represented by "I don't have to drink or drug." Many recovering persons never complete this stage, nor do they necessarily relapse. According to the psychoanalytic perspective, insight-oriented therapy is appropriate at this stage (Zimberg, 1978). However, because a recovering client's perception of the need for change is usually diminished at this point (life is relatively normal or manageable), few recovering persons pursue insight-oriented therapy.

Psychoanalytic Concepts in Clinical Practice Today

Psychoanalytic concepts are widely employed in the practice of substance abuse counseling. However, many practitioners are not aware that they are derived from psychoanalytic theory. For example, many attempt to identify clients' defense mechanisms in an effort to help the clients recognize their perceptual distortions. Denial, rationalization, and fantasy are typical protective mechanisms employed by clients with addiction problems. Closely intertwined with them is the unconscious, which is an indisputable influence on at least some classes of human behavior.

Despite a continuing reliance on psychoanalytic notions in clinical practice, *traditional Freudian psychoanalysis* is now largely dismissed as a

TABLE 5.1. A Contemporary Psychoanalytic View of Treatment Stages

Stages	Client status	Treatment
Stage I	"I can't drink or drug" (need for external controls)	Detoxification, directive psychotherapy, Antabuse, drug testing, AA/NA, family therapy
Stage II	"I won't drink or drug" (control becomes internalized)	Directive psychotherapy, supportive psychotherapy, AA/NA; Antabuse and drug testing may be discontinued
Stage III	"I don't have to drink or drug" (conflict over abstinence is resolved)	Psychoanalytic psychotherapy

Note. From Zimberg (1978). Copyright 1978 by Plenum Publishing Corporation. Adapted by permission of Springer Science and Business Media.

viable treatment approach for substance abuse (McCrady, Owens, Borders, & Brovko, 2015; Rothschild, 2010). More than a decade ago, Leeds and Morgenstern (1996) observed that "it is not hard to see why there is currently a crisis of confidence from within psychoanalysis in the efficacy of psychoanalytic understanding and treatment of substance abuse" (p. 80). More recently, respected American psychiatrist George Vaillant (2005) stated: "I think almost everything psychoanalysis has said about alcoholism has been (180 degrees) wrong" (p. 275).

This is not to say that psychoanalytic concepts have no place in conceptualizing client problems. As Leeds and Morgenstern (1996) have noted, there often has been confusion between the psychoanalytic *understanding* of addiction and the psychoanalytic *treatment* of the disorder. It should not be assumed that one necessarily leads to the other. In fact, the theory itself seems to predict that traditional psychoanalytic methods would not work well with substance abusers. Contemporary psychoanalysts have pointed out that individuals with substance dependence suffer from poor ego controls. This makes them poor candidates for psychoanalysis, a process that requires significant ego strength. Wurmser (1974), himself a leading psychoanalyst, stated that most compulsive drug users are relatively inaccessible by psychoanalysis. There are various reasons for this poor match. Many persons with substance dependence enter treatment with little initial motivation for personal change. Many others require assistance with the ordinary, mundane challenges of staying sober and "straight" a day at a time (e.g., remembering to take Antabuse and finding a ride to an AA meeting). Still others need strong guidance and structure to avoid relapse. These pressing reality-based concerns are not readily addressed in traditional psychoanalysis, with its emphasis on the intellect, the origins of problems, and protracted self-analysis.

In recent decades, psychoanalytically oriented clinicians have recommended that traditional psychoanalytic practice be modified for the treatment of persons with substance dependence in the following ways:

1. The initial stage of treatment should be supportive and didactic in nature.
2. Management issues must be emphasized in early phases of treatment (i.e., hospitalization, dangerous behavior, and withdrawal symptoms).
3. Sessions should be held once or twice a week.
4. The "couch" should not be used.
5. Interpretation should be minimized.
6. Abstinence should be encouraged.
7. AA attendance should be emphasized (see Yalisove, 1989).

In the past decade, the psychoanalytic community has made attempts to bridge the divide between their field and the field of substance abuse treatment (Matusow & Rosenblum, 2013; Rothschild & Gellman, 2009). Psychoanalysts have sought to rekindle interest in the psychoanalytic treatment of substance use disorders by integrating the approach with other helping strategies. One model employs *relational* psychoanalysis (Director, 2002). A second model represents an attempt to integrate relational psychoanalysis with *harm reduction therapy* (Rothschild, 2010; Rothschild & Gellman, 2009). These attempts represent an effort from within the psychoanalytic community to show that psychodynamic concepts continue to be relevant and have important contributions to make to helping persons with substance abuse problems (see Khantzian, 2012).

Relational psychoanalysis views chronic substance abuse as arising from unresolved conflicts in the organizing relationships of early adult life. These unresolved conflicts lead persons to view life as "a series of calculated sacrifices, made to achieve marital or material ends" (Director, 2002, p. 552). Such persons cope with these sacrifices by excessive drinking and/or drug use. Alcohol or drug intoxication allows the person to temporarily escape the everyday concessions and constraints of his or her unsatisfactory relationships and to feel alive again. Alcohol and drug use essentially become an outlet for feeling an array of intense emotions that are hidden within the relationship. They may include desires for power, passion, independence, dominance, pampering, defiance, and so forth. These temporary experiences of feeling alive reinforce the act of substance abuse. They also establish a relational dynamic in which the conflict remains unresolved, thereby providing a functional purpose for continued substance abuse. The goals of relational psychoanalytic treatment are to (1) help clients recognize the conflicts hidden in their relationships, (2) assist them with gaining insight into how their substance abuse is an expression of their relational binds, and (3) explore opportunities for change (Director, 2002).

Rothschild (2010) and Rothschild and Gellman (2009) extend relational psychoanalytic treatment of substance abuse by incorporating harm reduction principles (see Chapter 11). In contrast to traditional psychoanalysis, the therapist using a relational psychoanalytic harm reduction approach does not remain neutral or silent, but rather takes a more active approach by presenting discrepancies between the client's life goals and his or her substance abuse. The therapist and client are seen as partners. The therapist not only seeks to stimulate self-reflection, but also may teach relapse prevention skills. Interpretation focuses not only on the internal psychodynamics of the client, but on his or her external environment as well.

CHAPTER SUMMARY

At this time, it is unclear whether attempts by the psychoanalytic community to reinfuse their concepts into substance use disorder treatment will take hold. One question raised by the recent attempts to integrate psychoanalysis with other models is whether the new approach can be implemented in contemporary substance use disorder treatment settings where the number of treatment sessions is often limited and emphasis is given to brief interventions (Botelho, Engle, Mora, & Holder, 2011). Skeptics will likely be unswayed by these attempts to evolve psychoanalytically oriented treatment unless evidence from controlled trials is produced demonstrating the efficacy of the integrated approaches. The utility of psychoanalysis seems to be its ability to provide a deep understanding of the etiology of addiction. However, its concepts have little to offer in support of effective addiction treatment and prevention strategies.

REVIEW QUESTIONS

1. What are the major features of psychoanalytic therapy?

2. What are the chief characteristics of the id, ego, and superego? How do they interact?

3. How are defense mechanisms related to anxiety and the unconscious?

4. What is meant by *abuse as affect defense*?

5. Is the self-medication hypothesis of psychoanalysis supported by empirical research?

6. What specific affects are different drugs thought to correct?

7. Why do addicts not recognize the risks associated with their compulsive use?

8. What are the three stages of contemporary psychoanalytic treatment?

9. What are the criticisms of psychoanalysis as a treatment of addiction?

10. In the last decade, what approaches have the psychoanalytic community integrated into psychoanalysis to make it more useful in the treatment of substance use disorders?

CHAPTER 6

Conditioning Models and Approaches to Contingency Management

Dan is a 19-year-old college football player. After injuring his back one day in practice, the team physician prescribes an opioid pain medication for a week. Dan has very little experience with drug use and no family history of addiction. On occasion he drinks a beer; he has tried marijuana once but did not like it. Dan finds that the opioid medication not only manages his back pain, but also provides a euphoria he has never experienced. In hopes of experiencing that "high" or reward again, he returns to the team physician to request another prescription but is firmly told "no."

Determined to experience opioid-induced euphoria again, Dan shops around town for another physician who will provide another opioid prescription. He quickly finds several physicians willing to write prescriptions for these pills. Over time, Dan begins to ingest more and more pills.

The euphoria (or reward) that occurs *following* the ingestion of an opioid *reinforces* the act of drug self-administration, that is, swallowing pills. This is the fundamental principle of the conditioning models and contingency management approaches to treating addiction.

AIMS OF BEHAVIORISM

The principal aims of behaviorism are to elucidate the conditions of human learning and to develop a technology for behavior change. Behaviorists believe that most or all human behavior is learned, including not only adaptive but also maladaptive behavior (e.g., addiction). One of the major premises, then, is that certain fundamental laws (known and unknown) govern the initiation, maintenance, and cessation of human behavior. Alcohol or drug use is considered a behavior subject to the same principles of learning as driving a new car, acquiring job skills, or sending text messages from a newly purchased mobile device.

Behavioral psychology, for the most part, restricts itself to the study of overt behavior—behavior that is observable and measurable. There is a heavy emphasis on empirical evidence, as behaviorists are interested in building a true science of human behavior. For this reason, they often are not interested in internal "mentalistic" constructs, such as mental illness, self-esteem, affective states, thoughts, values, personality structure (e.g., the ego), defense mechanisms, or the unconscious. These concepts cannot be directly observed or measured, and there is no way to prove or disprove their existence. It is thus believed that they are not appropriate subjects for scientific inquiry.

CONDITIONED BEHAVIOR

Learned behavior is usually classified according to whether it is the result of *respondent conditioning* or *operant conditioning*. This distinction is an important one. However, the two types of conditioning do not represent different kinds of learning but, instead, different types of behavior (Domjan, 2015). Respondent behavior is under the control of a well-defined stimulus, whereas operant behavior appears voluntary and is not directly elicited by a stimulus situation. Most human behavior falls into the latter category.

Respondent Conditioning

Respondent conditioning is also known as *classical conditioning* or *Pavlovian conditioning*. It was the first type of learning to be studied systematically and was first investigated by the great Russian physiologist Ivan Pavlov (1849–1936). Respondent behavior is reflexive in the sense that it is under the control of well-defined environmental stimuli. Examples of respondent behavior include:

1. Blinking in response to a bright light.
2. Pulling one's hand away from a hot stove.
3. Salivating at the sight or smell of food.
4. Perspiring as the result of walking into a hot room.
5. Jerking one's leg forward when struck on the knee with a physician's hammer.

When a dog salivates at the sight of food, the salivation is considered respondent behavior, under the control of the stimulus of food. Pavlov found that if he paired the sight of food with a neutral stimulus such as a ringing bell, the bell alone would eventually elicit the salivation. Thus, the bell became a conditioned stimulus able to elicit salivation—a strange situation, indeed. Figure 6.1 diagrams the respondent or Pavlovian conditioning model.

Interestingly, research conducted by Siegel (1982) demonstrated that drug tolerance can become partially conditioned to the environment in which the drug is normally used via respondent conditioning procedures. If a drug is administered in the presence of usual cues (i.e., the paired stimulus situation depicted in Figure 6.1), the drug effect will become somewhat diminished over time. In behavioristic jargon, "the drug effect is reduced by these anticipatory conditioned compensatory responses" (Brick, 1990, p. 178). In other words, repeated drug use in the same environment will gradually produce diminishing effects. This is one process for building behavioral tolerance. Thus, although cellular adaptation (a biological process) is clearly involved in the development of drug tolerance, learning also plays an important role.

Operant Conditioning

Operant behavior is different from respondent behavior in that operant behavior appears to be voluntary. In most cases, it does not seem to be directly elicited, or caused by, a specific stimulus in the environment. Furthermore, operant behavior is conditioned if it is followed by a reinforcer. In other words, operant behaviors are those that are maintained by events occurring *after* the behavior, not before it. If a behavior is followed by a reinforcer, the behavior will probably appear again. The subsequent change in rate of behavior is considered *learning*.

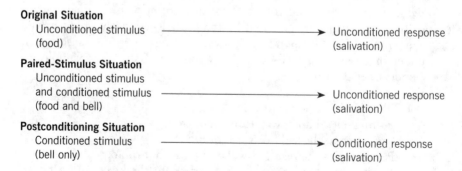

Original Situation
Unconditioned stimulus ——————————————→ Unconditioned response
(food)   (salivation)

Paired-Stimulus Situation
Unconditioned stimulus
and conditioned stimulus ——————————————→ Unconditioned response
(food and bell)   (salivation)

Postconditioning Situation
Conditioned stimulus ——————————————→ Conditioned response
(bell only)   (salivation)

FIGURE 6.1. Model of respondent or Pavlovian conditioning.

A *reinforcer* is best defined as any event that increases the probability or rate of a behavior (Miltenberger, 2016). Reinforcers can be any number of things. Some examples include alcohol, drugs, food, sex, verbal praise, money, a good grade, public recognition, and job promotion. Each person finds different things reinforcing. For example, actively drinking alcoholics find intoxication to be a potent reinforcer. Furthermore, the potency of a reinforcer is determined by an individual's state of deprivation. For instance, in all probability, a soldier who returns from 6 months of combat duty in a place where no alcohol was available is going to generate much more behavior to obtain a beer than a civilian who has ready access to alcohol.

The varying effectiveness of alcohol as a reinforcer is further illustrated by the ability of researchers to breed strains of alcohol-craving mice (McKim, 1986). Some strains show a strong fondness for alcohol; others demonstrate a dislike for the beverage. Alcohol-craving mice prefer alcohol to sugar water and will occasionally drink to drunkenness. For these mice, alcohol is a potent reinforcer. They will learn new behaviors and engage in high rates of a behavior to continue to get alcohol; in other words, they will work for it. Among the mice that do not care for alcohol, the drink cannot be used as a contingency to train them. For this group, alcohol has little reinforcement value.

An important distinction in operant conditioning involves the difference between *positive reinforcement* and *negative reinforcement*. In both situations, the rate or probability of a behavior increases. Furthermore, negative reinforcement is not punishment. A negative reinforcement procedure begins with an aversive stimulus; the behavior generated to remove the stimulus results in relief from the noxious stimulus. Thus, in a negative reinforcement procedure, *relief* is the reinforcer. The use of an alarm clock is a good example of negative reinforcement. The alarm sounds until one awakens in order to shut it off. The reinforcer in this case is silence (i.e., relief from noise), and the behavior change is reaching to turn off the alarm.

With addictive behavior, the classic example of negative reinforcement is withdrawal sickness. In alcoholic withdrawal, the symptoms include tremors, irritability, restlessness, anxiety, insomnia, and cravings. These symptoms are known by the alcoholic to almost disappear immediately upon taking a drink. Thus, in chronic alcoholism where an abstinence syndrome is present, drinking is reinforced by relief from the symptoms of withdrawal. Notice that the reinforcer is not alcohol or withdrawal itself but, rather, *relief from withdrawal.* In cases of alcohol dependence in which there is no withdrawal sickness (among teens, young adults, heavy episodic drinkers, etc.), drinking behavior is contingent upon positive reinforcers, such as euphoria and enhanced sociability.

Punishment can be defined as any event that decreases the probability or rate of a behavior (Miltenberger, 2016). Again, punishment and negative reinforcement have opposite effects: Punishment decreases behavior, whereas negative reinforcement increases it. Punishers can also be any number of things or events. They can include a disdainful look, ignoring a comment, all the way to physical abuse.

In regard to substance use and punishment, it is known that some people have particularly negative physical or psychological reactions to small amounts of alcohol or a drug. The examples of the person who becomes flushed, dizzy, and nauseated after one drink and the person who becomes extremely paranoid and panicky after a couple of puffs on a joint of marijuana illustrate this point. Such persons are essentially punished for substance use. The punisher (i.e., sickness or a panic attack) decreases the probability of future substance use. In cases such as these, there is little likelihood that substance dependencies will develop.

Generalization and Discrimination

Generalization and discrimination are two types of learning that are influenced by environmental stimuli as well as by reinforcement. *Generalization* can be defined as the tendency of an action to occur in a new setting because of the setting's similarity to the one in which the behavioral response was originally learned, with the likelihood of the response recurring being proportional to the degree of similarity between the settings (Miltenberger, 2016). For example, let us imagine that a cocaine addict, 4 years into recovery, goes on a business trip to a distant city. After arriving at the airport, he heads to the subway to catch a train for a downtown meeting. While riding on the subway train, he experiences intense cravings for cocaine. The last time he can remember having such an intense desire for cocaine was when he used to snort the drug with his buddies while riding the trains in his hometown. His cocaine cravings (and use) essentially generalized to all subway trains.

By contrast, *discrimination* can be defined as learning distinct responses to two or more similar but different stimuli due to differing benefits and costs associated with each one (Miltenberger, 2016). The *failure* to discriminate contributes to many relapses during early recovery. For example, let us suppose that an addict is discharged from an inpatient treatment facility. He has many new friends whom he has met through NA and many old friends with whom he used to get high. He insists that he can be with his old friends and not "pick up" or "slip." Unfortunately, he soon relapses, but he gradually learns that his old friends represent a stimulus condition that he must avoid. This gradual recognition is the process of *discriminative learning*. This learning process is also important for understanding the dynamics of controlled drinking—an issue discussed later in the chapter.

Extinction

Another conditioning principle is *extinction,* which is the absence or removal of a reinforcer. With regard to substance abuse, abstinence and treatment represent extinction procedures. Relapse can be considered evidence of an incomplete extinction procedure. However, the sheer availability of alcohol and drugs, and their ever-present potential for producing euphoria, make complete extinction of drug-seeking behavior difficult. Thus, from a behavioral perspective, a return to drug use (i.e., relapse) is always a possibility.

INITIATION OF ALCOHOL AND DRUG ABUSE

From a behavioristic perspective, the initiation of substance use is related to three factors: (1) availability, (2) lack of reinforcement for alternative behavior, and (3) lack of punishment for experimenting with alcohol or another drug. Clearly, use cannot begin if a substance is not available; this simple fact is the basis for the federal government's drug interdiction efforts. The second factor, lack of reinforcement, becomes operative when socially approved behavior (e.g., studying, working, attending church, and family recreational activities) that could take the place of drug-using behaviors is not sufficiently rewarded. In such cases, individuals are likely to engage in drug-taking behavior, which is accompanied by more potent or alluring reinforcers. Third, and perhaps most important, many people who experiment with a substance do not receive immediate punishment. Following the first use of a substance, few people get arrested, suffer an adverse physical reaction, lose a job, fail an exam, or receive harsh criticism from peers. The negative consequences of drug use are almost always delayed, sometimes for years or even decades (particularly with alcoholism and nicotine addiction). Not only are people unpunished immediately; usually, they are quickly reinforced by euphoria and peer acceptance. Initiation, then, is the result of the combination of availability, reinforcers, and the absence of punishers in the social environment.

ADDICTION

Some time ago, McAuliffe and Gordon (1980) offered the following behavioral definition of addiction: "an operantly conditioned response whose tendency becomes stronger as a function of the quality, number, and size of reinforcements that follow it" (p. 138). Each addict experiences his or her own set of multiple reinforcers. We can classify reinforcers into three categories: (1) euphoria, (2) desired social variables, and (3) elimination of withdrawal sickness. The combination of reinforcements from these categories will vary for each individual and each type of drug. For example, elimination of withdrawal sickness may be a more potent reinforcer for the heroin addict than for those addicted to cannabis. In addition, relief from withdrawal may be a stronger reinforcer for the physically dependent heroin addict than for one who is not physically dependent.

Euphoria is also important. For example, the euphoric consequence of cocaine ingestion may be more important to the maintenance of cocaine addiction than the euphoria that results from drinking alcohol. Furthermore, peer acceptance, a social variable, may be a more potent reinforcer for the adolescent marijuana smoker than for the 40-year-old marijuana user. Thus, the specific combination of reinforcing effects is that which "drives" each addiction.

For behaviorists, the difficulty of refraining from drug use merely indicates that a sufficient history of reinforcement has probably been acquired to impel a high rate of use. After a period of sustained drug use, abstinence should be expected to be challenging because self-administration is associated with immediate euphoria (and sometimes relief from withdrawal sickness), whereas nonuse leads to delayed (or "down-the-road") benefits (Dallery, Meredith, & Budney, 2012). Behaviorists do not believe that there is a single point at which an individual suddenly becomes "addicted." Rather, the word *addiction* is simply a term used to describe an operantly conditioned behavior that occurs at a relatively high rate. The individual's addiction develops gradually and varies continually in response to drug-related contingencies. The term *addict* merely refers to a person who engages in a high rate of drug use and who has a sufficient history of reinforced drug taking to outweigh the more socially acceptable rewards of life (e.g., career accomplishments, family interests, material possessions).

RELATIONSHIP BETWEEN ADDICTION AND PHYSICAL DEPENDENCE

For behaviorists, physical dependence on a drug is neither a necessary nor a sufficient condition for development of an addiction. This is consistent with the addiction criteria of the fifth edition of the *Diagnostic and Statistical Manual of Mental Disorders* (DSM-5; American Psychiatric Association, 2013). Physical dependence is simply a side effect of using certain classes of drugs at a high rate over a sufficient period of time. It merely sets the stage for experiencing withdrawal sickness and its relief. The relief is but one possible reinforcing effect that maintains addictive behavior. Euphoria and peer acceptance are equally potent, and in some cases, more potent reinforcers. Again, this is especially true of drugs that do not produce physical dependence or do so only minimally (e.g., hallucinogens, inhalants, marijuana).

It may be readily apparent that some addictions are not driven by the reinforcing effects of relief from withdrawal sickness (e.g., marijuana dependence). However, it should also be pointed out that physical dependence can exist in the absence of addiction. The most common example involves hospitalized patients recovering from surgery. Such patients are sometimes administered large doses of narcotic analgesics after surgery, over an extended period of time. When the patients are gradually weaned off the drug, they may experience some symptoms of withdrawal (e.g., irritability, diarrhea, headache, muscle ache, depression). However, because they are not "addicted," they typically do not engage in drug-seeking behavior or verbalize cravings for the drug. In fact, in many cases they do not even recognize the symptoms as those of withdrawal but simply as those of recovery from surgery.

Even in heroin addiction, relief from withdrawal is sometimes not an important reinforcing effect, in part because the severity of symptoms, which depends on the dosage administered, can be quite mild (Crevecoeur, 2009). Three situations involving heroin addicts illustrate the distinction between addiction and physical dependence:

1. Some heroin users, when administered a narcotic antagonist, experience no withdrawal symptoms. Yet, they claim they cannot stop using heroin, even though they want to, and they are adamant about continuing their use despite the known risks.
2. Many compulsive, long-term heroin addicts go for months, sometimes even years, without ever interrupting their use long enough to experience withdrawal. This indicates that physical dependence (i.e., relief from withdrawal) is not the reinforcer driving their addictive behavior.
3. Many detoxified heroin addicts continue to report that they still feel addicted to the drug many months after last using it. They often continue to express strong desires for heroin.

CESSATION AND RELAPSE

From a behavioristic perspective, cessation of alcohol and drug abuse occurs when the punishers that follow ingestion become less temporally remote. The immediate severity of punishment effects gradually builds over months or years of abusing a drug. Typically, alcoholics and addicts experience repeated brushes with the law, including perhaps longer and longer jail sentences; their sources of money become scarce, jobs become harder to find and keep, family members and friends become increasingly hostile, medical problems worsen, and so on. As these contingencies become more closely linked in time to the substance use, its rate gradually, or in some cases abruptly, ceases.

Behaviorists expect relapses to occur at relatively high rates among persons in early recovery because drugs are widely available in our society and always retain their ability to cause euphoria. Combined with these factors is the reality that many of the rewards (i.e., reinforcement) that come with abstinence and recovery are delayed. The unfortunate reality is that some abstinence-related reinforcers come only after months or years of sobriety. For example, to regain the trust and respect of family members and coworkers, addicts may have to maintain a year or more of abstinence. Some cocaine addicts have not been able to stabilize their financial affairs for years as a result of the debt they incurred using the drug. Drug dealers may not be able to make progress toward life or career goals because of jail time or simply as a result of their convictions. Whenever reinforcers such as these are delayed to some distant point in the future, their effectiveness in maintaining behavior consistent with recovery is diminished. For these reasons, relapses are always a possibility, especially during early stages of recovery.

DELAY DISCOUNTING

In the last two decades, there has been a great deal of interest in the maladaptive decision-making process known as *delay discounting* (Koffarnus & Kaplan, 2018). The central principle is that when behavioral consequences or reinforcers are delayed into the future, they often lose value and thereby become less effective in influencing behavior choices in the present (such as refraining from substance use or gambling). Consequences or reinforcers lose value in the decision-making process because the delay introduces uncertainty about future experience. Under such conditions, some individuals will make choices about consumable commodities that could be deemed to be less than rational; for example, choosing to take a $100 monetary reward today over waiting for a $1,000 reward 7 days in the future. This tendency to *defect* to smaller but immediate rewards may be implicated in the predisposition to addictive behaviors. Steeper discounting of delayed reinforcement is thought to increase vulnerability to addictive behavior (Frost & McNaughton, 2017; Hill, Yi, Spreng, & Diana, 2017). In many studies of alcohol use, drug use, and pathological gambling, delay discounting has been operationalized by measures of impulsiveness (Reynolds, 2006). Thus, delay discounting is sometimes treated as a personality trait characterized by impulsivity, which varies in strength across individuals and can predispose one to relapse.

Numerous studies have found that higher delay discounting is associated with alcohol use disorder. Gerst, Gunn, and Finn (2017) compared the rate of delayed discounting in three groups: persons with alcohol use disorder (N = 61), persons with alcohol use disorder and antisocial personality disorder (N = 79), and healthy controls (N = 64). The investigators used a computer-based tool that was designed to assess delay-discounting performance. The program prompted participants to make a series of choices between losing a specific amount of money immediately or losing $50 after one to six periods of delay. All participants understood that their choices about money/delay were imaginary and that the compensation they received for participating in the study was not affected by their performance. The immediate monetary values ranged from $2.50 to $47.50. Participants completed six randomly ordered delay blocks that represented different lengths of time. Ascending and descending value trials were presented in each block. The trials would switch when the participant chose the delayed option over the immediate option in the ascending sequence or in the descending sequence when the participant chose the immediate option over delayed option. Gerst and colleagues found that participants with alcohol use disorder only and persons with alcohol use disorder and antisocial personality disorder discounted delayed negative consequences at higher rates compared to the healthy controls. In other words, participants with alcohol use disorder, including those with co-occurring antisocial personality disorder, demonstrated, under experimental conditions, a decision-making style that favored larger future negative consequences over smaller, immediate negative consequences. This explains why persons with externalizing problems persist in injurious conduct, even though the pattern of behavior has long-term negative repercussions for themselves and others.

Over a 48-month period, Bernhardt and colleagues (2017) followed 114 treatment-seeking, alcoholic patients who had been abstinent at baseline for an average of 17 days. These patients were compared with 98 nonalcoholic controls matched on sex, age, and smoking status. Bernhardt and colleagues found that the alcoholic patients had significantly higher rates of delay discounting compared to controls. Although their study design could not provide definitive evidence, the investigators speculated that delay discounting may be a consequence of habitual heavy drinking rather than a case of alcohol disorder. Further research is needed on this question.

A large number of studies have demonstrated relationships between delay discounting and other addictive behaviors, including gambling. For example, MacKillop and colleagues (2011) conducted a meta-analysis of 46 delay-discounting studies that assessed alcohol, tobacco, stimulant, opiate, and marijuana use, and gambling. The investigators found that the associations of delay discounting with addictive behaviors were strongest in clinical samples, compared to nonclinical samples, and that the magnitude of these relationships did not differ across type of addictive behavior. In a subsequent and expanded meta-analysis of 64 delay-discounting studies, Amlung and colleagues (2017) also found strong associations between delay discounting and clinical diagnoses of addiction. However, the associations with quantity and frequency of drug use and gambling were statistically significant but less robust. Amlung and colleagues also noted that delay discounting did not differ by type of addictive behavior.

Moody, Franck, Hatz, and Bickel (2016) examined delay discounting across patterns of polydrug use. To assess the impact of delay discounting on non-, mono-, dual-, and tri-substance use, the investigators compared heavy smokers, and alcohol- and cocaine-dependent individuals to healthy community controls. They found that all drug-using groups were significantly more likely to engage in delay discounting than the community controls. Furthermore, groups that smoked cigarettes and had another substance dependence disorder were significantly more likely to engage in delay discounting than the group that only smoked cigarettes. Tri-substance users with both alcohol and cocaine dependence, and heavy smoking engaged in significantly more discounting than those who only smoked heavily. However, delay discounting appeared to have a ceiling effect because the tri-substance use group did not discount more than any dual-substance group (Moody et al., 2016).

In an earlier study, Petry (2002) examined the association between antisocial personality disorder (ASPD) and delay discounting. A question-based hypothetical measure of delay discounting (determining both $100 and $1,000 delayed standards) was used to compare three groups: (1) patients with a substance use disorder (alcohol, cocaine, and/or heroin abuse) and ASPD, (2) patients with a substance use disorder without ASPD, and (3) matched control participants with no history of substance use disorder or ASPD. For both delayed standard amounts, substance abusers with ASPD discounted more by delay than substance users without ASPD, and substance abusers without ASPD discounted more than controls. These findings suggest that ASPD adds to the delay-discounting effects observed in the population of substance abusers.

In summary, it appears that persons with addictive behaviors engage in more delay discounting than nonaddicted persons. This association has been observed across addictive behaviors, including gambling. Furthermore, the association between delay discounting and addictive behavior seems to be dose-dependent: High rates of delay discounting are linked to severe involvement in addictive activities. Future research needs to test interventions designed to alter the decision-making process that supports the steep discounting of delayed consequences.

BASIC PRINCIPLES OF CONTINGENCY MANAGEMENT

The application of learning principles to the helping process is called *behavior modification, behavioral contracting, contingency contracting,* or simply *contingency management.* Based on the premise that alcohol and drug use (and addiction) are learned, a clinical practitioner's role is to assist clients in learning more effective ways of behaving so that clients reach *their* goals. Contingency management consists of a functional analysis of behavior with four primary aims (Miltenberger, 2016).

1. *Specification of a target behavior.* What behavior is maladaptive? Specifically, which behaviors should be increased or decreased?
2. *Analysis of the current environmental events that control the behavior.* What contingencies currently maintain or support the behavior? As applied to addiction, what are the rewards that maintain the drug use? Are there punishers associated with avoiding use?
3. *Modification of current environmental events.* What changes in the immediate environment can be manipulated to alter the behavior?
4. *Measurement of behavior change.* What procedures will be used to assess the behavior before and after the environmental intervention?

In the contingency management approach, the development and maintenance of addictive behaviors are seen as involving the same components as the development and maintenance of any other behavior. This view has two important implications. First, addictive behaviors are not deemed inherently maladaptive; rather, they are defined as harmful as the result of labels that significant others assign to them. For instance, an alcoholic is simply a person whose drinking behavior has adversely affected a family member, friend, or coworker. The second implication is that addictive behaviors are maintained because other, more adaptive behaviors are not reinforced or are not possible. A typical example would include an alcoholic man in early recovery and his nonsupportive wife. As a result of several months of abstinence, he begins to demonstrate appropriate parenting behavior (e.g., helps his son with homework), which his wife criticizes. The lack of reinforcement for these new behaviors soon leads him back to drinking.

The contingency management approach is based on a somewhat unique view of human nature and the change process involving the following assumptions:

1. Human behavior is neither intrinsically good nor bad, but it is labeled as such by external observers.
2. Human behavior is both overt (observable) and covert (e.g., thinking).
3. Humans can learn to change and effectively manage their behavior.
4. Human behavior influences the behavior of others and changes the environment.
5. Human behavior is lawful, meaning that it is influenced systematically by environmental events (Miltenberger, 2016).

Contingency management approaches can be thought of as strategies that seek to teach clients to become more effective in managing their own behavior. In this collaborative process involving client and clinician, there are six steps.

1. The first step focuses on *specifying the problem behaviors*. With empathic understanding, the clinician assists clients in identifying their problems in behavioral terms.

2. The second step directs attention to *antecedent manipulations*. Here, the clinician and client explore ways to change the environmental/ social conditions in the client's life. For example, a person addicted to video gaming may be lonely and depressed, and may lack the social skills necessary for meeting new people. In teaching such skills, the clinician would assist the client in identifying the necessary stimulus and reinforcing conditions for meeting new friends.

3. The third step is *goal setting*, in which the clinician helps the client identify goals. The clinician does not impose goals on the client.

4. The fourth step is *arranging reinforcers and punishers*. Perhaps by making a behavioral contract, the clinician helps the client design a system for supporting his or her behavioral change, using predetermined rewards and penalties identified by the client. For engaging in recreational behaviors that replace time spent involved in video gaming, the schedule and system for providing rewards to oneself would be identified, established, and possibly monitored by significant others.

5. The fifth step involves helping the client develop a system of *social support* that will help him or her monitor progress and provide encouragement. Here, the client enlists the assistance of significant others in these change efforts, possibly by providing them with weekly progress reports on his or her attempts to reduce time spent video gaming.

6. The sixth step involves helping the client to *make a commitment to change*. Typically, there are barriers to making such a commitment, particularly when existing reinforcement is already in place that maintains problem behaviors, such as gaming addiction. The use of incentives to generate and maintain motivation to adopt new behaviors is critical. Ignoring this phase or giving it little attention would likely hinder client progress.

APPLICATIONS OF CONTINGENCY MANAGEMENT

The following discussion shows how contingency contracting has been applied to a number of treatment issues. These include efforts to (1) establish and maintain controlled drinking; (2) initiate and maintain abstinence and encourage the adoption of recovery behaviors (taking an Antabuse [disulfiram] tablet, attending AA each day, etc.); (3) promote positive change in a client's vocational, recreational, social, and familial functioning; (4) reduce cocaine and other illicit drug use; and (5) enhance compliance with methadone maintenance.

Moderation-Oriented Treatment

Among problem drinkers who do not demonstrate severe impaired capacity to control their alcohol intake, moderation-oriented treatment, managed by contingency contracting, is a viable alternative to abstinence (Stockwell et al., 2018; Storbjörk, 2017; Vallance et al., 2016; Witkiewitz et al., 2017). It should be emphasized that moderation-oriented treatment (also known as *controlled drinking*) is not an effort to encourage recovering alcoholics to "try drinking again." Rather, it should be considered an option to be negotiated at the *onset of treatment* for those who prefer it as a treatment goal (Adamson, Heather, Morton, Raistrick, & UKATT Research Team, 2010). Furthermore, it is important to point out that abstinence (not moderation) is usually the preferred drinking goal among those who seek treatment for alcohol problems. One study found that when presented with the two goal options of abstinence and moderation during screening for treatment, 54.3% expressed a preference for abstinence-oriented treatment (Heather, Adamson, Raistrick, Slegg, & UKATT Research Team, 2010). Nonetheless, there is evidence that alignment of the client's preferred goal (abstinence vs. moderation) with actual treatment services (abstinence vs. moderation) improves treatment outcomes for all clients (Adamson et al., 2010).

For more than 25 years, there have been calls for expanding the use of moderation-oriented treatment in the United States (see Sobell, Wilkinson, & Sobell, 1990). Interestingly, controlled drinking appears to be a frequent outcome of both moderation-focused and abstinence-focused treatments; for example, Sanchez-Craig and Lei (1986) and Adamson and colleagues (2010) found that many clients with positive outcomes adopted moderation in both goal conditions. Many successful clients benefit from abstinence-oriented treatment but apparently reject its basic goal, and at some point in their treatment or after their treatment, they successfully practice controlled use instead.

As a treatment strategy, moderation-oriented treatment has long been denounced in the United States (Allsop, 2018; Sobell & Sobell, 2006). Yet, in Canada, Britain, and the Scandinavian countries, it has had much greater acceptance for many years (Rosenberg, Melville, Levell, & Hodge, 1992; Walsh & Stuart, 2009). For instance, as early as 1989–1990, 75% of alcohol treatment agencies in England, Scotland, and Wales reported that moderation was an acceptable treatment goal (Rosenberg et al., 1992). About one-half of these providers thought it to be acceptable for 1–25% of their clients. At that time, the providers most frequently reported that their position on moderation-oriented treatment was based on their own professional experience rather than on research or agency policy.

Some time ago, Heather and Robertson (1983) identified six possible advantages of a controlled-drinking strategy:

1. In our society, abstinence from alcohol is deviant behavior. This is unfortunate. However, the stigma and the label of *alcoholic* pose significant adjustment problems for some people.
2. Among some alcoholics, abstinence may lead to overwhelming states of anxiety or depression that are unlikely to be managed in other ways.
3. Sometimes, overall improvement in life functioning does not result from abstinence.
4. In some alcoholics, abstinence is associated with severe psychosocial problems that lead to frequent relapse.
5. Abstinence during treatment rules out the possibility for changes in drinking behavior.
6. The demand placed on alcoholics to abstain deters many from seeking help until their problem is quite severe.

Behavioral self-control training (BSCT) is an extensively studied treatment strategy for alcohol problems (Hester, 1995; Marinchak & Morgan, 2012). As early as the late 1970s, Miller and Hester (1980) demonstrated an effectiveness rate for BSCT of 60–80% with selected candidates. In a later study, Harris and Miller (1990) reported that 78% of problem drinkers in a self-directed BSCT group and 63% of those in a therapist-directed BSCT group were rated as maintaining improvement 15 months after initiating treatment. The improved group consisted of abstainers (confirmed by collateral reports) and controlled drinkers. The criteria for being classified as *improved* included (1) on average, no more than 20 standard drinks weekly; (2) not exceeding blood alcohol levels of 0.08–0.10 on any occasion (verified by collateral reports); and for those who failed to meet the criteria for controlled drinking, (3) succeeding in reducing their weekly alcohol intake by 30% or more (confirmed by collateral reports).

BSCT consists of the following components (Miller & Hester, 1980):

1. A functional analysis of the drinking behavior is conducted. Together, the client and the helping professional determine specific and appropriate limits for alcohol consumption; these depend on body weight and safety concerns. Typically, limits for consumption range two drinks to perhaps four on one occasion.
2. The client monitors and records consumption.

3. Clients are trained to control the rate of their drinking.
4. Self-reinforcement procedures are created to maintain gains.
5. Emphasis is placed on stimulus-control training.
6. In place of alcohol, clients are taught a variety of coping skills for obtaining those outcomes they no longer derive from excessive alcohol use.

Numerous studies have demonstrated the effectiveness of BSCT in helping abusive drinkers to control their drinking. Unfortunately, it is probably not possible to apply BSCT to the broad spectrum of alcoholic clients who appear for treatment. In addition to not being appropriate for clients with certain medical conditions (discussed later), it may be ineffective for the large number of coerced clients (e.g., those who are more or less "forced" into treatment by employers, family members, the courts). Such clients often seek treatment to escape even more aversive sanctions and frequently have little interest in learning to modify their drinking behavior. The limited appeal of BSCT among many abusive drinkers is highlighted by the fact that many controlled-drinking studies have found it difficult to recruit clients (Cameron & Spence, 1976; Robertson, Heather, Dzialdowski, Crawford, & Winton, 1986). Furthermore, in the United States, community-based treatment providers have expressed relatively little interest in contingency management and behavioral approaches to treating substance abuse (Hartzler, Lash, & Roll, 2012). The reasons behind this lack of interest are complex and varied, but seem to involve barriers associated with the intervention itself, setting, clinician characteristics, and implementation impediments (Ruan, Bullock, & Reger, 2017).

It should be noted that even the proponents of controlled drinking have long contended that it is not a viable strategy for most alcoholics (Miller, 1982). Good candidates are generally young, motivated clients who have no biomedical impairment from alcohol abuse. Lewis, Dana, and Blevins (1988) developed criteria for ruling out controlled-drinking candidates; those who should not attempt it include:

1. Clients with liver dysfunction, stomach problems, an ulcer, or any other disease of the gastrointestinal tract.
2. Clients who have cardiac problems that would be adversely affected by alcohol.
3. Clients who have any physical illness or condition that would be negatively affected by alcohol.
4. Clients who have a diagnosis of alcohol idiosyncratic disorder intoxication (American Psychiatric Association, 1980, p. 132).
5. Clients who are committed to abstinence.
6. Clients who have strong external demands for abstinence.
7. Female clients who are pregnant or are considering pregnancy.
8. Clients who lose control of their behavior while drinking.

9. Clients who have been physically addicted to alcohol.
10. Clients using any medication or drug that is dangerous when combined with alcohol.
11. Clients who are abstaining from alcohol.
12. Those people with the following history—over 40, divorced and not in a supportive relationship, out of work—or with a family history of alcoholism.
13. Clients who have tried a competently administered moderation-oriented treatment and have failed. (p. 153)

Contracting for the Initiation and Maintenance of Abstinence

When abstinence has been chosen and initiated, certain behaviors are conducive to the maintenance of what is commonly called *recovery*. They include:

1. Attending AA/NA meetings.
2. Calling one's sponsor.
3. Reading self-help literature.
4. Getting to work on time.
5. Avoiding "slipping places."
6. Taking Antabuse as prescribed.
7. Socializing with fellow recovering addicts.
8. Practicing relaxation exercises or other coping skills.
9. Attending to one's family responsibilities.

Contingency contracting can be used to help clients initiate and maintain these behaviors and any others found to be conducive to recovery. Reinforcers and punishers are linked to the occurrence and absence of specified behaviors, as outlined in a written contract. Of course, the contract is not legally binding; even so, both client and counselor should sign it, and the client should receive a photocopy. Again, it is not forced on a client but, rather, is an agreement that a helping professional and client develop together.

Typically, contracts outline the rewards that clients give themselves if they engage in the specified behaviors. For example, if a client attends five AA meetings a week, he or she can go out for dinner on the weekend. If the client fails to make it to five meetings in a particular week, then he or she must forgo the restaurant outing. Likewise, a client may decide to "punish" him- or herself for neglecting to take Antabuse on a particular day. Such oversights can be self-penalized by arranging for donations (perhaps $5 or $10) to be given to a political or religious organization they dislike.

A number of important principles are involved in effective contingency contracting. Two of these are the temporal proximity of the reinforcer or punisher to the specified behavior and the potency of the contingency (Miller, 1980). First, in brief, reinforcers and punishers are most effective when they occur immediately after the specified behavior; those that are delayed are generally less effective. Second, individuals differ considerably in regard to rewards and punishers. For instance, ice cream might be a potent reinforcer for some recovering clients but completely ineffective for others. Thus, effective contracts will rely on contingencies that have special significance for the particular client.

Stitzer and Bigelow (1978) examined the desirability of reinforcers among a group of methadone maintenance patients (N = 53). Using a questionnaire, they found that the methadone "take-home" privilege was the most effective incentive available to methadone maintenance clinics. The second most effective reinforcer among this group was $30 per week, followed in descending order of desirability by $20 per week, opportunity to self-select methadone dose, fewer urinalyses, availability of a client representative or advocate, elimination of mandatory counseling, a monthly party, and finally the opportunity to play pool.

The Community Reinforcement Approach

In the 1970s, behavioral therapists recognized that the application of contingency management procedures to isolated aspects of substance abuse is a narrow approach. To enhance the effectiveness of behavioral treatment, Hunt and Azrin (1973) and Azrin (1976) developed a multicomponent treatment strategy that makes reinforcement in the patient's community contingent upon abstinence from alcohol and/or drugs. A system of contingencies is created for four areas of a client's life: vocational, recreational, social, and familial. As long as abstinence is maintained, the recovering client receives reinforcers in these areas. Typically, the client's significant others are involved in these contingency contracts, and their behavior may be shaped as well.

In an early study in this area, Hunt and Azrin (1973) compared a community reinforcement program for alcoholism to a standard hospital treatment program and found that the former approach produced significantly better patient outcomes over a 6-month period. Compared to patients in the standard hospital program, those in the community reinforcement program spent less time drinking alcohol, were less likely to be unemployed, and were less likely to be readmitted for treatment. In a second study, Azrin (1976) was able to replicate these findings using a 2-year follow-up assessment.

Recent research using the community reinforcement approach has shown that it is effective for treating substance use disorders in adolescents and young adults. For example, Henderson and colleagues (2016) conducted a randomized controlled trial of 126 adolescents with moderate to severe alcohol or drug problems. All of the adolescents were on legal probation. They were randomized to either an adolescent community reinforcement approach or a treatment-as-usual condition. The treatment in both conditions lasted 3 months. The adolescents were assessed at baseline and 3, 6, and 12 months after treatment. Although both groups showed significant reductions in alcohol and drug use and related problems following treatment, the adolescents assigned to the adolescent community reinforcement approach had better 12-month outcomes (Henderson et al., 2016).

Godley and colleagues (2017) tested the adolescent community reinforcement approach in treating those with a primary alcohol or marijuana problem or a primary opioid problem. Data were collected from 1,712 adolescents at treatment intake and at 3, 6, and 12 months following intake. Upon admission, the adolescents in the primary opioid problem group were more likely to be white, older, female, and school dropouts. In addition, adolescents in the opioid group were more likely to report severe substance use and mental health problems, and greater involvement in risk behaviors. There were no significant differences between the two treatment groups in treatment initiation, engagement, retention, and satisfaction. Substance use was significantly reduced in both groups. However, at the 12-month follow-up, the opioid problem group reported a greater rate of substance use and more days of emotional problems compared to the alcohol/marijuana group. Godley and colleagues concluded that the adolescent community reinforcement approach can feasibly be implemented in community settings and is accepted by adolescent substance abusers. In addition, they concluded that adolescent opioid users may need longer term care and medication to manage opioid withdrawal and craving.

Voucher-Based Treatment for Cocaine Dependence

During the 1990s, the failure to effectively treat cocaine dependence, based on pharmacological and psychosocial interventions, led to a resurgence of interest in research based on reinforcement principles (Higgins et al., 2004). Much of this research has relied on a voucher-based incentives approach, which involves "the delivery of vouchers exchangeable for retail items contingent on patients meeting a predetermined therapeutic target" (Higgins, Alessi, & Dantona, 2002, p. 888). Biochemically verified abstinence from recent cocaine use has usually been that target. The voucher-based approach has been found to increase treatment retention because clients must remain in the program to receive incentives. This is important because retention has been associated with positive treatment outcomes. In addition, a great deal of the research in this area has coupled the use of vouchers with the community reinforcement approach.

Higgins and colleagues (1991) conducted the first study testing the voucher incentive approach as a means to establish an initial period of abstinence in cocaine addicts in an outpatient setting. The investigation compared the efficacy of behavioral treatment to that of a traditional 12-step drug counseling program. A total of 28 patients participated in the study. The first 13 cocaine-dependent patients were offered the behavioral treatment program; all 13 accepted it. The following 15 patients were offered the 12-step drug counseling program. The authors note that 3 of the 15 patients refused this program option.

The two treatment regimens were quite different. In the behavioral program, patients and therapists jointly selected material reinforcers (Higgins et al., 1991). The specific goal of the behavioral program was to achieve abstinence from cocaine. The program's contingencies pertained only to cocaine use. Urine specimens were collected four times a week, and patients were breath-tested at these times as well; however, patients were not penalized for positive test results for drugs other than cocaine. The patients were informed of their urine test results immediately after providing their specimens.

Patients with urine specimens testing negative for cocaine metabolites were rewarded with points that were recorded on vouchers (Higgins et al., 1991). Each point was worth 15 cents. Money was never given directly to patients; rather, it was used to make retail purchases in the community. Staff members actually made the purchases and gave the items to the patients. The first negative urine specimen earned 10 points (i.e., $1.50), the second specimen was worth 15 points ($2.25); and the third one earned 20 points ($3). The value of each subsequent negative urine specimen was increased by 5 points. To bolster the probability of continuous abstinence from cocaine, patients were rewarded with a $10 bonus each time they provided four consecutive negative urine specimens. Patients who remained continuously abstinent throughout the entire 12-week treatment program earned points worth $1,038, or $12.35 per day.

When the patient tested positive for cocaine or failed to provide a specimen, the value of the vouchers dropped back to 10 points (i.e., $1.50). Items that had previously been purchased did not have to be returned. Higgins and colleagues (1991) reported that the items purchased were "quite diverse and included ski-lift passes, fishing licenses, camera equipment, bicycle equipment, and continuing education materials" (p. 1220). In the program, counselors retained the right to veto purchases. Purchases were approved only if their use was consistent with treatment goals.

The community reinforcement procedures focused on four broad issues: (1) reciprocal relationship counseling, (2) identification of the antecedents and consequences of cocaine use, (3) employment counseling, and (4) development of recreational activities. These issues were addressed in twice-weekly 1-hour counseling sessions throughout the 12-week program. The emphasis appeared to be placed on the first issue, relationship counseling. Eight of the 13 patients in the behavioral program participated in reciprocal relationship counseling. This counseling consisted of procedures "for instructing people how to negotiate for positive changes in their relationship" (Higgins et al., 1991, p. 1220). Higgins and colleagues describe how this system worked:

> To integrate the community reinforcement approach and contingency management procedures, the patient's significant other was telephoned immediately following each urinalysis test and informed of the results. If the specimen was negative for cocaine, the spouse, friends, or relative engaged in positive activities with the patients that had been agreed upon beforehand. If the result was positive for cocaine use, he or she refrained from the agreed-upon positive activities but offered the patient assistance in dealing with difficulties in achieving abstinence. (1991, p. 1220)

The 12-step drug treatment consisted of either twice-weekly 2-hour group therapy sessions or once-weekly group sessions combined with 1-hour individual therapy sessions (Higgins et al., 1991). In both formats, the 12 steps of NA were emphasized. The patients were informed that cocaine addiction was a treatable but incurable disease. They were required to attend at least one self-help meeting a week and to have a sponsor by the final week of treatment. The counseling sessions provided both supportive and confrontive therapy, as well as didactic lectures and videos on vital recovery topics. In the ninth week of treatment, attempts were made to involve family members in the treatment process. Finally, aftercare plans based on 12-step principles were created in the latter weeks of treatment.

After 12 weeks, the two groups (i.e., behavioral treatment vs. 12-step drug counseling) were compared on a variety of outcomes. Across all these measures, the patients in the behavioral treatment showed better outcomes than those in the 12-step group (Higgins et al., 1991). For example, 11 of the 13 patients in the behavioral treatment completed the 12-week program, compared to just five of 12 in the 12-step treatment. In the behavioral treatment group, one patient dropped out at week 9 and returned to cocaine use, and the other one had to be admitted to an inpatient unit because of "bingeing." Six of the seven unsuccessful patients in the 12-step treatment were terminated for the following reasons: (1) lack of regular attendance; (2) refusal of group counseling; (3) refusal to abstain from marijuana; (4) failure to return after being denied a prescription for antianxiety medication; (5) following a relapse, entry into inpatient rehabilitation; and (6) decision that treatment was no longer needed. The seventh unsuccessful patient was murdered.

Patients in behavioral treatment were also more likely than those in the 12-step treatment to have longer periods of continuous abstinence from cocaine (Higgins et al., 1991). Of 13 behavioral therapy patients, 10 achieved 4-week periods of continuous abstinence; of the 12-step patients, only three of 12 did the same. Furthermore, six of the behavioral therapy patients achieved 8-week periods of continuous abstinence, whereas none of the 12-step patients accomplished the same. In the behavioral treatment group, 92% of all collected urine specimens were cocaine-free, whereas 78% were "clean" in the 12-step group. This occurred even though many more urine specimens were collected from the behavioral treatment group (N = 552) than from the 12-step group (N = 312).

The results from this initial study were provocative for a number of reasons. First, the findings suggested that reinforcers could be found to compete with cocaine's intoxicating effects. At the time, the popular perception was that cocaine is so rewarding that food, sex, and all other sources of reinforcement could not compete with the drug; the Higgins and colleagues (1991) study suggested that money (in the form of vouchers) could be an effective alternative reward. Second, the findings suggested that polydrug abusers need not be required to stop use of all drugs at the same time. Contrary to traditional drug treatment philosophy, perhaps it is possible, even preferable, to work on eliminating use of one drug at a time. Finally, the Higgins and colleagues study demonstrated how important incentives are in motivating clients to stay in treatment and to adopt and maintain abstinence. It appeared that many clients drop out of traditional 12-step programs too early (i.e., before completing 3 months) because they either do not receive or do not anticipate receiving significant rewards for staying in treatment. Thus, the initial Higgins study raised the possibility that incentives may be the key to providing effective treatment for cocaine dependence.

Over the next two decades, Higgins and colleagues conducted a series of randomized clinical trials to further test the efficacy of the combined community reinforcement training (CRT)–voucher intervention (see Garcia-Fernandez et al., 2011; Garcia-Rodriquez et al., 2009; Higgins et al., 1993, 1994, 1995, 2000, 2003). Three of these trials were designed to assess the independent ability of specific intervention features to produce positive treatment outcomes (Higgins et al., 1994, 2000, 2003). The purpose of attempting to decompose the intervention was to make the treatment more efficient to aid in its transfer to conventional treatment settings.

One trial tested CRT in combination with voucher incentives against CRT alone (Higgins et al., 1994). Retention in treatment and abstinence from cocaine were significantly greater in the CRT–vouchers condition than in CRT alone. This finding indicates that the voucher component of the intervention made an active contribution to the positive outcomes produced by the combined CRT–vouchers treatment. In addition, these intervention effects were observed 6 months after the termination of treatment (Higgins et al., 1995). Another trial in this research program (1) provided further support for the active contribution of the voucher program to cocaine abstinence and (2) demonstrated that the positive effects of the voucher incentives could be detected 1 year following treatment termination (Higgins et al., 2000). The purpose of a third trial was to determine whether CRT combined with voucher incentives improves treatment outcomes above and beyond that produced by voucher incentives alone (Higgins et al., 2003). Compared to voucher incentives alone, the CRT–voucher combination was found to independently contribute to improved treatment retention and decreased cocaine use, but only during the treatment period. Thus, it appears that posttreatment abstinence from cocaine is more closely associated with the voucher incentives than with CRT.

Subsequent research further extended knowledge about the use of vouchers to treat cocaine dependence. For example, Higgins and colleagues (2007) showed that higher incentives are positively associated with longer abstinence during and following cocaine addiction treatment. In Spain, Garcia-Fernandez and colleagues (2011) documented that adding vouchers to the community reinforcement approach improved cocaine addiction treatment outcomes 6 months after the incentive program ends.

The research based on CRT vouchers presented here suggests that drug dependence is essentially a "reinforcement disorder" (Higgins et al., 2002, p. 907). Although there is clear evidence supporting the approach, the major obstacle to its widespread dissemination as a treatment option is how to cover program costs. The pioneering work done by Higgins and colleagues and other research groups is typically supported by federal research grants. Thus, the unresolved issue is how a funding mechanism can be created to support incentive-driven treatment programs for persons with substance use disorders. In the public policy arena, this issue would generate a great deal of controversy.

Enhancing Compliance with Methadone Maintenance

Methadone is a relatively long-lasting synthetic opiate that prevents opiate withdrawal symptoms for 24–36 hours (Center for Substance Abuse Treatment, 2012). In proper doses, methadone does not produce sedation or euphoria and therefore has been used for several decades as a treatment for heroin addiction. Although the positive outcomes of methadone maintenance are well established (Mueller & Wyman, 1997), one common problem is that many clients continue to use a variety of illicit drugs while receiving methadone from a clinic (Center for Substance Abuse Treatment, 2012).

Contingency contracting has been found to be an effective approach to this problem. A variety of contingencies have been used to increase the rate at which methadone clients produce drug-free urine samples. Money and program privileges have been used as positive reinforcers (e.g., Stitzer, Bigelow, & Liebson, 1980). Aversive consequences, such as contracting for the termination of methadone treatment, also have been found to be effective in reducing positive urine samples (Dolan, Black, Penk, Robinowitz, & DeFord, 1985). Another effective approach has been to make access to methadone maintenance contingent upon cocaine-free urine samples during the initial phase of treatment (Kidorf & Stitzer, 1993).

The combination of a *take-home* incentive (a positive reinforcer) and a *split-dosing* contingency (an aversive consequence) appears to boost the rate of drug-free urine samples among chronic polysubstance abusers who do not comply with conventional methadone treatment (Kidorf & Stitzer, 1996). A take-home incentive allows a client to leave the clinic with a dose of methadone. This is a convenience for the client because it reduces the frequency with which he or she must travel to the clinic. A split-dosing contingency requires clients to make two daily visits to the clinic to receive their full dose of methadone. Kidorf and Stitzer (1996) implemented split dosing following a positive urine test. They found that the combined use of positive reinforcers and aversive consequences had a marked effect on 28% of a previously noncompliant sample.

China introduced methadone maintenance treatment to address the related problems of increasing prevalence rates of HIV and intravenous opiate use (Sullivan & Wu, 2007). However, high rates of methadone maintenance dropout and relapse have plagued these programs. Hser and colleagues (2011) designed and tested a contingency management intervention to improve methadone maintenance retention and reduce drug use in Shanghai and Kunming, China. A total of 319 methadone maintenance participants were randomly assigned to usual care with or without incentives during a 12-week trial. In exchange for opiate-negative urine samples or consecutive attendance, participants earned the opportunity to draw for a chance to win prizes. Compared to those in the treatment-as-usual (control) group, participants in the incentive condition had better retention at the Kunming site (75% vs. 44%) but not at the Shanghai site (90% vs. 86%). Submission of negative urine samples was more common among the incentive group than the usual care (74% vs. 68% in Shanghai and 27% vs. 18% in Kunming). Hser and colleagues concluded that the contingency management system improved methadone maintenance retention and drug abstinence. However, there were considerable differences in effects across the two sites. The differential effects were attributed to uneven training of staff members, methadone dosing practices, and participant economic status.

CHAPTER SUMMARY

An examination of the findings from behaviorally oriented treatment indicates that contingency contracting is an effective strategy for helping those with alcohol and drug problems. The strength of interventions based on operant principles is that they are grounded in *science*. Indeed, this is a principal concern of behaviorally oriented practitioners. Another strength is that these procedures rely on *incentives* to motivate clients. Many conventional treatment programs have failed to incorporate incentives into their intervention strategies as a means of enhancing client motivation. This is understandable because cost considerations make it a very challenging proposition.

Interest in behaviorally based interventions is likely to remain strong as long as public officials demand to know "what works." This emphasis on accountability, evidence, and outcomes is inherent to the behavior technology approach.

REVIEW QUESTIONS

1. How do respondent and operant conditioning differ?

2. What is the difference between positive reinforcement and negative reinforcement?

3. What are the three general classes of reinforcers in addiction?

4. Why should relapse be expected among those in early recovery (in behavioral terms)?

5. Why is steeper discounting of delayed reinforcement thought to increase vulnerability to addictive behavior?

6. What are the four aims and six steps of contingency management?

7. What is behavioral self-control training? Who are good candidates?

8. How can contingency contracting be used to structure and support abstinence?

9. What is the community reinforcement approach?

10. How are voucher-based procedures used to treat cocaine dependence?

11. What are the strengths of contingency management as a strategy for helping substance abuse clients?

CHAPTER 7

Cognitive Models

Jackie is 25 years old and is in recovery from cocaine addiction. She has not used cocaine for almost 12 months. She recently got a job and hopes the court will soon allow her to regain custody of her young daughter. Although she has severed all ties with her drug-using friends, Jackie begins to drive by the houses and apartments where she used to get high. She visits corner stores and restaurants that were frequented by her old friends who used cocaine. When questioned by her mother about these activities, Jackie vehemently denies that she is using cocaine again. Although this is true, she persists in visiting these locations.

One evening Jackie encounters an old friend, Reggie, at a gas station. He suggests she get in his car. She hesitates because she knows Reggie will probably offer her cocaine. Reluctantly, Jackie joins him, and he soon pulls out his crack pipe. Her mind is racing about what to do. She does not want to lose all she has gained during the past year, but she does not believe she has the *self-efficacy* to resist. Jackie takes one hit from the pipe and instead of stopping there and leaving the car, she spends the rest of the night smoking with Reggie. The next day, terribly depressed and feeling horrible, she calls in sick to work. Old beliefs resurface from Jackie's former using days when she felt her life had no value and she was not being worthy as a mother. Later, feeling hopeless, she gets together with Reggie again to get high.

FUNDAMENTAL SOCIAL-COGNITIVE CONCEPTS

Substance use and misuse can be explained within a cognitive-behavioral framework. *Cognitive* in this context refers to covert mental processes that are described by a number of diverse terms, including *thinking, self-talk, internal dialogue, expectancies, beliefs,* and *schemas.* These "hidden" variables mediate the influence of external stimuli in the production of observable human behavior. Because they represent "behaviors" that are not readily observable, cognitive models are usually distinguished from those that are strictly behavioral. This chapter draws on constructs from a number of cognitive-behavioral approaches, including self-efficacy theory (Bandura, 1997; Rotgers, 2012) and alcohol and other drug expectancy theory (Goldman, Brown, & Christiansen, 1987; Hendricks, Reich, & Westmaas, 2009). The discussion shows how cognitive constructs have been used to explain the initiation and maintenance of addictive behavior; they have also been used to guide the development of relapse prevention strategies based on enhancement of coping and social skills.

Albert Bandura is recognized as a leader in cognitive psychology. In his early work, he used the term *social learning theory* (SLT), but as the theory became increasingly focused on cognition, he adopted the term *social-cognitive theory.* As the theory continued to evolve, the construct of self-efficacy became central, sometimes leading to use of the term *self-efficacy theory.* These propositions about human behavior grew out of dissatisfaction with the deterministic views of human beings as expressed by both psychoanalysis and behaviorism several decades ago. In the orthodox psychoanalytic perspective, humans are considered to be under the control of the unconscious, whereas in the behaviorist camp, behavior is seen as controlled by external contingencies (i.e., rewards). In both of those theoretical systems, self-regulation plays no part. Bandura (1977) rejected this view and insisted that humans can create and administer reinforcements (rewards and punishers) for themselves and to themselves. He described it this way:

> Social learning theory approaches the explanation of human behavior in terms of a continuous reciprocal interaction between cognitive, behavioral, and environmental determinants. Within the process of reciprocal determination lies the opportunity for people to influence their destiny as well as the limits of self-direction. This conception of human functioning then neither casts people into the role of powerless objects controlled by environmental forces nor free agents who can become whatever they choose. Both people and their environments are reciprocal determinants of each other. (p. vii)

Note that Bandura indicates that self-direction is possible within limits. These limits vary by both person and environment. For example, a cocaine addict in early recovery who lives in a suburban neighborhood is probably going to have much more control over drug-taking behavior than a similar addict who lives in an inner-city, cocaine-ridden neighborhood. Bandura's (1977) reasoning is apparent in the following passage:

If actions were determined solely by external rewards and punishments, people would behave like weathervanes, constantly shifting in different directions to conform to the momentary influences impinging upon them. They would act corruptly with unprincipled individuals and honorably with righteous ones, and liberally with libertarians and dogmatically with authoritarians. (p. 128)

In SLT, the consequences of behavior (i.e., reinforcements and punishments) do not act automatically to shape behavior in a mechanistic manner. Rather, these external, environmental contingencies influence the acquisition and regulation of behavior. Internal cognitive processes, such as efficacy and outcome expectancies, are also important because they mediate the influence of environmental contingencies (Rotgers, 2012). These cognitive processes are based on prior learning experiences and serve to determine (1) which environmental influences are attended to, (2) how these influences are perceived (e.g., as "good" or "bad"), (3) whether they will be remembered, and (4) how they may affect future behavior. Within this paradigm, human behavior is produced by learning processes; genetic traits are not thought to be essential to understanding most forms of conduct (Rotgers, 2012).

SLT stresses that individuals are actively involved in appraising environmental events. The acquisition and maintenance of behavior are not passive processes. Furthermore, Bandura (1977) maintains that the conditions for learning are facilitated by making rules and consequences known to potential participants. By observing the consequences of someone else's behavior, an individual can learn appropriate actions for particular situations. Bandura indicates that people create symbolic representations from these observations and rely on them to anticipate the future outcomes that will result from their own behavior. This cognitive process (i.e., symbolic representation) assists in generating motivation to initiate and sustain behavior.

Self-Regulation

Another central concept in SLT, and one of particular importance to the problem of substance use, is *self-regulation* (Abrams & Niaura, 1987). This concept refers to the capability of humans to regulate their own behavior via internal standards and self-evaluative assessments (Rose & Walters, 2012). The concept helps explain why human behavior can be maintained in the absence of external environmental rewards and why externally coerced behavior is often not sustained upon the removal of punitive contingencies. In the process of self-regulation, humans make self-rewards (and self-punishments) contingent upon the achievement of some specific internal standard of performance. If a discrepancy develops between one's internal standards and one's behavioral performance, the individual will be motivated to change standards, behavior, or both. The internal standards are thought to be the result of one's history of modeling influences and differential reinforcement (Wilson, 1988).

In SLT, alcoholism and addiction are not thought to be conditions characterized by a lack of self-regulation but, rather, forms of self-regulation that are deemed problematic by society (and possibly the family). In other words, the disease model's concept of *loss of control* is disputed by SLT. The alcoholic's or addict's lifestyle is seen as regulated (i.e., organized) around the consumption of alcohol or drugs. The person's behavior is not random or unpredictable; it is purposeful and goal-directed. The high degree of self-regulation is clear when consideration is given to the amount of time and effort needed (often daily) to obtain the drug, use the drug, conceal its use, interact with other users, and recover from the drug's effects. Many persons with substance use disorders manage these lifestyles for years, even while holding jobs and having families.

In this context, it should be noted that *self-regulation* does not imply *healthy*, which is a value-laden term that is, by definition, subjective. Furthermore, SLT maintains that in some cases addiction may be a means of coping (i.e., regulating the self) with internal performance standards that are too extreme or unrealistic. For example, an alcoholic may cope with long work hours by consuming many martinis. For other addicts, their evaluation of self is not "activated" by other persons' opinions of their substance use; that is, criticism from others has little impact on how they perceive themselves. Thus, they easily engage in behavior (alcohol/drug abuse) for which there is little external reward and perhaps much punishment (social/family ostracism, arrests, financial debt, health problems, etc.).

Reciprocal Determinism

In Bandura's (1977) view, person, behavior, and environment are continually engaged in a type of interaction called *reciprocal determinism*. That is, each of the components is capable of changing the nature of the interaction at any time. Individuals are thought to be capable of reassessing their behavior, its impact on the environment, and the environment's impact on themselves and their behavior. In a given situation, one of the three components may gain momentary dominance. Figure 7.1 illustrates the relationship among these components, where it can be seen that individuals are not driven by internal forces alone, nor do they passively respond to external forces. Instead, a set of interlocking forces is involved. Wilson (1988) describes it this way: "A person is both the agent and the object of environmental influence. Behavior is a function of interdependent factors. Thus, cognitions do not operate independently. In a complete analysis

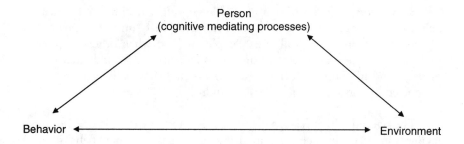

FIGURE 7.1. Interactive schema of person, behavior, and environment.

of the cognitive control of behavior, mediating processes must be tied to observable action" (pp. 242–243).

MODELING AND SUBSTANCE USE

Modeling, which is vicarious or observational learning, is an important concept in social-cognitive paradigms. Wilson (1988) defines it in the following manner:

> In this form of learning people acquire new knowledge and behavior by observing other people and events, without engaging in the behavior themselves and without any direct consequences to themselves. Vicarious learning may occur when people watch what others ("models") do, or when they attend to the physical environment, to events, and to symbols such as words and pictures. (pp. 240–241)

Bandura (1977) identified three types of effects on behavior that can result from observing a model:

1. *Observational learning effects.* These refer to behaviors acquired through observation of a model that did not previously exist in the individual's behavioral repertoire (e.g., smoking marijuana from a "bong").

2. *Inhibitory–disinhibitory effects.* These refer to increases or decreases in the intensity of a previously learned inhibition. Such behaviors usually result from observing a model being rewarded or punished for some specific action. Thus, a teenage boy may drink a beer—an action he had previously inhibited—when he observes an admired friend (i.e., a model) receive a reward for doing so. In this case, the "reward" may be any number of social consequences (e.g., other peers voice their approval; the admired friend becomes more sociable, funny, or easy to talk to).

3. *Response facilitation effects.* These refer to the appearance of behaviors that are not novel and were not previously inhibited. Examples of such behaviors are as follows: "People applaud when others clap; they look up when they see others gazing skyward; they adopt fads that others display; and in countless other situations their behavior is prompted and channeled by the actions of others" (Bandura, 1977, p. 6).

The pace at which friends drink beer is another example of a response facilitation effect. In such a group, drinking beer is not a new behavior and it is not inhibited, but the pace of an individual's drinking is influenced by that of the group. If most group members are sipping slowly, it is also likely that a particular individual will match that pace. Consider a wine-tasting event in which small amounts are consumed for taste and food is eaten to cleanse the mouth. In such cases, individuals rarely become drunk, as models of such behavior do not normally exist at such events. In contrast, consider a typical college fraternity party, in which models of heavy drinking abound. Again, SLT asserts that the models in both of these two drinking situations facilitate the pace of the group's drinking behavior. The models do not cause or require others to increase or decrease their drinking; they simply influence it.

Controlled experiments using a bogus taste-rating task have systematically examined the influence of modeling on alcohol consumption. In this procedure, participants are manipulated by the investigator's deception. They are deceived into believing that they are participating in a procedure to evaluate the *taste* of alcoholic beverages. The story is concocted to provide study participants with a rationale for consuming alcoholic beverages in a laboratory setting.

In one seminal study, Caudill and Marlatt (1975) assigned heavy drinking, male college students ($N = 48$) to one of six groups in a 3 × 2 design. Without their knowledge, the participants were exposed to different types of confederate models who had been trained by the investigators. The participants were exposed to one of three types of drinker models: heavy, light, or nondrinker. In addition, prior to the taste-rating task, they had a brief interaction with a model who was trained to act either "warm" or "cold" toward the participant. The findings showed that participants exposed to heavy drinking models consumed significantly more alcohol than those exposed to light drinking and no drinking models. The latter two groups did not differ from one another. Although the prior social interaction conditions (warm vs. cold) did not influence consumption, these experimental findings indicate that modeling can be an important social determinant of alcohol consumption (Caudill & Marlatt, 1975).

Later, Collins, Parks, and Marlatt (1985) conducted two similar experiments to study modeling effects. Using male undergraduates who were moderate and heavy drinkers, students were recruited under the pretense of assessing the realism of an on-campus barroom laboratory. They were told that the assessment would involve consumption of alcohol. In one experiment, confederates, under the control of the investigators, acted in a sociable or unsociable fashion while modeling either light or heavy alcohol consumption. Heavy drinking was produced in the participants by exposure to three types of models: sociable heavy drinking, unsociable heavy drinking, and unsociable light drinking. The sociable light drinking models tended to produce light drinking in confederates. The investigators interpreted these findings in context of the camaraderie and rivalry that exist among young men under differing social conditions. In the second study, the confederates adopted different roles indicating three levels of social status: "transient laborer," "typical college student," and "30-year-old medical resident." Whereas the alcohol consumption of the participants matched that of the confederates, level of status did not influence drinking behavior (Collins et al., 1985). Regardless, the findings from this study offered further support for the hypothesis that modeling can influence alcohol consumption in small groups.

SELF-EFFICACY AND TREATMENT OUTCOMES

Self-efficacy has become the unifying construct of the social-cognitive framework (Bandura, 1997). Previously, it tended to be described as a minitheory within the larger framework of SLT (e.g., Wilson, 1988). Regardless, self-efficacy has been defined as "a perception or judgment of one's capability to execute a particular course of action required to deal effectively with an impending situation" (Abrams & Niaura, 1987, p. 134). Efficacy beliefs have been shown to play an influential role in many classes of human behavior, including coping with stress (Burger & Samuel, 2017; Loton & Waters, 2017; Wahlberg, Nirenberg, & Capezuti, 2016), educational attainment (Putwain, Remedios, & Symes, 2015; Schneider & Preckel, 2017; Sitzmann & Ely, 2011; Zahodne, Nowinski, Gershon, & Manly, 2015), career development (Jiang, Hu, & Wang, 2018; Suh & Flores, 2017; Troesch & Bauer, 2017), health-related behavior (Christy, Winger, & Mosher, in press; Hamilton & Hagger, 2018; Matthews, Doerr, & Dworatzek, 2016; Náfrádi, Nakamoto, & Schulz, 2017), and addictive behavior (Clingan & Woodruff, 2017; Lac & Luk, 2018; Roberts & Fillmore, 2017; Takamatsu, Martens, & Arterberry, 2016).

The two components of self-efficacy are outcome expectations and efficacy expectations. An *outcome expectation* is a person's estimate that a particular outcome will occur. In other words, an individual assesses the situation and the various factors involved in his or her own performance and formulates an expectation of the probability that a specific course of action will lead to a particular outcome (Monte, 1980). Of particular relevance here are alcohol and drug expectancies. The next section of this chapter discusses these beliefs more fully.

An *efficacy expectation* is a person's belief that he or she can carry out the necessary course of action to obtain the anticipated outcome (Bandura, 1997). Thus, an outcome expectation is knowledge of what to do and of what will be obtained, whereas an efficacy expectation is the belief (or doubt) that one can do it. Bandura (1995, 1997) contends that people who are healthy, personally effective, and successful tend to have a high sense of perceived self-efficacy. In other words, they believe that they can achieve what they set out to do. Furthermore, people with high self-efficacy are likely to interpret life problems as challenges rather than as threats or unmanageable situations.

Psychosocial interventions can alter behavior to the extent that they affect efficacy expectations (Sheeran et al., 2016). Prevention, treatment, and brief intervention services that enhance a person's sense of personal competence and autonomy are likely to lead to improved functioning. About 30 years ago, Wilson (1988) recognized this cornerstone of behavior change:

> Unless treatment creates strong expectations of efficacy, coping behaviors may be easily extinguished following the termination of therapy. The phenomenon of relapse is a problem for all methods of psychological treatment, including behavior therapy. Self-efficacy theory is a means of conceptualizing the relapse process and suggests procedures for facilitating the long-term maintenance of behavior change, especially in the addictive disorders. (p. 243)

According to Bandura (1977), efficacy expectations are based on (and can be altered by) four sources of information. The most powerful influence is thought to be that of *performance accomplishments* in previous mastery situations. Past failure experiences will undermine efficacy beliefs, whereas success will boost them. The second source of efficacy expectations consists of *vicarious experiences*—that is, observation of others' success and failures. A third source is *verbal persuasion*; here, a person is told that he or she can master a task. This source has a relatively weak influence on efficacy expectations because it provides no personal experience of success or failure. The fourth and last source of efficacy expectations is the *emotional arousal* that stems from attempting a demanding task. The experience of anxiety is a powerful cue to people regarding their possibilities for success (or failure) and the amount of effort they will have to exert to achieve mastery. High levels of anxiety and fear are likely to have a debilitating effect on a person's attempts at mastery.

As applied specifically to substance use, Marlatt, Baer, and Quigley (1995) identified five specific types of self-efficacy. *Resistance self-efficacy* concerns judgments about one's ability to avoid the initial use of a substance. This type of self-efficacy is important for understanding the onset of substance use, particularly in adolescents. *Harm-reduction self-efficacy* involves perceptions of one's ability to avoid harm following initial use of a substance. *Action self-efficacy* pertains to one's perceived ability to achieve abstinence or controlled use. This type is important for understanding initial behavior change efforts among people who have intensified involvement with substance use. *Abstinence* (or *coping*) *self-efficacy* is concerned with one's anticipated ability to cope with relapse crises. Finally, *recovery self-efficacy* is composed of judgments about one's ability to return to recovery following lapses and relapses.

Efficacy expectations are particularly important in relapse prevention. Persons with substance dependence who doubt that they can maintain the tasks necessary for recovery (i.e., abstinence self-efficacy) are likely to relapse. Furthermore, the sources of efficacy expectations suggest specific relapse prevention strategies. Successful efforts will be those designed to ensure success (i.e., performance accomplishments) by first providing simple tasks and gradually building to more difficult ones. Successful efforts will also expose an addict to other successfully recovering addicts (i.e., vicarious experiences) and will teach ways to cope with negative affective states (emotional arousal). Finally, the sources of efficacy expectations suggest that verbal persuasion (e.g., "I know you can do it") is an inadequate intervention by itself. Outcome studies have examined the associations between abstinence self-efficacy and substance use lapses while in treatment.

Shaw and DiClemente (2016) conducted a secondary analysis of data from Project MATCH, a multisite, randomized clinical trial that matched patient characteristics to three different treatments for alcohol use disorder. In this analysis, they examined the responses of 627 patients (337 in outpatient treatment and 290 in aftercare). These patients had no alcohol use during the last 7 days of the 12-week end-of-treatment assessment period, but then had a lapse and reported drinking at some point during a follow-up period. In addition to demographic, alcohol consumption, and alcohol use outcomes, the patients' alcohol abstinence self-efficacy and temptation to drink self-ratings were analyzed to closely examine the relationship between self-efficacy and temptation to drink. Shaw and DiClemente (2016) found that abstinence self-efficacy predicted time to first drink, temptation predicted number of drinks on first drinking day of the follow-up period, and temptation minus abstinence self-efficacy predicted both of these outcomes. From a clinical perspective, these findings assist with treatment planning in clients who have established an initial period of abstinence from drinking. Both counselors and clients should be aware that drinking temptations and confidence to remain abstinent will fluctuate, sometimes on a daily basis. For example, when experiencing negative emotions, clients with higher temptation than self-efficacy may be provided with services that focus on coping.

Blevins, Farris, Brown, Strong, and Abrantes (2016) conducted a 12-week telephone-delivered smoking cessation treatment trial designed to help daily smokers to stop smoking. The study sample consisted of 61 smokers with an average age of 47.3 years. Two-thirds of the smokers were women. The screening procedure required the participants to smoke at least 10 cigarettes per day for the past 12 months and to exercise less than 60 minutes a week in the 6 months before study enrollment. In addition, participants were excluded if they had a co-occurring psychiatric disorder, current suicidal/homicidal ideation, or a physical issue that would prevent aerobic exercise, and they could not be using a pharmacological aid for smoking cessation. Participants were randomized to either a 12-week aerobic exercise intervention or a 12-week health education intervention. All participants were provided an intervention based on the cognitive-behavioral approach by telephone over the course of 8 weeks. Nicotine replacement therapy was provided to all participants as well. Participants were assessed on smoking behavior and urges, smoking cessation self-efficacy, and adaptive coping at baseline, end of treatment, and two follow-ups that were 6 and 12 months after baseline.

Blevins and colleagues (2016) found that levels of both smoking cessation self-efficacy and adaptive coping significantly increased during the course of treatment, with decreases in smoking urge, regardless of the intervention condition of the participant. Importantly, increases in smoking cessation self-efficacy were related to decreases in smoking at each follow-up assessment. Furthermore, reductions in posttreatment urge were mediated through self-efficacy. The investigators concluded that the key to effective smoking cessation treatment is increasing self-efficacy.

ROLE OF OUTCOME EXPECTANCY IN ALCOHOL AND DRUG USE

Cognitive models of substance abuse rely heavily on the *outcome expectancy* and *efficacy expectancy* constructs. The outcome expectancy concept has been used to predict and explain drinking behavior and other drug use, whereas both play a role in relapse (and its prevention). This section provides a detailed discussion of both alcohol and other drug outcome expectancies.

Expectancy refers to a cognitive variable that intervenes between a stimulus and a response. Goldman and colleagues (1987) defined *outcome expectancy* as the "anticipation of a systematic relationship between events or objects in some upcoming situation" (p. 183). The construction implies an "if–then" relationship between a behavior, such as drinking, and an anticipated outcome, such as relaxation.

Expectancies are dynamic cognitive variables, for they embody a person's accumulated lifetime experience of direct and vicarious exposure to stimuli of all kinds (Janssen, Treloar Padovano, Merrill, & Jackson, 2018). Thus, expectancies result from family experiences, exposure to media and marketing, observations of peers' behavioral consequences, news events, culture, and so on. Prior experiences with the euphoria produced by alcohol and other drugs are important influences on the generation of substance use expectancies.

Expectancy theory maintains that drug self-administration is largely determined by the reinforcements an individual expects to obtain as a consequence of self-administering a drug (Goldman et al., 1987). Hence, expectancy theory focuses on the *anticipated* reinforcement of drug use.

Alcohol and other drug expectancies vary in strength from person to person, and their strength can change over time within individuals. A lack of positive alcohol expectancies should lead one to abstain from alcohol, whereas heavy drinking can be predicted by a variety of strongly held expectancies. Thus, those drinkers who consume abusively may strongly expect alcohol to make them more relaxed, more sexual, or possibly more aggressive. Moderate and light drinkers may hold weaker expectancies in these areas or expect no positive outcomes in some of them. Expectancies associated with drugs operate in much the same manner. The intriguing aspect of alcohol expectancy theory, in particular, is that it is not necessary to assume that the outcomes of drinking (tension reduction, enhanced sexuality, aggression, etc.) are produced by the pharmacological actions of ethanol. Instead, in expectancy theory, drinkers' moods and behaviors are changed largely (during intoxication) by their *beliefs* about the ability of alcohol to transform them. Whether the same can be said to be true for drugs such as marijuana and cocaine is less clear.

Expectancy and Human Adaptation

Early formulations of expectancy theory came close to ignoring the genetic and neuroscience aspects of substance use and abuse (Goldman et al., 1987). Today, the expectancy concept has become woven into our neurobiological understanding of addictive behavior. In this contemporary view, addiction is not thought to be a unique pattern of behavior or a disease, but instead represents a malfunction of human neurobehavioral adaptation (Calvey, 2017). This particular adaptation, involving multiple biological and cognitive systems, is seen as expectancy-based (Goldman, 2002). Evolutionary pressures are thought to have fostered the development of a human brain and nervous system that could store information about past experiences in memory to establish a means of anticipating and navigating future events and threats that often require an immediate response. As Goldman (2002) observes:

> The evolutionary pressure that led to this adaptive approach derives from a little appreciated, but inexorable, feature of existence, namely, that time always moves forward. Hence, no situation, no environment, and no context in which a living organism finds itself is static. It instantly changes into the next circumstance, and that circumstance, into the subsequent one. (pp. 738–739)

In the human ancestral environment, a brain that could generate expectancies was adaptive because survival often depended on reacting to threatening events, securing food, and having sex. Memory of past events facilitated upcoming efforts in these behavioral situations, particularly in conditions of uncertainty and incomplete information. It seems that our neurobehavioral system evolved to store information (memory) about past events to allow for judgments to be formed about whether newly encountered circumstances match memories. If they do match, then the prospect for efficient and effective behavior is maximized, at least in situations that require immediate action (Goldman, 2002).

Unfortunately, this expectancy-based adaptation that served early humans well facilitates addictive behavior today. Observations of others engaged in alcohol and drug use, as well as other addictive behaviors, and past personal experiences engaging in them, produce expectancies that often focus attention on immediate rewards and not long-term consequences. In essence, expectancies *lock in* memory that can trigger automatic behavioral response sequences that maintain addictive behavior (Goldman, 2002).

Early Laboratory Research

Empirical support for the alcohol expectancy hypothesis comes from laboratory research using placebo and balanced-placebo designs. In early laboratory research on alcohol use, placebo designs were used to control for the effects of expectancy. This was done, for the most part, as a control formality, following customary practice in pharmacological research (Goldman et al., 1987). It was not hoped that the placebo condition would produce effects similar to that of the actual condition.

One early placebo study tested the concept of loss of control in the disease model (Merry, 1966). According to this concept (which was discussed in detail in Chapter 2), alcoholics experience intense, probably biologically induced cravings for alcohol after having consumed just a small amount; this intense need for alcohol (once consumed) leads to a loss of control over drinking behavior. Merry (1966) tested this hypothesis by administering alcohol to nine inpatient alcoholics without their knowledge. During an 18-day period, each patient was given an orange-flavored beverage at breakfast. The patients were told that the beverage contained a mixture of vitamins that would help them remain abstinent from alcohol. The beverage was alternated every 2 days such that the patients received either a totally nonalcoholic drink or one that contained 1 ounce of vodka. As a routine part of their treatment regimen, patients were asked to rate their level of alcohol craving later each morning. There was no relationship between their ratings and the beverage consumed, indicating that the basis for alcohol cravings was not pharmacological. Other studies have yielded consistent findings.

In the 1970s, the placebo effects themselves increasingly became the focus of research. Investigators expanded the placebo design and developed a balanced design that included four cells:

   I. Told alcohol, given alcohol.
   II. Told alcohol, given only tonic.
   III. Told no alcohol, given alcohol.
   IV. Told no alcohol, given only tonic.

In this balanced-placebo design, an *antiplacebo* condition (III) is added; this condition assesses alcohol effects in the absence of the usual drinking mindset (Goldman et al., 1987).

Using the balanced-placebo design, Marlatt and his colleagues conducted pioneering research on the relationship between alcohol expectancies and drinking behavior. In one landmark study, Marlatt, Demming, and Reid (1973) investigated the loss-of-control hypothesis by presenting separate groups of male alcoholics and social drinkers with the bogus alcohol taste-rating task (as described in the discussion of modeling in this chapter). Both drinker groups had 32 members. The alcoholics (mean age = 47) were actively drinking with no intention to quit. They met at least one of the following criteria: (1) history of alcoholism treatment, (2) five or more arrests for "drunk and disorderly conduct," and/or (3) previous membership in AA or a vocational rehabilitation program for alcoholics. Most of the alcoholics (25 of 32) met more than one of these criteria. The social drinkers (mean age = 37) did not meet the aforementioned criteria, and they were screened out if they described themselves as "heavy" or "problem" drinkers (Marlatt et al., 1973).

The subjects were told that the beverages were either vodka and tonic or tonic only. The actual beverage contents were systematically varied to be either consistent or inconsistent with the instructional set. It was found that both alcoholic and nonalcoholic men drank significantly more when they thought their drinks contained alcohol, regardless of the actual contents. This finding seriously challenged the loss-of-control hypothesis of the disease models, which held that alcoholic drinking is mediated by a physiological mechanism that can be triggered by the introduction of alcohol to the body. Rather, it appears that the subjects' *beliefs* (expectancies) about beverage content were the crucial factors in determining amount of alcohol consumed.

Psychometric Research Linking Expectancy and Substance Use

A large body of psychometric research has specified the different types of expectancies that are held by humans (Monk & Heim, 2013). The seminal research was conducted by Sandra Brown, Mark Goldman, and their colleagues, who developed the original Alcohol Expectancy Questionnaire (AEQ). This 90-item self-report questionnaire assesses whether alcohol, when consumed in moderate quantities, produces specific positive effects (Brown, Christiansen, & Goldman, 1987). The AEQ was derived from an initial pool of 216 verbatim statements collected from 125 people, who were interviewed individually and in groups. They ranged in age from 15 to 60, and their drinking behavior varied from total abstinence to chronic alcoholism. When the items were factor-analyzed, the following six alcohol expectancy factors emerged:

1. Global positive change
2. Sexual enhancement
3. Physical and social pleasure
4. Increased social assertiveness
5. Relaxation and tension reduction
6. Arousal with power

These factors represent relatively distinct domains of anticipated drinking outcomes. For example, the common belief or expectation is that alcohol consumption helps a person "unwind"; that is, it facilitates relaxation and tension reduction. Again, in alcohol expectancy theory, outcomes such as relaxation and tension reduction are not thought to be pharmacological effects but instead are produced by cognition in the form of expectancy.

The six expectancy factors were subsequently used in a large number of survey research studies as variables to predict various drinking practices. In general, the research has consistently linked these expected consumption outcomes to actual use, abuse, and related problem behavior. For example, Brown, Creamer, and Stetson (1987) found that alcohol abusers expected more positive outcomes from drinking than did their nonabusing peers. Similarly, Critchlow (1987) found that heavy drinkers held stronger expectations of positive consequences of alcohol use than did light drinkers and that they generally evaluated all drinking outcomes more positively.

Furthermore, Brown (1985) and Thombs (1991) reported that alcohol expectancies were better predictors of heavy and problem drinking than the demographic characteristics of the drinkers.

Among young adolescents, alcohol expectancies have been shown to predict the initiation of drinking behavior 1 year later (Christiansen, Roehling, Smith, & Goldman, 1989). Among college students, one study found that problem drinkers expected more relaxation/tension reduction than did social drinkers, whereas the latter group expected more social enhancement (Brown, 1985). Another study of college students found that the expectancy profile that distinguished female problem drinkers from female nonproblem drinkers was relatively distinct from the profile that separated these drinker types among males (Thombs, 1993). In this same study, the AEQ factor that had the strongest discriminating value among the women problem drinkers (and thus provided the clearest indication of what they sought through drinking) was arousal with power, whereas for the men it was physical and social pleasure (Thombs, 1993).

In the 2006 Hispanic Americans Baseline Alcohol Survey, Mills, Caetano, Ramisetty-Mikler, and Bernstein (2012) examined alcohol expectancy variation in U.S. Hispanic subgroups. Data were collected from 5,224 randomly selected persons, ages 18 and older, representing four ethnicities: Puerto Ricans, Cuban Americans, Mexican Americans, and South/Central Americans. Mills and colleagues found that Hispanic alcohol expectancies could be characterized by three factors: emotional or behavioral impairment, emotional fluidity, and social extraversion. Emotional or behavioral impairment expectancies involved drinking outcomes related to losing self-control and becoming emotional or argumentative. Emotional fluidity expectancies were represented by feeling relaxed, romantic, friendly, and sexually aroused. Social extroversion expectancies described becoming talkative and laughing. Overall, Hispanic men expected more emotional fluidity than Hispanic women as a result of drinking. Puerto Ricans and Mexican Americans generally expected greater emotional fluidity than Cuban Americans and South/Central Americans. Gender differences in emotional fluidity were greatest among Puerto Ricans, followed by South/Central Americans and Cuban Americans. Among Mexican Americans, there was no gender difference in emotional fluidity expectancy. These results highlight how culture and life experience influence beliefs about the effects of alcohol, and they also illustrate that the pharmacological effects of ethanol alone do not account for the range of human responses to alcohol.

In addition to alcohol, a body of psychometric research has generated evidence in support of a 10-factor model of cigarette smoking expectancies (Brandon & Baker, 1991; Rash & Copeland, 2008). Smoking expectancies include both immediate and distal positive and negative anticipated consequences of cigarette use. The 10 smoking expectancies factors are:

1. Negative affect reduction
2. Stimulation/state enhancement
3. Health risks
4. Taste/sensorimotor manipulation
5. Social facilitation
6. Appetite/weight control
7. Craving/addiction
8. Negative physical feelings
9. Boredom reduction
10. Negative social impression

These expectancy scales have adequate to good reliability. They distinguish between current smokers and ex-smokers such that current smokers have higher scores on positive smoking expectancies and lower scores on negative expectancies, compared to ex-smokers (Rash & Copeland, 2008).

In a study of 1,262 monozygotic and dizygotic young adult, female twins who were regular smokers, Kristjansson and colleagues (2011) examined the relationships between cigarette smoking expectancies and nicotine dependence, as well as the heritability of cigarette smoking expectancy. The research team found that nicotine dependence was associated with the following six smoking expectancies: negative affect reduction, boredom reduction, weight control, taste manipulation, craving/addiction, and stimulation/state enhancement. In addition, Kristjansson and colleagues found some evidence of familial transmission of smoking expectancy. However, about 70% of the phenotypic variance in smoking expectancy was attributable to individual-specific influences. The smoking expectancy factor that appeared to be most strongly associated with heritability was boredom reduction.

As the legal context of marijuana use and it public acceptance has changed in the United States, recent research has focused more attention on marijuana expectancies and their relationship with marijuana use. The increased research activity appears to be driven by a desire to better understand motivations to use marijuana and a recognition of the need to build a base of knowledge for identifying risk factors that predict cannabis use disorder. In one interesting study, Loflin and colleagues (2017) sought to determine whether edible forms of cannabis could induce placebo effects. When consumed, edible cannabis products are commonly expected to have about a 30-minute delay in onset of intoxication. Thus, in a study relying on deception, Loflin and colleagues informed a sample of 20 study participants that they would receive a cannabis lollipop containing a high dose of tetrahydrocannabinol (or THC). However, this was not the case. THC was absent from the lollipop. The investigators assessed marijuana intoxication and mood at baseline, 30 minutes, and 60 minutes following the ingestion of the placebo lollipop. The analyses revealed statistically significant changes across time in marijuana intoxication and negative mood. There were no observed changes across time in positive mood. The investigators concluded that edible cannabis products can induce a placebo effect when participants are informed that they are receiving active THC (Loflin et al., 2017).

Foster, Ye, Chung, Hipwell, and Sartor (2018) prospectively investigated the associations between marijuana expectancies and marijuana use in groups of African American and European American girls in Pittsburgh. The study sample included 2,173 girls (56.2% of whom were African American) who were assessed by annual assessments from the age of 12 to 17. The investigators found that across all years, the African American girls reported somewhat higher levels of negative marijuana expectancies than did the European American girls. The African American group also reported greater intentions to use marijuana. However, there were no significant differences between the groups on positive marijuana expectancies. The evidence indicated that the relationship between negative marijuana expectancy and marijuana use was not causal but reciprocal; that is, the two variables had a bidirectional influence on one another. Reciprocal relations between positive marijuana expectancies and marijuana use was limited to African American girls and only for a subset of ages. Foster and colleagues concluded that the differences between the African American and European American girls were not great. Overall, these findings suggest that the expectancy–marijuana association is different from the expectancy–alcohol relation in that stronger expectations of negative consequences appear to facilitate marijuana use, whereas stronger positive expectations of outcomes prompt alcohol use.

In a study of 357 college students who had a lifetime history of smoking marijuana, Brackenbury, Ladd, and Anderson (2016) examined associations between marijuana expectancies and marijuana use. The investigators used an online survey to assess both marijuana use expectancies and marijuana *cessation* expectancies. The latter variable was a measure of expectations that cutting down or quitting future marijuana use would lead to positive social, health, and other outcomes. The investigators found that both marijuana use expectancies and marijuana cessation expectancies were independently associated with marijuana use frequency, quantity, and related problems. The findings suggest that strongly held marijuana expectancies are risk factors for high-frequency marijuana use and cannabis use disorder in young adults.

Evidence in Support of Causality

A fundamental question is: Does expectancy influence alcohol and other drug use, or is it merely an artifact of existing substance use? This question has important implications for both prevention and treatment of substance abuse. Evidence clearly indicates that expectancy is a causal determinant of drinking behavior and possibly smoking cannabis (Goldman, 2002). For example, Miller and colleagues (1990) sought to determine whether alcohol expectancies could be detected in a sample of 114 elementary school children, grades 1–5. The investigators developed an assessment procedure that relied on hand puppets to collect expectancy data from the first to third graders. For fourth and fifth graders, the adolescent version of the AEQ was administered in addition to the use of hand puppets. Although they were less differentiated than those of adolescents and adults, it was found that alcohol expectancies were present in this age group. As age increased, expectancies about drinking tended to increase as well. Most of the increase occurred during third and fourth grades (children ages 8½–10 years). Because these children presumably had little or no personal drinking experience, it can be assumed that their expectations were the result of exposure to family drinking models, commercial advertising, and other media messages.

In a prospective study, a sample of 422 preteens and teens (mean age at baseline = 12.8 years) were assessed twice at a 12-month interval (Reese, Chassin, & Molina, 1994). Baseline alcohol expectancies were found to prospectively predict drinking consequences (problems) 12 months later. This relationship was observed even after the effects of the following variables were controlled for: baseline drinking consequences, parental alcoholism, and age. However, expectancies did not predict alcohol use, perhaps because of the relatively high number of abstainers and light drinkers among younger participants. Another prospective study assessed 461 participants, ages 12–14, over a 2-year period (Smith, Goldman, Greenbaum, & Christiansen, 1995). A baseline assessment was followed by two 12-month follow-ups. The purpose of the study was to examine the relationship between expectancy for social facilitation and alcohol use. The investigators found that teenagers' expectations for social facilitation had a reciprocal relationship with their past drinking behavior. In other words, the greater their expectation for social facilitation, the greater their drinking level, followed by the greater expectations, and so on. Two other directional models were not supported by the data: (1) expectancy influences alcohol use and (2) alcohol use influences expectancy.

In a third prospective study, Stacy, Newcomb, and Bentler (1991) assessed alcohol and marijuana expectancies among 584 participants as they moved from adolescence to young adulthood. The primary purpose of the research was to determine the nature of the relationship between drug expectancy and drug use. Three possibilities were tested by structural equation models: (1) expectancies predict future drug-taking behavior; (2) expectancies result from drug use, that is, they merely reflect personal experience with a substance; and (3) the relationship between expectancy and drug use is reciprocal.

Stacy and colleagues (1991) assessed their sample twice at a 9-year interval. At the first assessment interval, the cohort's mean age was about 18. The investigators found that the adolescent measures of expectancy were predictive of adult drug-taking behavior. Furthermore, the data suggested that expectancy is not a consequence or artifact of existing drug use but, rather, a determinant of these behaviors. Little evidence was found to support the social learning proposition that expectancy and drug use have a reciprocal or bidirectional relationship (Stacy et al., 1991).

Expectancy and Treatment Outcomes

Young, Connor, and Feeney (2011) examined the degree to which alcohol expectancies and self-efficacy expectancies were associated with alcohol dependence treatment outcomes. A total of 298 alcoholic clients (207 males) were administered the Drinking Expectancy Profile (DEP) at intake and upon completion of a 12-week alcohol abstinence program based on cognitive-behavioral therapy. They found that baseline measures of alcohol expectancy and self-efficacy were not strong predictors of treatment outcome. However, among the 164 patients who completed treatment, all alcohol expectancy and self-efficacy factors showed change over the course of treatment. Analysis of the variables that significantly discriminated treatment completers from noncompleters revealed that the former group had positive changes with regard to social pressure drinking refusal self-efficacy, sexual enhancement alcohol expectancies, and assertion alcohol expectancies. Young and colleagues concluded that treatment response may be bolstered by giving greater attention to the social functions of alcohol in clients' lives.

Weinberger, McKee, and George (2010) examined changes in cigarette smoking expectancies during the course of an 8-week smoking cessation trial. This study evaluated the safety and efficacy of the monoamine oxidase B inhibitor selegiline hydrochloride compared to placebo. The investigators classified clients into three groups: "quit" (N = 18), "reduced" (N = 34), or "not quit" (N = 49) by 1-week point prevalence abstinence at the end of treatment. Smoking expectancies were assessed at three points in time: randomized assignment pharmacological treatment, 7 days after the target quit date, and at the end of treatment. Weinberger and colleagues found that smoking expectancies assessed prior to the quit attempt were not related to cessation outcomes. However, among clients who quit smoking, reductions were observed in expectations that smoking would reduce negative affect, boredom, and cravings, and facilitate social interactions. Among clients who did not quit smoking, expectancy increases were detected in negative social impression beliefs. Some gender differences were also observed. Medication did not change expectancies. Weinberger and colleagues recommended that attention be given to designing smoking cessation treatments that are tailored to clients' beliefs about smoking outcomes.

Research has also tested social-cognitive variables for their ability to predict cannabis disorder treatment outcomes. Gullo, Matveeva, Feeney, Young, and Connor (2017) followed 221 cannabis-dependent patients who participated in a 6-week treatment program based on cognitive-behavioral therapy. Data were collected at five intervals during the treatment program. The investigators assessed both positive and negative marijuana expectancies. An example of a positive expectancy was: "Smoking cannabis makes me feel outgoing and friendly." An example of a negative expectancy was: "Smoking cannabis makes me feel confused." In addition, the investigators assessed cannabis refusal self-efficacy, which consisted of three subscales: emotional relief, opportunistic, and social facilitation. Examples of the survey items used to measure these variables include: "I am very sure I could *not* resist smoking when I feel sad," "I am very sure I could resist smoking when I am at a party," and "I am very sure I could *not* resist smoking when I want to feel more accepted by friends." Gullo and colleagues found that stronger negative cannabis expectancies at the beginning of treatment were associated with abstinence, whereas stronger positive expectancies were associated with lower emotional relief self-efficacy, thereby mediating its relationship with treatment outcomes. In addition, patients with lower levels of emotional relief self-efficacy (confidence in their ability to resist cannabis during negative emotional states) were less likely to abstain from cannabis and had more days of use and greater quantities of use. These findings point to specific social-cognitive variables that should be the focus of treatment planning designed to treat cannabis disorder.

TIFFANY'S MODEL OF DRUG CRAVINGS

The construct of *urge* or *craving* is central to many explanations of addictive behavior. It is used to explain the maintenance of a high rate of use as well as relapse. The notion that urges or cravings prompt substance use seems to be taken for granted by laypersons, addicts themselves, and many professionals.

Many years ago, Marlatt (1985) proposed a distinction between *urge* and *craving,* noting that an urge is an *intention* that motivates use, whereas craving represents the *anticipation* of a positive drug effect (i.e., an outcome expectancy). Regardless of whether this distinction is accepted, Marlatt's conception represents a positive reinforcement model of urge–craving. In contrast, an even earlier model by Jellinek (1955) proposed that cravings represented the anticipation of relief from withdrawal—in essence, a negative reinforcement model.

Tiffany (1990) contends that neither Marlatt's nor Jellinek's model is an accurate explanation of the relationship between craving and substance use. Tiffany's longstanding position is based on an examination of the relationship between drug urge and actual use (Tiffany & Wray, 2009). Across both self-report and physiological measures, correlations between urges and drug use were only of modest or moderate magnitude (Tiffany & Conklin, 2000). This finding suggests that *drug use occurs frequently without being prompted by urges*. Furthermore, *many relapses were not provoked by urges and cravings*. In such cases, these episodes can be characterized as "absentminded relapses" (Tiffany, 1990, p. 163). To account for these observations, Tiffany created the following cognitive model to explain drug urges and cravings.

Human cognitive processing includes both *automatic* and *nonautomatic* processes (Shiffrin & Schneider, 1977). According to Tiffany (1990), an automatic cognitive process is "a relatively permanent sequence of tightly integrated associative connections in long-term memory that always become active in response to a particular input configuration" (p. 152). Among humans, across many classes of behavior, automatic processes are revealed by the following: (1) the task is performed speedily; (2) the behavior is executed without intention and is elicited by specific stimuli; (3) under eliciting stimuli, the behavior is difficult to inhibit or curtail; (4) the behavior is easy and nondemanding to carry out; and (5) the behavior can be conducted without much conscious awareness. The common example of automatic cognitive process is driving a motor vehicle to a familiar destination, such as work. Operation of the vehicle occurs automatically and without much conscious awareness.

The same processes may guide compulsive drug self-administration, whether it be smoking, alcohol consumption, or drug injection. Tiffany and Conklin (2000) assert that with repeated practice, drug acquisition and consumption become behaviors that are produced by automatic cognitive processing. He employs the concept of *drug use action plans* to emphasize that, over time, the sequence of behaviors involved in using alcohol and/or drugs becomes integrated, efficient, and effortless. In typical situations in which drug use occurs unimpeded, urges do *not* accompany the process. It is on this point that Tiffany's model departs significantly from traditional views of urges–cravings. To explain how urges are generated, Tiffany points to an opposite set of cognitive processes.

Nonautomatic cognitive processing is slow, and it depends on careful attention and effort. Other features of nonautomatic processing include (1) identification of strategies, (2) conscious decision making, (3) planning, and (4) monitoring of task performance. In Tiffany's (1990) model, *both* abstinence–avoidance and abstinence–promotion urges are produced by nonautomatic processes. Abstinence–avoidance urges occur when drug use action plans are blocked or obstructed by external barriers (e.g., when one runs out of cigarettes late at night), whereas abstinence–promotion urges are produced when the individual is attempting to change drug use or to maintain abstinence (e.g., while the individual is in treatment). Tiffany hypothesizes that stress and other negative emotional states give rise to both types of urges, which generate competing nonautomatic processes that can influence drug use action plans. This competition tends to inhibit the impact of abstinence–promotion urges and thereby increases the likelihood of individuals executing their automatic drug use action plans.

This cognitive processing model continues to challenge the addiction treatment community (Tiffany & Wray, 2009). It seems that some researchers and practitioners have difficulty accepting that cravings and substance use are not always closely linked. Others are perhaps concerned that describing addiction as an automatic process trivializes the problem and fails to give proper emphasis to important features of the disorder.

COGNITIVE DYNAMICS OF RELAPSE

A *relapse* can be defined as a return to excessive alcohol and/or drug use following a period of sustained abstinence. It is probably the most significant issue in treating chemically dependent clients. It is often puzzling that individuals who seem to recognize the seriousness of their addiction, who appear committed to recovery, and who have gained some mastery over their drinking or drug-taking behavior often have tremendous difficulty in remaining abstinent.

Historically, views on relapse have tended to be moralistic. Such views still predominate in many segments of our society. Relapsed alcoholics or addicts are scorned: They are thought of as lazy, irresponsible, or possibly weak-willed. Essentially, they are viewed as having a defect of character. Unfortunately, such views, especially when held by legislators, government officials, and other key decision makers, impede progress in treatment approaches by depriving treatment and research centers of much-needed financial support.

Interestingly, the disease model of addiction has traditionally had little to say about relapse prevention. AA folklore, and especially its slogans, provide various messages of caution about "slippery places" and direct members to call their sponsors, but little is provided in the way of skills. Moreover, the disease model has not elaborated on the meaning of relapse. The loss-of-control concept in alcoholism has, in fact, been cited for inadvertently contributing to full-blown relapses. The assertion that alcoholics cannot stop drinking once alcohol enters their bodies seems to establish an expectation that one drink must lead to 20. Thus, when many alcoholics and other drug addicts do relapse, they often seem to go on extended binges.

An Analysis of Relapse and Its Prevention

SLT offers a perspective on relapse that differs from the one put forth by the traditional disease model. Some time ago, Lewis and colleagues (1988) stated: "The social learning perspective . . . looks at a return to substance use as a learning experience that can be successfully used to bolster gains previously made in treatment" (p. 200). In fact, clients are taught to view "slips" in just this way. Relapse is not viewed as something that is "awful" or "terrible," and clients are not taught to fear it. Instead, they are encouraged to understand it as a response to environmental cues that constantly impinge upon them. It is not evidence that they are incompetent, stupid, or worthless. The experience of relapse can provide clients with the opportunity to learn about their high-risk situations, or *triggers,* and to identify strategies that they can use to prevent them.

Much of the work done in relapse prevention was carried out by Marlatt and Gordon (1985). They view relapse as the result of *high-risk situations* combined with the tendency to engage in *self-defeating thinking.* High-risk situations are those that may trigger a slip; they may include visiting a friend at a bar, attending a wedding reception, returning to an old neighborhood, or the like. In AA parlance, as noted, they are referred to as *slippery places.* Relapse prevention strategies teach clients how to cope better with high-risk situations. Thus, this approach can be viewed as an attempt to enhance coping skills. Client self-efficacy is a critical factor.

Marlatt and Gordon (1985) believe that self-defeating thinking emerges from lifestyle imbalances. These lifestyle imbalances occur when the external demands on an individual's time and energy interfere with his or her ability to satisfy desires for pleasure and self-fulfillment. In this imbalance, recovering clients feel pressure to "catch up" for lost time and thus feel *deprived* of pleasure, enjoyment, fun, and so on. As a result, they come to feel that they deserve indulgence and gratification. During this state of perceived deprivation, cravings for their preferred substance tend to arise, and they begin to think very positively about the immediate effects of the drug. In other words, they generate positive alcohol or drug expectancies in which substance use is anticipated to make their immediate situation better. At the same time, they deny or selectively forget about all the negative consequences that go along with a reinitiation of use. There is often the tendency to rationalize the return to using (e.g., "I owe myself this drink").

Apparently Irrelevant Decisions

In this process of covert cognitive change, recovering persons may find themselves in more and more high-risk situations prior to the first slip. As this movement begins, they start making apparently irrelevant decisions (AIDs; Marlatt & Gordon, 1985). According to Lewis and colleagues (1988):

These AIDs are thought to be a product of rationalization ("What I'm doing is OK") and denial ("This behavior is acceptable and has no relationship to relapse") that manifest themselves as certain choices that lead inevitably to a relapse. In this respect AIDs are best conceptualized as "minidecisions" that are made over time and that, when combined, lead the client closer and closer to the brink of the triggering high-risk situation. (p. 203)

Figure 7.2 illustrates the sequence of covert cognitive events that precede a relapse.

Examples of AIDs abound. Following is a list of typical ones as they apply to recovery:

1. A recovering alcoholic begins to purchase his cigarettes at liquor stores, insisting that the liquor stores are more conveniently located than other sales outlets.
2. A recovering alcoholic begins taking a new route home from work, saying that she is bored with the old way. The new route is somewhat longer; it also has several liquor stores along the way.
3. A husband in early recovery begins to offer to run to the store for groceries. His wife is pleased. He regularly goes to the supermarket with a liquor store next door, even though it is further from home. He says that this market has better prices.
4. A recovering substance abuser goes to an old drug buddy's house to borrow a hammer.
5. A recovering alcoholic offers to go alone on out-of-town business trips. Her supervisor says that it's not necessary that she always go, but she says she likes to travel by herself.
6. A recovering alcoholic refuses to get rid of his liquor cabinet, saying that he needs it when entertaining friends and relatives.
7. A recovering substance abuser transfers to a new job within the company. It is not a promotion, but it happens to have little direct supervision.

The Abstinence Violation Effect

In the SLT perspective, there is a significant difference between a *lapse* (or a *slip*) and a full-blown *relapse* (Abrams & Niaura, 1987). A *lapse* is seen as a return to drinking that is brief, involves ingesting a small amount of alcohol or another drug, and has no other adverse consequences. By contrast, a *relapse* involves a return to heavy use (perhaps a prolonged binge) and is accompanied by a host of emotional and physical complications. The aim of relapse prevention is to prevent lapses from turning into relapses (Abrams & Niaura, 1987).

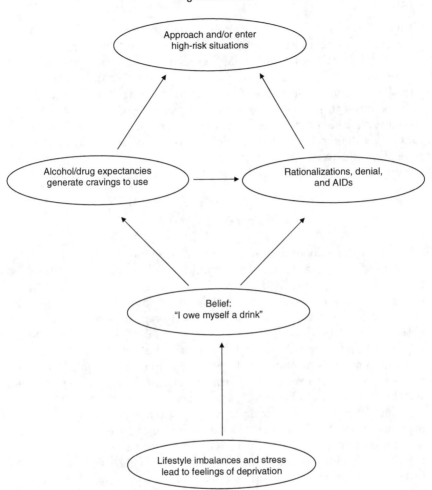

FIGURE 7.2. Covert (cognitive) events leading to a relapse. AIDs, apparently irrelevant decisions.

The *abstinence violation effect* is the experience of intense shame, guilt, and embarrassment that frequently occurs following a lapse or a slip (Marlatt & Gordon, 1985). It increases the likelihood that a slip will turn into a full-blown relapse. Among those recovering persons who are committed to abstinence, the slip may be interpreted as evidence of personal inadequacy or incompetence. The person can be overwhelmed by intense negative emotion directed at self. One recovering alcoholic told me (D.L.T.) that he recalls saying this to himself after he slipped: "I can't believe I did this. I'm so stupid. What I've done is horrible. My wife will have no respect for me. This shows that I really am nothing but a no-good drunk—just a piece of shit. I might just as well keep drinking. It don't matter no more."

Early in treatment, prior to lapses, clients need to be educated about the meaning of slips and relapses. It is important that they not think of relapse as personal failure. This type of cognitive restructuring teaches that a slip is only a mistake, not evidence of inadequacy or worthlessness. Furthermore, it is helpful for the clients to attribute the slips to environmental cues rather than to themselves. By doing this, they place the focus properly on dealing effectively with the trigger situations. Such a focus tends to build self-efficacy as clients learn skills for coping with high-risk situations.

CHAPTER SUMMARY

The cognitive-behavioral models provide a sound conceptual base for understanding substance use. The initiation of substance use is influenced by outcome expectancies and by modeling. Young people initiate substance use as a result of observing others. They imitate parents, peers, media figures, and others because they anticipate deriving the same rewards they observe others obtain.

Alcohol and drug abuse are self-regulated behaviors. The high degree of self-regulation is demonstrated by the time and effort required to maintain a lifestyle organized around drinking and/or drug use. The view that such behavior is "out of control" is probably inaccurate.

The concept of *self-efficacy* is an extremely important one in assisting persons with substance use disorders. Evidence suggests that a crucial determinant of whether treatment will be successful is the client's belief in his or her ability to master the various tasks of recovery. Without this belief, treatment is likely to fail. In addition, research indicates that self-efficacy is most likely to be enhanced by *performance accomplishments*. Thus, it is imperative that clients initially be given small tasks at which success is virtually assured, before they attempt more difficult ones.

Cognitive models have shed light on how drug outcome expectancies influence drug use and related behavior, including treatment outcomes. Some of this work has attempted to tie expectancy formation to cognitive processing. These important advances in cognitive science have added precision to our understanding of such nebulous topics as alcohol use and stress and drug urges and cravings.

Relapse is often related to an inability to cope with environmental stressors (i.e., high-risk situations). It often appears to result from negative emotional states, social pressure, and interpersonal conflicts, rather than being evidence of a character flaw. Effective relapse prevention strategies anticipate these events by teaching clients specific coping skills tailored to their individual needs.

Finally, cognitive-behavioral relapse prevention considers lapses (and even relapses) to be opportunities for learning. Instead of viewing them as events to be feared and as evidence of treatment failure, treatment providers should assist clients in analyzing their high-risk situations and covert cognitive processes. Helping clients to think differently about the meaning of relapse can result in a reduction of the abstinence violation effect and thus in fewer subsequent full-blown relapses.

REVIEW QUESTIONS

1. As it relates to determinism, how does social learning theory (SLT) differ from both psychoanalysis and conditioning theory?

2. How are expectancies and modeling related to one another?

3. What is *self-efficacy*? How is it influenced?

4. With respect to substance use, what types of self-efficacy exist? Has research found self-efficacy to be related to treatment outcomes?

5. What are alcohol and drug expectancies?

6. How are placebo conditions used to study alcohol expectancies?

7. In Tiffany's model, when do drug urges appear in cognitive processing?

8. How has relapse been viewed historically?

9. What cognitive patterns lead to relapse? What is the significance of feeling deprived?

10. What are *apparently irrelevant decisions* (or AIDs)? How do they lead to relapses?

11. What is the *abstinence violation effect*?

CHAPTER 8

The Family System

Systems theory and family therapy have been linked for several decades; however, the two are not synonymous. *General systems theory,* which emerged from such disciplines as physics, engineering, mathematics, and biology, is concerned with the structure and operation of whole entities, such as machines and organisms (von Bertalanffy, 1968). Rather than focusing on individual units or parts in isolation, systems theory explains the organization, composition, or network as a whole, in its entirety. This is accomplished, in part, by studying the dynamics of a particular system; that is, examining the connectivity and reciprocal influences within the system and how the system maintains itself over time. In the social and behavioral sciences, including the fields studying addictive behaviors, the connections of interest are social (among people) and ecological (interactions between people and their environment). These systems include culture-based traditions and practices (discussed in Chapter 9) and communities such as neighborhoods and schools. The public health model discussed in Chapter 3 is a type of systems theory in its focus on population health, rather than just individual-level health.

The family is only one system represented under the umbrella of systems theory. Early application of systems theory to the family unit was done by Bateson, Jackson, Haley, and Weakland (1956), who studied how families with mentally ill members, namely, schizophrenia, functioned on an ongoing basis. They focused on communication patterns among members, specifically "double-bind" communications, or contradictory messages from the same person (e.g., parent) to another (e.g., child) that result in a guaranteed failure to please the speaker (Kaslow, Bhaju, & Celano, 2011). Bateson and colleagues proposed that double-bind and other distorted communication patterns among family members *caused* schizophrenia.

Although this etiological explanation is no longer supported, Bateson and colleagues' focus on the family unit rather than the individual to explain human behavior paved the way for the emergence of family therapy as a distinct discipline (see Mangelsdorf & Schoppe-Sullivan, 2007).

The family system typically includes the subsystems of spousal or other adult couple dyads, parent–child units, and siblings; it also can span several generations as multigenerational families. Falloon (2003) describes the family as "the intimate social network that provides both emotional and physical support for an individual on an everyday basis" (p. 154) and is not necessarily confined to people who share a living space or are related by birth. Regardless of the proximity or biological connection among members, the family operates as a multilevel social system rather than simply as a collection of members who work independently (Bandura, Caprara, Barbaranelli, Regalia, & Scabini, 2011).

FAMILY SYSTEM PRINCIPLES

Kaslow and colleagues (2011) discuss several principles of systems theory that are integral to family therapy. Four of these principles are:

1. *Wholeness,* meaning that families are organized wholes with interdependent components, and that the whole is greater than the sum of its parts.
2. *Anamorphosis,* an evolutionary concept referring to the complex changes that occur in the family unit's composition and function over time (e.g., births, deaths, separation).
3. *Homeostasis,* a regulatory function that seeks equilibrium or stability in patterns of family member interactions, patterns that often are not amenable or responsive to change.
4. *Circularity* or *circular causality,* the principle that patterns of interaction are bidirectional, reciprocal, and circular, rather than linear, and that there is no identified beginning or end in the sequence of events in these interactions.

To help understand these and other family system concepts in this chapter, we borrow the analogy used by Miller and colleagues (2011)—the analogy of a mobile that hangs over a baby's crib. Think of this mobile as a family unit. Just as any family has more than one member, the mobile has several parts. These different parts hang separately but they are all connected and held together by a fulcrum or central organizing point. In some families, this fulcrum is an authority figure (e.g., parent) or a belief system (e.g., religious faith). When the baby's mobile is turned on, all the parts move in the circular and steady motion for which it was designed;

each part may twirl in different ways, but all the parts move together. This interconnectivity may be described by some families as "the ties that bind." When the baby tugs at one of the hanging parts on the mobile, there is a disruption in the circular motion. And, if one part is pulled too hard, the mobile becomes lopsided; it is no longer balanced.

Addiction can disrupt familial equilibrium. The entire unit may be thrown off-kilter and become imbalanced; cohesion is then compromised, and chaos and unpredictability are prominent. Notable stressors reported by family members include living in a relationship that has become disagreeable and sometimes aggressive, conflict over money and possessions, and sensing that home and family life are threatened (Orford, Velleman, Copello, Templeton, & Ibanga, 2010). The family system's fulcrum may no longer operate, triggering, in its dysfunction, what Jackson (1962) described some time ago as "a cumulative crisis for the family" (p. 482).

A cumulative family crisis is exemplified in the case of the Rowan family presented in Box 8.1. As you read the case, consider the factors that contributed to the family's imbalance—their cumulative crisis: How (1) events outside of any member's control and (2) each member's responses to these events may have magnified an already simmering or latent crisis and toppled the fulcrum of the family's equilibrium.

BOX 8.1. CASE EXAMPLE: THE ROWAN FAMILY

The case of the Rowans is based on actual events as described in a feature story published in their Midwestern city's newspaper. Names and a few other details have been altered here.

The Rowans are unfortunately one of many families swept into the opioid epidemic of the United States. They have lived through a cumulative family crisis—at least the family members who are still alive to talk about it. The exact beginnings are unknown, as is the case for many families. Mike's alcoholism certainly was a precursor to the crisis. His wife Anne insisted he get sober before they got married. He did and stayed sober for the first few years of their marriage, holding down a good-paying job. When their daughter Kaitlyn was born after their sixth wedding anniversary, Mike started drinking again. This continued for another 5 years and worsened when their son Aiden was born, around the time Mike's doctor prescribed him pain pills. He soon became addicted to opiates and alcohol, and Anne divorced him when Aiden was 10 years old. She retained custody of Kaitlyn and Aiden.

Three years later, Anne remarried and soon after was diagnosed with a rare form of cancer. In the early stage of her medical treatment, Mike died inside his parked car from an accidental overdose of the painkiller oxycodone, the antianxiety medication diazepam, and alcohol. In the wake of his father's sudden death, shy and bashful Aiden, now 13, refused to return to school, saying he wanted to stay home to take care of his sick mother. Anne reluctantly signed him up for online school. Her extensive medical treatments became a blur; she doesn't know when Aiden began using marijuana or starting using her pain pills. Even though she got a lock box, he still managed to access her medication. His use escalated, parallel to his mother's recovery. She was cancer-free; Aiden was in the throes of drug addiction.

Aiden turning 18 signaled another crisis point for the Rowans. He now was of age to access the $70,000 in Social Security death benefits from his father. He took the lump sum. It was in the next month that he overdosed on heroin for the first time; frightened by this experience, he was adamant that he would never use again. Meanwhile, Kaitlyn did her best to look after her younger brother. However, he soon became bored and still had inheritance money to spend. The surge of heroin and now fentanyl available in their Midwestern town was a magnet for Aiden. His friends knew he had the cash, too. He was arrested and overdosed a second time 2 days after being released from jail. Anne decided it was time for some "tough love." She sent him to her mother's house 45 minutes away and told him he couldn't return home until he had completed treatment for his addiction.

Aiden tried treatment twice. He was scared of dying like his father did and as he feared his mother would during her cancer treatments. He told his mom to clean out his stash at home before he was released from treatment the second time. He never made it back. He overdosed on heroin a third time, and his mother refused to let him return home. Instead, Aiden went to his grand-mother's house where Kaitlyn was now living. He stayed clean for 3 months, during which time he turned 19. There was some hope. One mid-morning after she woke up, however, Kaitlyn found him in their grandmother's garage. This fourth overdose was fatal. Aiden's body was cold, although his hand still clasped his mobile phone. When the police arrived, they used his thumb print to unlock the security code on his phone.

Anne and Kaitlyn no longer speak. They disagree over whether a family friend supplied Aiden with heroin and cocaine. Although Anne remains can-cer-free, she now is estranged from her daughter and has lost her son to a drug overdose, the same manner of death as his father. She wonders what more she could have done to protect Aiden from his father's inheritance, money and otherwise.

Effects of Addiction on the Family System

As illustrated in the Rowan family's case, addiction affects all members, not just the person or persons who have a substance use problem or other addictive disorder. (Later in the chapter, we use the term *relative* to refer to a member of the family struggling with substance use.) Persons who have grown up in a family affected by addiction, such as Kaitlyn Rowan, know this all too well. In one study (Hussaarts, Roozen, Meyers, van de

Wetering, & McCrady, 2011), the family member of a patient in outpatient addiction treatment reported that about four other family members or friends were directly affected by the patient's addiction-related problems (patients reported less than three affected family members or friends). Addiction affects not only a person's family of origin (biological and adoptive); it also affects the adult's nuclear and extended family unit—families related by blood, marriage, legal, or life partnership, and/or shared residence. As reported by Rowe (2012), the initiation and maintenance of drug use are products of multiple interacting factors in the individual as well as in the family and other systems (e.g., peer network, community). In turn, family functioning is significantly compromised by a family member's drug use, "maintaining a corrosive and often multigenerational cycle of addiction and related problems" (p. 60).

Addiction, however, does not necessarily "tear apart" every family. It can function, somewhat ironically, as a homeostatic or stabilizing force. This often happens over time and subtly. It is as if the family member's substance abuse fuels or maintains, rather than disrupts, the circular motion of the baby's mobile; it is the fulcrum that regulates family functioning. According to Steinglass (1981), many families maintain their "structural, emotional, and economic integrity" (p. 578) over the course of at least one member's addiction. From a systems point of view, the abusive drinking or drug use has adaptive consequences. That is, it functions to keep the family "in balance"—not a "healthy" balance, but a relatively stable one nonetheless. This pathological equilibrium or rigidity is preferred over continual chaos and crisis. In essence, such families opt for low-level discomfort and "put up" with the substance abuse in order to avoid grappling with even more painful and sensitive issues. When the drinking or drug use is stopped (e.g., an attempt is made at recovery), the family becomes dysregulated or is thrown off balance.

It should be noted that dysfunctional families are not forever locked into maladaptive patterns of interaction. The early research of Steinglass (1981) identified phases of alcoholism in the family and cycles or periods of transition from active addiction to sobriety and vice versa (i.e., relapse). The concept of homeostasis therefore describes the tendency to regulate change; it does not describe an unalterable pattern of maladaptive interaction.

Whether addiction serves to stabilize or disrupt the family system, what explains its effects? How can addiction have so many and seemingly contradictory effects on families? This chapter responds to these questions by consulting the work of clinical practitioners and scientific investigators. Three models of family theory in addictions are presented and corresponding approaches are described, with emphasis on evidence-based practices. We begin with a synopsis of how addiction influences the family system.

GENETIC AND ENVIRONMENTAL INFLUENCES

Two primary sources of influence in any family system are genetic factors and environmental conditions. As described in Chapter 2, genetic factors may explain as much as 40–60% of the etiology of substance use disorders. In a Swedish adoption study, Kendler and colleagues (2012) found the risk for drug abuse among adopted children with at least one biological parent with drug abuse (8.6%) to be more than twice the risk for adopted children who did not have a biological parent with drug abuse (4.2%). This difference was statistically significant, and the risk for drug abuse increased significantly if both biological parents had a drug abuse problem (11.9%) compared to only one parent (8.2%). Note that, in this study, the large majority of children with one or more biological parents with a drug problem did not develop a drug problem themselves.

Genetic factors also may explain disordered gambling. After controlling for shared environments among American twins, genetic influences were found to account for about 49% of disordered gambling in men and women (Slutske, Zhu, Meier, & Martin, 2010). In a separate study (King, Keyes, Winters, McGue, & Iacono, 2017), this rate was higher among a sample of 25-year-old Caucasian twins (57%) and had increased significantly from when they were 18 years old (21%). Shared environmental influences in this same twin sample decreased from 55% at age 18 to 10% at age 25.

Environmental influences on the family system include within-family or intrafamilial interactions (e.g., parenting practices, parental substance use, level of family cohesion) and extrafamilial exchanges or ways in which an individual member or the entire system is affected by forces external to the family (e.g., incarceration of a family member, adolescent involvement with deviant peers). Of course, there is significant overlap between intrafamilial and extrafamilial influences: Parental implementation of rules, for example, is impacted by events that take place outside the family, such as adolescent involvement with friends who smoke cigarettes; the reverse also is true. Both types of environmental influences are associated with addictive behaviors. In one study of male twin offspring (McCutcheon et al., 2013), having a mother who inconsistently applied rules and having friends who smoked cigarettes while growing up were found to significantly increase the likelihood of developing not only alcohol use disorders, but also comorbid disorders (e.g., alcohol dependence and major depressive disorder).

In a more recent and expanded Swedish adoption study that included stepfamilies, Kendler and colleagues (2015) found that an adopted child's risk for an alcohol use disorder (AUD) significantly increased when at least one adoptive parent had an AUD. Other environmental conditions also predicted an adoptee's risk for AUD: adoptee criminal behavior and adoptive parental criminal history, low socioeconomic status, divorce, and death.

When stepfamilies were considered, similar risk factors predicted AUD in stepchildren: step-parental AUD, criminal history, low educational level, and premature death.

In addition, parental gambling and approval of their children's gambling practices are associated with adolescent gambling and gambling-related problems (McComb & Sabiston, 2010). In a longitudinal study of over 1,200 low-income minority children from inner-city Chicago (Artega, Chen, & Reynolds, 2010), the two factors that significantly predicted substance dependence by age 26 and exemplified intrafamilial and extra-familial influences were (1) frequent family conflict at ages 5–10 and (2) involvement in the child protective system by age 9. Although not tested, it is highly likely that early intrafamilial conflict contributed to later child protective service involvement.

Adverse Childhood Events/Experiences (ACEs)

What is clear is that trauma and other forms of adversity experienced early in life contribute significantly to subsequent substance use problems. Zimić and Jukić (2012) found that compared to adults without substance use disorders, adults with addictions experienced more psychological trauma, parental divorce and death, and poor parent–child communication (particularly with the father) in early childhood. Adults with addiction problems also reported receiving relatively low levels of parental monitoring as children.

Four adverse childhood events/experiences (ACEs) were assessed in the National Epidemiologic Survey on Alcohol and Related Conditions (NESARC, a national probability sample). The only ACE significantly associated with lifetime alcohol dependence was parental divorce before age 18 (Pilowsky, Keyes, & Hasin, 2009). The other ACEs were death of a biological parent, living with foster parents, and living in an institution outside the home. Experiencing any of these four ACEs, however, increased the likelihood of adult alcohol dependence. In a separate 14-year-longitudinal study, LeTendre and Reed (2017) found that three other ACEs were strongly associated with adolescents developing a drug use disorder in adulthood: emotional abuse, physical abuse, and sexual abuse.

These and four other ACEs are associated with subsequent alcohol problems for male and female adults: witnessing domestic violence (e.g., having a battered mother), household drug use during childhood, mental illness in the home, and parental separation (not just divorce). In a recent study of over 21,000 Canadian adults, Fuller-Thomson, Roane, and Brennenstuhl (2016) found that three types of ACEs were independently associated with increased rates of lifetime alcohol and drug dependence: sexual abuse, physical abuse, and exposure to domestic violence. Compared to their female and male counterparts who reported no ACEs, Strine and colleagues (2012) found that women who reported four or more ACEs were 2.7 times more likely to report alcohol problems as an adult, and men reporting four or more ACEs were 1.9 times more likely to report alcohol problems as adults.

Caregiver Substance Abuse and Child Maltreatment

There is extensive and convincing empirical evidence supporting the strong association between parental or other caregiver substance abuse and child maltreatment (Berger, Slack, Waldfogel, & Bruch, 2010; Dube et al., 2001; Dunn, Mezzich, Janiszewski, Kirisci, & Tarter, 2001; Fuller & Wells, 2003; Larrieu, Heller, Smyke, & Zeanah, 2008; Scannapieco & Connell-Carrick, 2007). In 2015, approximately 25% of child maltreatment cases involved caregiver drug abuse; another 10% involved caregiver alcohol abuse (U.S. Department of Health & Human Services, 2017). Higher rates have been reported elsewhere. For example, Besinger, Garland, Litrownik, and Landsverk (1999) found that among a sample of 639 children who had been removed from their home for substantiated maltreatment incidents, caregiver substance abuse was present in 79% of the cases. This problem may be disproportionately concentrated in African American caregivers (Small & Kohl, 2012; Vanderploeg et al., 2007).

For the 273,539 children placed in foster care in the United States in 2016, 34% were removed from their home because of parental drug abuse, second only to parental neglect (61%; Administration for Children and Families, 2017). Turney and Wildeman (2017) reported that 54% of children placed in foster care or adopted from foster care in 2011–2012 were exposed to at least one household member with substance abuse. Although evidence is lacking, child welfare experts suspect that opioids are increasingly these substances of abuse. Lloyd, Akin, and Brook (2017) suggest that parental or other caregiver opioid use may explain the annual increases in children placed in foster care in the United States since 2012. They also report that foster care entry because of parental substance abuse decreases the likelihood of reunification or exit to guardianship for younger children (ages 0–3 years) compared to older children or those who entered foster care for other reasons. Their analysis of 32,680 child welfare cases tracked over 10 years in one state found that children ages 0–3 who had been removed from their home for caregiver substance abuse were less likely to reunify with their custodial parent and less likely to exit foster care to guardianship than the other two groups. These are "troublesome" findings, Lloyd and colleagues state, because "children 0–3 are typically the most 'adoptable' age group compared to older children" (p. 183).

Although alcohol often is implicated in child maltreatment, caregiver methamphetamine use also places children at high risk for neglect and abuse. Messina and Jeter (2012) studied 99 children who had been removed from home-based methamphetamine laboratories in Los Angeles County during the years 2001–2003. Child neglect was documented in 93% of the cases. It was also alarming that 80% of the children received a medical diagnosis, which in most cases was related to exposure to the chemicals used to manufacture methamphetamine in their homes.

The relationship between caregiver substance abuse and child maltreatment is correlational and not necessarily causal. In some cases, alcohol and drug use may facilitate child maltreatment among caretakers who have a prior proclivity for such behavior; in other cases, certain mechanisms may mediate between substance use and maltreatment of a child. Abusive caretakers are often stressed by multiple life problems, including poverty, inadequate social support, and a personal history of child maltreatment (Young-Wolff, Kendler, Ericson, & Prescott, 2011). It also is important to note that many caretakers who misuse substances do not neglect or abuse their children (Scannapieco & Connell-Carrick, 2007). Regardless, the problem of child maltreatment attributable to caretaker substance misuse has not been adequately addressed.

When both genetic vulnerability and adverse environmental stressors appear in families, addiction is likely to occur. It is the *confluence* of these influences within the family context that fosters addictive behavior. That one or both biological parents have problems with addictive behavior does not guarantee that their offspring will have such problems as adults. Their child's vulnerability to addiction is higher than that in persons without parental addiction, but genetic susceptibility is not destiny. Similarly, familial environmental influences can increase a child's susceptibility to addictive behaviors, but these influences, even any number of ACEs, do not cause addiction for an adult. How addiction is transmitted and maintained among family members, such as the Rowan family described in Box 8.1, is explained in many ways. This includes its transmission and maintenance over generations and even during end-of-life care (Bushfield & DeFord, 2010). Three explanations are discussed in the following sections.

THREE FAMILY TREATMENT MODELS IN ADDICTIONS

McCrady, Ladd, and Hallgren (2012) identify three models that dominate contemporary family addiction treatment: family disease models, family systems models, and behavioral models. We believe these models apply to the range of addictive behaviors (e.g., substance dependence, gambling), not just substance abuse. Each of these models is described in the following sections. Although the three models overlap, we highlight characteristics that are more illustrative of one model than another. There is more empirical support for the family systems models and the behavioral models than for the disease models, the last-named having developed in early substance abuse treatment settings. In the second half of the chapter, several evidence-based or empirically supported family-based approaches are discussed, each of which is informed by either the family systems models or behavioral models.

Family Disease Models

The earliest model of family theory in the addictions is the family disease model. It had its beginnings in the 1950s when the accounts of wives of alcoholics and the stages of family adjustment to an alcoholic member were explored (Jackson, 1954). This represented a shift in focus from the individual alone (i.e., the person with a substance use problem) to the relationships with this individual. Addiction was no longer thought of as confined to one person, but rather as a condition shared among all family members. As Jackson (1962) observed, "Members of the alcoholic's family are no longer regarded simply as innocent victims but may be seen, for instance, as etiological agents or as complicating the illness" (p. 472). This also was a time when family members of alcoholics established their own support groups, namely, Al-Anon, the autonomous arm of AA for the spouse and relatives of an alcoholic, established in 1951.

The familial network of interest at this time in history consisted of a male alcoholic husband and father and his wife and children. Thus, the initial focus was on husband–wife, father–children, and mother–children relationships; sibling relationships also were explored (Steinglass, Weiner, & Mendelson, 1971). The families studied were primarily white and middle to upper-middle class, and were characterized as *alcoholic families* or *alcoholic systems* (Steinglass et al., 1971). Research involving direct observations of daily interactions among family members at home (Steinglass, 1981) or in laboratory conditions (Steinglass et al., 1971) revealed distinct and predictable patterns of within-family regulatory behavior over time, such as considerable time spent in separate rooms, rarely being equally drunk simultaneously (i.e., a relatively sober member protecting the drunken family member), and lack of extrafamilial engagement (i.e., few or no visitors to the home). From these observations, an *alcoholic family identity* (Steinglass, 1987) could be discerned.

Specific reference to alcoholism or addiction as a family disease did not occur until the 1980s, concurrent with the burgeoning research on family systems, the growing acceptance of addiction as an illness or a disease, the growth of Al-Anon, and the development of the Adult Children of Alcoholics (ACOA) movement (see Brown, 1991) that espoused the "damage model" that "all children are affected" by parental alcoholism (Black, 1982, p. 27). Although Steinglass (1981) described chronic alcoholism as "a unique disease" for families (i.e., unique in its "tenacity and its fluctuating, cyclical life course" [p. 583]), it is Wegscheider-Cruse (1989) who is credited with popularizing the concept of addiction (namely, alcoholism) as a family disease. She described it as "both *personal* and *systemic*; it affects each family member as an individual and the family system as a whole" (p. 80; italics in original). As a family disease, it is not so much that addiction is a member of the family; rather, it is that *all* members share in addiction and are "afflicted with complementary and interlocking illnesses" (Miller et al., 2011, p. 201). It is manifested in how members interact with one another—how their roles, responsibilities, and communication styles develop and adjust when at least one family member has an addictive disorder. In this way, addiction in the family also can be considered "a disease of lifestyle" (Kumpfer, Alvarado, & Whiteside, 2003, pp. 1760–1761).

Codependency

One interactional style that fits with the family disease model is *codependency* or *codependence* (or *co-alcoholism,* when alcoholism is involved). It describes an unhealthy relationship pattern typically between two adults; often, one of these persons has substance use problems and the other does not (the *codependent*). Children of alcoholic parents can exhibit what Greenleaf (1984) termed *para-alcoholism.* The codependent person protects the alcoholic or addict from the natural consequences of substance use. This behavior is known as *enabling.* Examples of enabling are calling in sick to a spouse's employer when that spouse has been out drinking or using drugs all night, and cleaning up after a spouse or parent has vomited during the night from too much alcohol. Enabling also can apply when a family member excuses an addict's drug use and does not intervene to prevent further drug-using behavior. An example of this behavior is continuing to give filled prescriptions for narcotics or benzodiazepines to a family member when those medications are not intended for that person. *Codependency* is considered an unhealthy relationship pattern, whereas *enabling* is a common behavior arising from it.

From their systematic analysis of the literature on codependency, Dear, Roberts, and Lange (2005) identified four key features of it. First, the person who is codependent (often female) has an *excessive external focus* and is overly involved with other people, namely, a significant other (often male) with substance use problems. There is an abnormal reliance on this other person's approval and acceptance, resulting in *self-sacrificing* behavior on the part of the codependent person, the second core feature of codependency. The codependent person neglects his or her own needs in order to please the partner and, in the process, loses all sense of self or identity. It is as if the codependent person has become emotionally dependent on the addict. The addict's mood dictates the codependent person's mood, implying that the codependent person has great *difficulty experiencing emotions* for him- or herself. This is the third defining feature of codependency.

In a sense, the codependent becomes an appendage to the addict and the substance abuse. Both share an addiction-like condition. In the words of Conyers (2003), it is as if the codependent person has become "addicted to the addict," exhibiting denial, obsession (i.e., preoccupation with family member's actions, feelings), and compulsion to control the family member's behavior. This *controlling* behavior is the fourth core feature of codependency. It is as if the codependent person has assumed full responsibility for resolving the problems of the other.

According to Beattie (1992), the concept of codependency was coined in the late 1970s or early 1980s by clinicians in the addictions field. It resembled earlier and more sophisticated concepts used in family systems theory to describe dyadic relationships lacking emotional maturity or healthy differentiation (e.g., an adult child's inability to attain independence from his or her family of origin). Scaturo, Hayes, Sagula, and Walter (2000) noted several of these concepts: *pathological complementarity, interlocking pathology,* and *overadequate–inadequate reciprocal functioning.* These concepts describe the dysfunctional relationship of two partners who do not hold equal positions of power, but remain rigidly intertwined in a system that maintains equilibrium or balance over time.

The term *codependence* may have gained a wide audience among family members in addiction treatment because of its brevity, its use of a recognizable addiction-related word, and its promotion by clinicians (many of whom were in recovery from a substance use problem or had a family member with an addictive disorder). Codependency remains a popular term today in self-help groups and in the self-help literature, as well as in some clinical settings, even though one of its staunchest proponents acknowledged its "fuzzy definition" (Beattie, 1992, p. 47).

The vague definition of codependency is but one of its many long-standing criticisms. A "psychosocial condition . . . manifested through a dysfunctional pattern of relating to others" (see Fischer, Spann, & Crawford, 1991, p. 88) is nonspecific, as is the 16-item scale developed to measure the construct. And despite their identification of four core features of codependency, Dear and colleagues (2005) were adamant that "this does not mean that we have established that a syndrome of codependency actually exists" (p. 203). It is important to note that codependency has never been included in standard medical taxonomies, such as the *Diagnostic and Statistical Manual of Mental Disorders* (DSM). It is *not* a pathological condition or disorder, despite recent claims that it is (see Knudson & Terrell, 2012).

Calderwood and Rajesparam (2014) noted several other criticisms of codependency. One criticism is its lack of empirical support, despite the claims of others (e.g., Fischer et al., 1991; Knudson & Terrell, 2012). Other criticisms are (1) the pejorative label of "codependent" that defines a person only in relation to another person, (2) the failure of its proponents to affiliate with and practice according to family systems theory, and (3) its failure to explain complex and current family dynamics such as same-sex partnerships. The spousal relationship is only one family subsystem, and the person identified as codependent may be a part of healthy systems outside of the spousal relationship or family unit.

Practitioners with little training in family systems theory who use the terms *codependency* or *codependence* with clients as jargon or in a cavalier fashion may underestimate or overlook entirely the complexities involved in a severely dysfunctional family system. According to Scaturo and colleagues (2000), this kind of practice can have "deleterious effects" (p. 65). One of these effects is that continued reference to a person and an unhealthy relationship as codependent "often encourages the person to excuse his or her own behavior in relations with others rather than trying to find solutions" (Sandoz, 2004, p. 37). Another is that labeling someone as codependent (or not refuting a client's self-label as codependent) can prevent healthy self-exploration, thus inhibiting the process of emotional growth (Scaturo et al., 2000). Calderwood and Rajesparam (2014) encourage practitioners to use the phrase "people in a relationship with someone with an addiction" rather than the term *codependent,* and Van Wormer and Davis (2013) recommend the terms *survivor* or *caring family member.* These references are consistent with Miller and colleagues' (2011) *stress-coping hypothesis* and the *stress–strain–coping–support model* (Orford, Copello, Velleman, & Templeton, 2010). These are alternatives to the disturbed family or codependence hypothesis. We discuss these alternative models later in the chapter as part of behavioral models of addiction treatment for families.

Family Roles

Over the years, therapists in addiction treatment have created a variety of schemes for classifying the types of role behavior in the chemically dependent family. For example, based on her work with children, Black (1982) proposed three roles that children of an alcoholic parent adopt: the very responsible child (often the oldest or only child); the adjuster (follows directions, adjusts to circumstances of the day); and the placater (the family comforter, tries to make others in the home feel better, feels responsible for the pain of others). Wegscheider-Cruse (1989) later developed five family roles: the enabler, hero, scapegoat, lost child, and mascot.

As with the concept of codependence, these family role typologies were derived from clinical practice, not from research. Therefore, they are not empirically validated (Sher, 1997). They have been criticized because they assume a rather stable pattern of family functioning and have not been applied across cultures (Vernig, 2011). Nevertheless, family role typologies continue to be relied upon in clinical settings because of their heuristic appeal to clinicians and clients alike. Vernig (2011) acknowledges that these typologies have "entered into the folk wisdom of the field of substance abuse counseling and self-help support groups" (p. 535). Because they remain well recognized and applied in clinical settings, we believe that addictions practitioners should have an understanding of these concepts. The following discussion presents one of the common classification typologies.

This typology is based on a nuclear family comprising two parents and four or more children. This depiction of family may be considered outdated, which is one criticism of this scheme of family roles. Because one of the parents is assumed to struggle with problematic substance use, the scheme emphasizes the adaptive roles of the children in the family. It should be noted that although some families who experience addiction have members who clearly fall into a specific role, other families have members who exhibit characteristics of more than one role; others have members who shift from role to role as time passes; and in the life of some families, certain roles never appear. Thus, the roles are probably too "neat" for most families with a member or two who struggle with addiction. For the sake of discussion, we describe each family role using stereotypical roles and functions. We agree with van Wormer and Davis (2013) that these roles and their descriptions should be regarded with appropriate skepticism.

THE CHEMICALLY DEPENDENT PERSON

From a family systems perspective, the chemically dependent member is not diseased; he or she is playing a role, and that role is to act irresponsibly. This role has a homeostatic function. Typically, it serves to suppress spousal conflict or to divert attention from more threatening family issues.

An important aspect of the chemically dependent role is emotional detachment from the spouse and the children. One consequence of this distancing is that parental power is abandoned and is then adopted by the nondependent spouse and an older child. The "first love" of the alcoholic or addict becomes the substance itself. Over time, the self-administration of the substance becomes the central activity in this person's life; family life diminishes in importance.

THE FAMILY MANAGER

The second role is the *chief enabler* or simply the *enabler*. Van Wormer and Davis (2013) use the less pejorative term, *family manager,* which we adopt. It is common in this scheme for there to be numerous enablers or managers in a family; however, the chief manager is usually the nondependent spouse. As mentioned earlier, enabling is a behavior that inadvertently supports the addiction process by helping an alcoholic or addict avoid the natural consequences of irresponsible behavior. Most addicts have at least one enabler in their lives, and many have three, four, or more who help maintain their addiction.

From a family systems perspective, the family manager reduces tension in the family (i.e., maintains family balance) by "smoothing things over," that is, making things right. The manager often faces a dilemma: If he or she (and more often it is she) continues a pattern of enabling behavior and does not intervene in potentially dangerous situations (e.g., taking car keys away from a drunk spouse), the substance abuser could do serious harm to self or others. A wife of an alcoholic once told one of us that she knew she was enabling her husband by picking him up from their snow-covered yard, but she had no choice, as otherwise he would have frozen to death. The family manager may decide on a course of action in the interest of self-preservation. For example, going to several pharmacies to refill pain medications for a spouse who no longer medically needs them may protect the family manager from her spouse's wrath. "At least this keeps him from yelling at me and the kids," she may say.

In many cases, family managers are unaware that their enabling behavior is contributing to the progression of addiction in their spouse and perhaps increasingly unhealthy patterns of behavior among other family members, such as their interactions with children. Managers believe they are simply being helpful and holding their families together, even though anger is their primary feeling (Wegscheider-Cruse, 1989). They may feel stuck and helpless. It therefore is not surprising that family members in this role can experience physical, emotional, mental, and spiritual difficulties (Wegscheider-Cruse, 1989).

THE FAMILY HERO

The role of the *family hero* is usually adopted by the oldest child. References to this role include the *parental child*, the *superstar*, and the *goody two shoes* (Deutsch, 1982). This child attempts to do everything right. He or she is the family's high achiever, and as such appears quite ambitious and responsible. Given the family circumstances (i.e., a chemically dependent parent), the child is often admired for excelling under difficult conditions.

The family hero often takes on parental responsibilities that the chemically dependent parent gave up. He or she provides care for younger siblings by cooking for them, getting them ready for school, putting them to bed, doing laundry, and so on. The nondependent spouse (i.e., the chief enabler) usually does not have much time for these chores because his or her time is divided between working and caring for the alcoholic or addicted spouse.

Family heroes often do well academically and in athletic pursuits (Deutsch, 1982). They may be class presidents, honor students, starters on the basketball team, or the like. They are achievement oriented and frequently develop well-respected professional careers. Their achievements, however, are not to satisfy their own needs, but to fill the self-worth deficit of their parents or other family members (Wegscheider-Cruse, 1989). This exemplifies the self*less* heroism of the hero. The family hero reduces tension in the family simply by doing everything "right." The hero is the source of pride for the family, inspiring hope and giving the family something to feel good about.

THE SCAPEGOAT

The scapegoat role often is adopted by the second oldest child. The scapegoat can be viewed as the reverse image of family hero (Wegscheider-Cruse, 1989). This child does very little right and is quite rebellious. Scapegoats may be involved in fights, theft, or other trouble at school or in the community; they are often labeled *juvenile delinquents*. Male scapegoats may be violent, whereas female scapegoats may express themselves by running away or becoming sexually promiscuous. Scapegoats of both genders most often abuse alcohol and drugs themselves.

A child in the scapegoat role seems to identify with the chemically dependent parent, not only in terms of substance abuse but in other ways as well (e.g., attitude toward authority, attitude toward the opposite sex, vocational interests). The scapegoat typically feels inferior to the family hero; still, the two of them are usually very close emotionally, despite the differences in their behavior. This special bond may continue throughout adulthood.

This child is referred to as the *scapegoat* because he or she is the object of the chemically dependent parent's misdirected frustration and rage. The child may be abused both emotionally and physically by this parent. This is especially true when the chemically dependent parent is the father and the scapegoat his son. In effect, the scapegoat becomes, in common parlance, "his father's son." Although the son may despise his father, the father is his role model and the son adopts his father's self-destructive and antisocial tendencies.

The scapegoat expresses the family's frustration and anger. The child in this role maintains family balance by directing some of the blame from the chemically dependent parent to him- or herself. This allows the chemically dependent parent to blame someone else for his or her own drinking and drug use. It also shields the chemically dependent parent from some of the blame and resentment that would have been directed at him or her.

THE LOST CHILD

Even in functional families, the middle children are thought to get less attention than their siblings, and they seem less certain of their contribution to the family. This tendency is exacerbated in chemically dependent families (Deutsch, 1982). The *lost child* may be a middle child but may also be the youngest. The chief characteristic of the lost child is his or her objective to avoid conflict at all costs. These children maintain balance in the family by simply disappearing; that is, by not requiring any attention. In essence, the youngster in this role supports the family equilibrium by causing no new problems and requiring minimal attention. Such children tend to feel powerless and are described as *very quiet, emotionally disturbed, depressed, isolated, withdrawn,* and so on. These children tend to be forgotten, as they are very shy. Indeed, this role is often referred to as the *forgotten child* (Wegscheider-Cruse, 1989). They are followers, not leaders. They engage in much fantasy. If they stand out in school in any way, it is by virtue of poor attendance (Deutsch, 1982). These behaviors point to a great deal of insecurity.

According to Deutsch (1982), the lost child is probably the most difficult child in a dysfunctional family to help. This child has never felt close to either parent and has been deprived of healthy adult role models (Wegscheider-Cruse, 1989). He or she may not have close friends or other supports outside the family. Also, the child's behavior is usually not disruptive in school; hence, teachers and counselors do not identify this child as needing intervention services.

As adults, lost children exhibit a variety of mental health problems. They may complain of anxiety and/or depression and may seek counseling. They have difficulty with developmental transitions because they fear taking risks; thus, they may put off making life decisions. They also may back out of intimate relationships when someone gets too close.

THE MASCOT

The last commonly described role is the *mascot* or the *family clown*. The youngest child in the family often adopts the role of the mascot, arriving in the family after circumstances have deteriorated considerably (Wegscheider-Cruse, 1989). Everyone in the family likes the mascot and is comfortable having him or her around. The family usually views the mascot as the most fragile and vulnerable; thus, he or she tends to be the object of protection. Deutsch (1982) noted that even the chemically dependent parent treats the mascot with kindness most of the time.

Mascots often act silly and make jokes, even at their own expense. The clownish behavior acts as a defense against feelings of anxiety and inadequacy. They often have a dire need for approval from others. As adults, they are very likable but appear anxious.

The child in the mascot role helps maintain family homeostasis by bringing laughter and fun into the home. By "clowning around" and making jokes, the mascot brightens the family atmosphere, becoming a counterbalance against the tension that is prevalent and oppressive in dysfunctional families. The mascot may be the one family member no one complains about.

Family Systems Models

Unlike the disease models, the family systems models in addiction treatment originated from family systems theory. Whereas the disease models developed in addiction treatment, the family systems models developed in mental health treatment, specifically couple and family therapy. Although the two share some similarities, such as family members operating according to certain roles, they differ with respect to the prominence of paradigms, differences attributed to their separate origins. For the disease models, addiction is the starting point; what is primary is the concept of addiction as a disease—a disease that happens to be relational in nature or a disease shared by all family members, but a disease or a chronic condition first and foremost. By contrast, the family systems models start with the structure, network, assemblage, or unit of the family. It is these interconnections and relationships that are primary; addiction is somewhat secondary, and it is not necessarily a disease or a chronic condition.

There are quite a few family therapy models, several of which Kaslow and colleagues (2011) have reviewed. Among them are *psychodynamically informed and intergenerational-contextual family models* that emphasize past rather than present interactions and intrapsychic more so than interpersonal dimensions. The *Bowen family model,* named after the work of Murray Bowen (1976), also considers multigenerational patterns, but its primary construct is *differentiation* of the self. People who are differentiated are able to distinguish emotional states from intellectual processes, both within themselves and from their experience of family members. People whose emotional and intellectual functioning is relatively well separated are more autonomous, more flexible, and better able to cope with stress; they demonstrate more independence of emotions. In essence, they possess a high level of emotional maturity. The opposite of differentiation is fusion. *Fusion* is the state of nondifferentiation; that is, no differentiation exists between the emotional and the intellectual self. Emotion, at this extreme, completely dominates the self. Persons who are *fused* are extremely dominated by automatic emotional reactions. Their relationships with other family members, namely, a spouse, are characterized as *emotional stuck-togetherness* (Gurman, 2011), similar to the concept of codependency.

Experiential and humanistic family models define dysfunctional systems as those that have prevented members from fulfilling their personal growth. This applies to the well-being of parents as well as children. An only child's longstanding alcohol and drug addiction, for example, can delay or interrupt his parents' retirement because of the emotional and financial support they have invested in him for more than 40 years. Important in these models is direct, open, and immediate communication among family members in an atmosphere of healthy spontaneity and respect for the contributions of each member. *Strategic and structural family models* are two separate models, but both focus on communication patterns and strategies used among members. The strategic family model considers the metacommunication strategies, symbolic communication patterns, or rituals used among members, and how these covert, nonverbal messages (e.g., shoulder shrugs, isolating behavior) exaggerate or change the meaning of verbal communication. In the structural family model, the focus is on the organizational structure of relationships and the source, function, and manifestation of power in the family unit. Concepts such as *boundaries, hierarchy, alignment* (e.g., who spends time with whom), and *coalitions* are integral to this model.

All family systems models operate according to the four principles described at the beginning of this chapter: (1) wholeness, (2) anamorphosis, (3) homeostasis, and (4) circular causality. When addiction is present, it serves a specific role (or has several roles) and influences the entire system. For example, substance use may serve as a lubricant, keeping the family unit assembled, operating, and relatively stable over years or even over generations.

Boundaries

Across all of the family systems models, not just the structural family model, the focus is on the organization of the family system. This organization is consistent with the systems principle of wholeness. Several concepts typically are used to describe the nature of the organization. One is *boundaries,* understood as invisible lines that define and separate one subsystem from another. Although certain demographic variables can determine boundaries (e.g., age, sex), from a family systems perspective, boundaries often are established and maintained through behavioral interactions and other forms of communication. In this way, they can be thought of as *rules of engagement* and *methods of functioning.* This is true in most cultures.

Like visible walls and fences, boundaries can be clearly delineated, highly restrictive or impenetrable, and therefore *rigid.* The spoken or unspoken messages sent to family members operating within these boundaries include "Do not enter," "Stay away," and "Leave me (or us) alone." Similar messages can be conveyed to persons outside the family. The purpose of these rigid boundaries is to prevent change and to maintain the status quo. In families where addiction is present, rigidity is evident in specific commands that govern family functioning. These include the rules that Black (1982) first identified: "Don't talk, don't feel, and don't trust." Lawson and Lawson (1998) observed three related, though slightly different, rules: (1) "Do not talk about the alcoholism," (2) "Do not confront drinking behavior," and (3) "Protect and shelter the alcoholic so that things don't become worse" (p. 58).

The result of such messages and rules is isolation and separation— among family members as well as within the entire family unit and with people outside the family. Another result is stagnation. Unfortunately, rigid boundaries enable the family member struggling with substance use to keep drinking or using drugs and inadvertently contribute to the progression of addictive behavior. A vicious cycle develops in which the isolation imposed by the three rules perpetuates the alcohol or drug abuse, and, in turn, the substance abuse maintains the need for isolation. This is an example of the principle of circular causality.

Far different from rigid boundaries are loose and permissive boundaries; these are known as *diffuse* or *enmeshed* boundaries. Relationships that operate according to these boundaries are characterized by overinvolvement. Differentiation of self from others is minimized. There is no room for separateness or individual uniqueness; an overemphasis is placed on sameness and unity (Lawson & Lawson, 1998). Families with very diffuse or enmeshed boundaries do not allow adolescents to pull away from the family. They discourage the development of exceptional or unique talents. Some adolescents may rebel against this "smothering" by abusing alcohol or drugs. Others may acquiesce, believing that a strong connection with their substance-using parent is their duty. They, too, may adopt the substance use practices of their parent (see Bartle-Haring, Slesnick, & Murnan, 2018). When spousal relationships are characterized by overinvolvement, the individuality of each partner is "sacrificed" for the "sake of the marriage" (Lawson & Lawson, 1998, p. 58).

Boundaries have been described on a continuum from *very diffuse* to *very rigid*; in the middle of this continuum lie *clear* boundaries. Within most family systems, boundaries lie at some point in the middle, although they may be closer to one extreme or the other. Optimally functioning family relationships are characterized by clear boundaries that support autonomy and yet promote intimacy; the members show genuine love and concern for one another without attempting to control or coerce one another. These relationships evince mutual respect; freedom and flexibility are evident, and communication patterns are clear and direct. Clear boundaries denote healthy separateness and serve as a protective factor (Bartle-Haring et al., 2018).

When one spouse is misusing substances, the spousal relationship may be disengaged at a fixed distance. That is, the partners may remain together, but they lead relatively separate lives. The alcoholic or addict may work and spend much time with drinking or drug-using affiliates rather than at home. The nondependent spouse may carry the full parenting load and pursue other interests without the chemically dependent spouse. Children of these disengaged families typically feel rejected and unloved. They may develop emotional problems or "act out." Either way, their maladaptive behavior represents a plea for help.

The three types of boundaries or rules of engagement are depicted in Figure 8.1. They are placed on a continuum, with rigid and diffuse boundaries on either end, as opposites, and clear and healthy boundaries in the middle. On the left end of the continuum, notice the thick lines around the two circles that illustrate rigid boundaries. There also is distance between the circles, corresponding to distance (physical, emotional) between family members. The circles on the right end of the continuum illustrate diffuse or enmeshed boundaries between family members. Their roles overlap and are blurry, and lines of separation are indistinct; who is responsible for whom is not clear. In the middle of the continuum lie clear boundaries, signifying healthy rules of engagement. Family roles are clear, and methods of interaction are healthy.

As a practitioner, you might consider using the continuum in Figure 8.1 with families, including adult couples and parent–child dyads. Ask each member of the family or couple to assess the type of boundaries present in their family and how they communicate with one another or each other. Ask them to define clear, healthy boundaries and how each may practice new behaviors (or do so consistently) within the relationship in the next week. Give each family member an opportunity to speak with the other family member listening quietly.

Subsystems and Hierarchies

Subsystems and *hierarchies* also contribute to the organization of the family system. There are several subsystems within the family, three of which are depicted in the pyramid in Figure 8.2. The original subsystem at the top of the pyramid is the spousal one. Within this subsystem, certain privileges, communication patterns, and behaviors are appropriate (e.g., financial decisions, career decisions, sexual relations). When children are brought into this subsystem through adoption, birth, or marriage (e.g., stepchildren), a new subsystem is created—the parental subsystem, which falls below the

  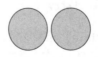

Rigid Boundaries   Clear and Healthy Boundaries   Diffuse Boundaries

FIGURE 8.1. Rigid, diffuse, and clear/healthy boundaries.

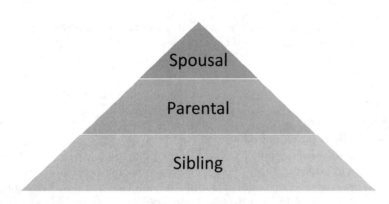

FIGURE 8.2. Hierarchy of family subsystems.

spousal subsystem in the pyramid. Within this subsystem, decisions about how to raise the children are made. This power rests with the parents; thus, a hierarchy appears in which parents have more power than the children. When one of the parents is struggling with addiction, the other parent typically assumes most of the parental power. The addicted spouse gives up or turns over power as a parent. This shift in role obligations places a heavy burden on the nondependent spouse and usually creates feelings of resentment. Sometimes a grandparent or older sibling may assume some parental power (e.g., by cooking meals, shopping, doing laundry), thereby shifting subsystems and blurring boundaries.

A sibling subsystem also evolves. This is the bottom rung in Figure 8.2. According to Lawson and Lawson (1998), the complexity of this third subsystem (and the entire family hierarchy) depends on the number of children, their age differences, their gender, their common interests, and their familial relationship to one another (e.g., step-, half-, or adoptive sibling). Kendler and colleagues (2012) studied over 18,000 adopted children born between 1950 and 1993 and over 51,000 adoptive parents and siblings. They found that the risk for drug abuse in adopted children was more strongly predicted by drug abuse in the adoptive *siblings* than in the adoptive parents. They concluded that "social influences (e.g., peer deviance and drug availability) shared with adoptive siblings are more potent environmental risks for [drug abuse] than direct psychological transmission of [drug abuse] from parent to child" (p. 695).

Sibling subsystems may distinguish sons from daughters, the oldest from the youngest, or the athletic from the nonathletic. In functional families, these subsystems remain somewhat fluid and dynamic as time passes and the children mature. In dysfunctional families, the subsystems may remain static as the children are required to assume inappropriate roles, such as that of a parent. Forcing a child into the spousal subsystem (e.g., incest) is another example in which subsystems are likely to remain static (Lawson & Lawson, 1998).

Family Rules

Another characteristic of family organization pertains to the rules that govern interactions between and among members. Several of these rules were mentioned in the previous section. Often these rules are implicit rather than explicit; however, most or all members somehow seem to know them. They define appropriate conduct within the family system and function to provide order, stability, consistency, and predictability in family affairs. They also serve to restrict behavioral options (e.g., "incest is unacceptable"). Families usually have rules governing the manner in which different emotions are expressed. Anger is not allowed in some families, whereas in others, shouting is permissible. In some families, affection is demonstrated with hugs and kisses, whereas in others, physical contact is minimized.

In families where active addiction is present, certain family rules are typical. For example, it usually is prohibited to talk openly about a family member's substance use, to reveal family secrets and break confidences and loyalties. Two rules often found in families where problematic alcohol use is present are that (1) anger can only be expressed when the alcoholic is drinking and (2) affection and intimacy can only be expressed when one or both partners has been drinking (Lawson & Lawson, 1998).

Behavioral Models

Behavioral models of family substance abuse treatment are primarily based on the principles of operant conditioning discussed in Chapter 6. These include the principles of positive and negative reinforcement, as well as punishment. As mentioned earlier, these are principles of learned *behavior*, not simply principles of learning, and consistent with operant conditioning, they describe volitional or proactive behavior. This means that the behaviors of family members serve a purpose, whether or not they are aware of it; there is a payoff to the family system, not just to an individual. The payoff to the family unit may be homeostasis or balance, keeping all the parts of the family "machinery" intact and working in sync. This payoff may be preferred to any type of family disruption, such as divorce, separation, or other forms of estrangement (e.g., shunning, disowning). As discussed earlier in this chapter, for families in which addiction is present, disruption also may include the initiation of abstinence and the beginning of recovery for one of its members because the system had accustomed itself to that family member's substance abuse over a considerable period of time. In this instance, sobriety would not reinforce family cohesion.

The focus of behavioral models is the *observed behaviors* of family members, including nonverbal and verbal forms of communication. Although social learning or social-cognitive models (e.g., expectancies, self-efficacy) and other cognitive models (e.g., rational-emotive) apply, it is the effect of these belief systems on family behaviors that is of interest. It is the influence of family rules on family roles, for example, or the effect of shared values on family traditions, that is the focus. Think of observed, concrete, and measurable behaviors as the visible "evidence" of rules, values, and other beliefs and cognitive processes. The behaviors are the verification of beliefs. Behavioral models thus give primacy to what is seen and heard, not simply to what is implied. Take, for instance, the words *resistant* and *manipulative,* words often used to describe interpersonal behaviors. From a behavioral perspective, these are not behaviors because they do not describe specific observable, measurable, or verifiable activities; instead, they describe the intent of another person (e.g., to influence or control another person) and an intent assumed by someone else that may lack empirical support. In these two examples, the demonstrable behaviors might be disagreement ("No, I'm not going to do that"), failure to complete a particular task, or repetition of a specific behavior (e.g., drinking in the garage) because it has been negatively reinforced (e.g., "calms me down and gives me peace and quiet after another stupid argument in the house with my girlfriend").

The focus on observed and measurable behaviors explains the empirical or scientific strength of behavioral models. Compared to the family disease and the family systems models, behavioral models are the most robust, informed by a strong research base. Of the attributes of a good theory described in Chapter 1, it is the attribute of empirical support that makes behavioral models a good theory.

Behavioral models are the most recent of the three models. Only in the past 15–20 years have they received increased attention since their introduction in the early 1970s. Dattilio (2001, 2010) provides three explanations for their slow start. First, the behavioral approach has been perceived by some practitioners as being too rigid and rigorous in its implementation to capture the nuances of family interaction. The focus on observable behaviors more so than feelings, for example, might be considered stringent and limiting by some. Highly specified intervention plans, such as those involving parents monitoring the daily activities of their adolescent and then following a strict system of reward and punishment, might also be considered too "sterile" or "laboratory-like" for many practitioners. Second, the popularity of family systems approaches (e.g., strategic, structural) has overshadowed the more empirically tested behavioral approaches. Research data can be less compelling than the charismatic style of family systems therapists such as Murray Bowen. Third, the traditional view that behavioral approaches are linear in perspective is thought to be contrary to systemic constructs, such as circular causality. This is one myth that Dattilio (2001) dispels. He acknowledges, however, that the strength of behavioral approaches is their ability to address specific behavior problems rather than to explain the comprehensive system of family dynamics. Behavior problems targeted include inadequate stress reduction skills, poor communication, and emotional dysregulation. Some of the first behavioral interventions applied to families were for the problem behaviors of bedtime tantrums and bedwetting among young children (Falloon, 2003).

Reinforcing and Protective Family Behaviors

When behavioral models are applied to the family system, a system affected by addiction, the behaviors of family members are the antecedents to substance use, and they also reinforce its consequences (McCrady et al., 2012). The consequences can be either negatively or positively reinforcing, meaning that the behaviors of family members can either increase or decrease the likelihood of a family member's future substance use. For example, the behavior of a non-substance-abusing partner (often referred to as the *concerned significant other* or *CSO*) can inadvertently reinforce ongoing substance use in his or her partner (Fals-Stewart, Lam, & Kelley, 2009). These behaviors include avoiding conflict with the relative when he or she is intoxicated or assuming the role of caretaker during or after drinking or drug use episodes.

For the remainder of this section, we use the terms *CSO* and other *affected family members* (AFMs) to refer to family members who are *not* struggling with substance use or other types of addictive behaviors. We use the term *relative* to refer to the family member who *is* struggling with addiction. For us, these are nonpejorative terms. They also are consistent with family member designations used by behavioral practitioners and researchers, including Orford and colleagues (Orford, Copello, et al., 2010; Orford, Velleman, et al., 2010), proponents of the stress–strain–coping–support model.

Reinforcing behaviors, however, are not limited to the CSO and other AFMs. The reverse is also true. The relative's behaviors can reinforce the behaviors of AFMs. As McCrady and colleagues (2012) note, behavioral models conceptualize couple and family relationships in terms of the *balance* and *exchange* of reinforcers in the relationships. Reinforcing behaviors are thus *reciprocal* in family relationships, consistent with family systems principles. The relative's behavior may reinforce caretaking behaviors in the CSO, for example. An adult child's substance misuse also may reinforce continued caretaking behavior in parents, such as paying off their child's jail and court fines and assuming responsibility for raising their grandchildren. Templeton (2012) conducted a qualitative study of 21 grandparents raising their grandchildren because of parental substance abuse. She reported that several grandparents believed their increased involvement in their grandchildren's care had actually worsened the substance abuse of their adult child, the parent of their grandchildren. This is another example of reciprocal and positive reinforcing behaviors in families.

The reciprocity of reinforcing behaviors in a family unit may explain several of the findings in the study conducted by Hussaarts and colleagues (2011) of 32 family dyads. Each pair comprised a patient in substance abuse treatment (i.e., relative) and an AFM, a first-degree relative, spouse or intimate partner, or someone living with the relative who was described as the CSO. One major finding of this study was that CSOs reported distress and dissatisfaction with their quality of life, and, compared to their relative, they were discontented with their intimate relationship. The second major finding was that relatives reported satisfaction with two areas of their spousal relationship—engaging in joint, pleasant activities and affection—and these were positively correlated with their years of substance use. This latter finding goes against extensive anecdotal and empirical evidence that continued substance abuse and its increasing severity are associated with increased problems in many life areas. Certain reinforcing behaviors of family members therefore can shield the relative from adverse consequences of the substance abuse and, as a result, make it possible for him or her to enjoy and be satisfied with life. This is one example of family system homeostasis at the expense of AFMs.

Specific family behaviors can serve to protect against problematic substance use. For example, maintaining family rituals, such as eating together at set times and attending religious activities together, is associated with reduced substance use (Fife, McCreary, Brewer, & Adegoke, 2011). This is true across cultural groups, including Asian American families with early-adolescent girls (Fang, Barnes-Ceeney, & Schinke, 2011) and rural African American adolescents (Nasim, Fernander, Townsend, Corona, & Belgrave, 2011). A recent study (Caetano, Vaeth, & Canino, 2017) found that a felt sense of family pride and cohesion (e.g., shared values) protects Puerto Rican family members against alcohol use disorders.

Other family practices that serve as protective factors include parental monitoring of child and adolescent behaviors. Some have suggested, however, that parental monitoring may not be the best indicator of caregiving quality for culturally diverse families. For disadvantaged Hispanic/Latino immigrant parents, for example, Bacio, Mays, and Lau (2013) explain that their "often-taxing work demands . . . may interfere with their ability to be present in their homes to closely supervise the activities of their offspring" (p. 19). However, the perception among both European American and Mexican American adolescents of strong parental control (i.e., their parents set rules and monitor their behavior) has been identified as a key protective factor in reducing the probability of alcohol and other drug use problems (Kopak, Chen, Haas, & Gillmore, 2012).

Functional Analysis and Family Coping Responses

Dattilio (2010) maintains that family systems models have focused almost exclusively on intrafamilial dynamics, viewing extrafamilial influences (e.g., stressors outside the family unit) as almost irrelevant. This focus also may characterize family disease models. Behavioral models, by comparison, offer a more contextualized approach to family functioning, examining dynamics occurring beyond or outside the boundaries of the family system (e.g., school behavior, natural disasters, neighborhood crime). The family system, therefore, is regarded as an open system rather than a closed system in the behavioral models.

Identifying all influential intrafamilial and extrafamilial dynamics for a particular family unit is the primary task of behavioral family therapists. This is known as conducting a *functional analysis* or a *behavioral analysis*. Its goal is to determine all of the systems operating on each spouse or family member that contribute to presenting problems (Dattilio, 2010). This approach includes determining the probability or the likelihood of behavioral patterns under certain conditions, and it begins with the basic question "What happens when . . . ?" (Drossel, Rummel, & Fisher, 2009, p. 16). In the case of substance abuse, the goal is to understand how all systems affecting family behaviors contribute to and maintain the addictive behavior of a family member.

Take, for example, the case of a single working mother raising three children. What is the effect of this mother's intermittent employment and three part-time jobs on her 15-year-old son's truant behavior and recent drug-trafficking charges? What happens when she is not home and is not able to share in mealtimes with him and his two younger siblings? What happens when school officials or the probation department contact the mother? Furthermore, how does their subsidized housing environment, repeated school levy failures, lack of funding for a community sports league, and recent factory closings in the area function to reinforce her teenage son's problematic behavior? What function does his behavior serve for his two younger siblings and their maternal grandmother? How is the family system responding to these intra- and extrafamilial dynamics and for what purpose? What is the probability of family behavior patterns continuing or being altered now that school officials and a probation officer are involved in the family system? The purpose of these and other questions asked during a functional analysis is to target potential interventions for the family (Falloon, 2003).

The first step in a functional analysis is to identify "patterns within the reciprocal relationship of behavior and context" (Drossel et al., 2009, p. 16). For a family unit, *context* broadly refers to the family's history and current circumstances, including cultural conditions and the involvement of people external to the family unit (e.g., employer, drug and alcohol counselor, school counselor). According to Falloon (2003), patterns of family behavior observed at any point in time represent the optimal response or the best attempt of each family member to resolve an existing problem. He writes: "Even when chaotic, distressing responses are observed, every family member is attempting to resolve the problem (or achieve the goal) in the manner he or she considers most rewarding (or least distressing), given all the constraints imposed by the biopsychosocial system at that time" (p. 157).

In a family system where addiction is present, these responses or behaviors are referred to as *coping responses*. From their interviews with 29 persons with one or more relatives with an addiction, Moriarty, Stubbe, Bradford, Tapper, and Lim (2011) identified four AFM coping strategies:

1. Minimizing or normalizing the addiction, viewing heavy drinking as acceptable.
2. Making allowances by continuing with their daily tasks.
3. Turning away from the relative by emotional distancing or physical relocation.
4. Carrying on with their own lives as if prior experiences had been forgotten and attempting to demonstrate their resilience or ability to overcome the negative influences of their family member's addiction.

Orford, Velleman, and colleagues (2010) and McCrady (2006) identified three general coping responses to addiction that family members assume, regardless of their age, sex, and other cultural variables (e.g., race, ethnicity):

1. "Putting up with it" is *tolerant coping* that accepts the substance use.
2. "Standing up to it" is *engaged coping* that attempts to change the behavior of the relative.
3. "Withdrawing from it" is *withdrawal coping* wherein the AFM withdraws from the relative and spends considerable time in separate activities and with other people.

Think of each of these general coping responses as an AFM's best effort at any given time to resolve the problem of addiction in the family. Orford, Velleman, and colleagues further noted specific behaviors AFMs can take that correspond to one or more of the three general coping responses, such as sacrificing and compromising (related to tolerant coping) and refusing, resisting, and being assertive (associated with engaged coping). Orford, Velleman, and colleagues' names for the three general coping responses and specific coping behaviors are depicted in Figure 8.3 on the next page.

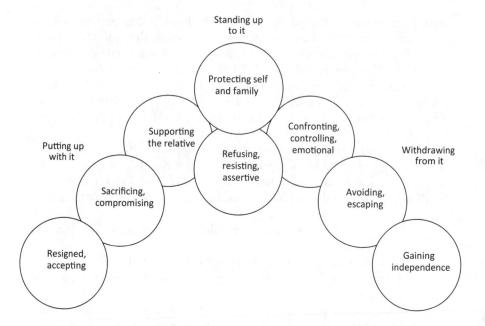

FIGURE 8.3. Three general and eight specific coping responses of a family member toward a relative's substance use. From Orford, Velleman, Capello, Templeton, and Ibaya (2010). Reprinted by permission of Taylor & Francis Ltd.

The case of the O'Connor family is presented in Box 8.2. It is a fictional case that illustrates several reciprocal, reinforcing, and coping behaviors. We invite you to read through the case and conduct your own functional analysis, noting such factors as extrafamilial and intrafamilial dynamics and the function or purpose of the behaviors of the four family members. Identify any of the three general coping behaviors used by family members. We offer our own functional analysis at the end of the chapter.

FAMILY-BASED APPROACHES TO ADDICTION TREATMENT

Involving family members in the prevention and treatment efforts of an adolescent or adult who is struggling with problematic substance use is now standard practice in the addictions field (O'Farrell & Fals-Stewart, 2008). In their meta-analysis of 15 studies investigating the effects of drug abuse treatment programs for adults and adolescents, Stanton and Shadish (1997) found that family-based approaches demonstrated more favorable results (i.e., reduced drug use) when compared to individual counseling or

BOX 8.2. CASE EXAMPLE: THE O'CONNOR FAMILY

Early in their 35-year marriage, Marge believed that Hank's regular and often heavy drinking was in response to her emotional instability and "clingy-ness." She never complained about his drinking and did what she could to keep the house in order. Once their children were in school and Marge learned that Hank's job at the university would allow her to go to school for free, she enrolled in a bachelor's degree program. Going to classes helped Marge gain new independence, and once she earned her degree, she got a full-time job for the first time. She now leaves the house every weekday at 7:30 A.M. and doesn't return until 6:00 P.M. Hank wasn't thrilled at first with Marge working full-time because she was no longer thorough in housecleaning or meal preparation, but he did like the extra income. Now that he's retired from the university, he thinks Marge should retire, too, because he doesn't like being home most of the time by himself. Although he is bored, he's relieved to no longer have anyone telling him what to do during the day.

Pam, their oldest daughter, stops by most days with her young son, Todd, and fixes Hank lunch and does some light cleaning. Hank enjoys playing with Todd and doesn't drink as much on the days that Pam and Todd stop by. Pam knows that her dad still drinks (she can sometimes smell it on his breath when she and Todd arrive in the late mornings or early afternoons), but she hasn't said anything to him or to her mother. It's a relief to Hank that no one has said anything to him about his drinking, something he believes he "deserves" to do now in retirement anytime he wants. Pam wants Todd to have contact with his grandfather (his paternal grandfather is deceased) and she wants her dad to spend time with Todd, the "only son" she says her dad will "ever have." Marge loves her job (she's been working full-time for 10 years now) and has established a strong support system among her coworkers. Since Hank's retirement, she has been spending more time away from home on weekends with friends. She is grateful that Pam helps out at home during the week and that Pam provides her dad with company so that Hank isn't as "grumpy" and "critical" when she returns home during the week.

---

therapy, peer group therapy, or family psychoeducation. In a recent study (Bartle-Haring et al., 2018), children (8–16 years of age) who participated in a 12-session family therapy condition with their substance-using mothers reported less alcohol and tobacco use over 18 months than children who did not attend an education-only intervention condition with their mothers.

Most family-based approaches reflect a combination of two or all three of the family models described in the previous sections of this chapter. There are commonalities across the family models with respect to family member roles and rules, as well as their terminology. Similar interventions are also used, such as training in coping, communication, and parenting skills, and spending time together in non-substance-abusing activities.

The majority of family-based approaches have addressed either solely or primarily problematic alcohol use within a family unit. However, a considerable number of approaches targeting drug abuse (beyond and including alcohol) have been developed over the past 30 years. These are reviewed by Rowe (2012). Whether alcohol or other drug use is the problematic behavior in a family system, the fourfold purpose of family-based interventions is generally to (1) engage the partner or other family members in a plan for systemic change, (2) clarify and reinforce family roles and responsibilities (e.g., parental discipline), (3) achieve and maintain abstinence, and (4) improve relational dynamics and satisfaction.

Not all persons are amenable to, or will benefit from, family-based approaches. In a study of 158 women with an alcohol use disorder (Hunter-Reel, McCrady, Hildebrandt, & Epstein, 2010), individual cognitive-behavioral therapy (CBT) rather than couple CBT was associated with greater motivation to change drinking at 3 months posttreatment. More women also chose the individual format at treatment entry. McCrady (2006) explains, however, that successful family-involved treatment is more likely when (1) the family has at least some members who do not have alcohol or drug problems themselves, (2) the individual client is experiencing more severe alcohol or drug problems, (3) there is a certain level of stability in social functioning (e.g., employment) and relational commitment (e.g., no threats of divorce or abandonment), and (4) counseling has been initiated following a crisis (e.g., arrest for drug-related offense), especially when the stability of the family unit has been threatened. For indigenous populations (e.g., Native American/Alaska Native), it is recommended that treatment not automatically exclude family members who are themselves problem drinkers (Calabria, Clifford, Shakeshaft, & Doran, 2012). In a predominantly white sample, Schumm, O'Farrell, and Andreas (2012) found that abstinence rates of "dual-problem couples" (i.e., couples in which both partners have a substance use problem) improved after completing 5–6 months of weekly couples counseling. Couple or family counseling clearly is *not* appropriate when there has been domestic violence that has resulted in injury or the need for medical assistance.

In the following sections, we review six evidence-based practices for working with couples and families in which problematic alcohol or drug use is present. The first two approaches are reviewed more extensively and separately; the remaining four are reviewed as a group because they all address adolescent substance abuse and related behavioral problems. Of the first two, one is a comprehensive approach designed for families in which there is an adult or adolescent with a substance use problem; the other is for adult couples only. All six approaches—to varying degrees—have considerable research support and are informed by one or more of the three family treatment models of addiction presented in this chapter.

Community Reinforcement and Family Training

Community reinforcement and family training (CRAFT; Smith & Meyers, 2004) is an evidence-based practice for family members (first-degree relative or intimate partner) or friends of individuals with substance use problems who refuse to get help from peers (e.g., AA) or from professionals. It is an adaptation and an extension of the community reinforcement approach (CRA) described in Chapter 6. CRAFT was developed from research on the CRA that identified family members, or concerned significant others (CSOs), as influential reinforcers of their family member's behavior (Meyers, Villanueva, & Smith, 2005; Miller, Meyers, & Tonigan, 1999). It thus was proposed that prevention and treatment methods target CSOs rather than intervene directly with the family member with the substance use problem. This is a form of unilateral family therapy because it is designed to work with family members *other than* the relative with the identified problem, such as substance abuse (Smith, Meyers, & Austin, 2008).

Roozen, de Waart, and van der Kroft (2010) describe CRAFT as "a rigorous treatment package" (p. 1730). CRAFT practitioners work directly with CSOs in individual sessions, teaching them behavioral skills to alter their interactions with their loved one, designated in CRAFT as the identified patient (IP). CSOs also are taught self-care practices. Specifically, CRAFT teaches CSOs how to (1) influence the IP to get help, preferably by entering a drug and alcohol treatment program, (2) help the IP reduce his or her substance use, and (3) procure and maintain psychological well-being for themselves, whether or not the IP reduces or abstains from substance use or enters treatment. The eight major components of CRAFT (Smith & Meyers, 2004) are teaching motivational strategies, conducting a functional analysis (i.e., learning the purpose of the IP's substance use behaviors from the perspective of the CSO), addressing potential for violence in the CSO–IP relationship, providing communication training, providing reinforcement training (e.g., reinforcing *non*-substance-using behavior, removing a reinforcer for substance use behavior, allowing natural consequences of substance-using behavior to occur), engaging in self-reinforcement training (i.e., self-care practices), and preparing the CSO to encourage his or her loved one to enter treatment.

CRAFT follows operant conditioning principles, and, although CRAFT practitioners do not meet jointly with the CSO and the IP, they endorse family systems principles, such as reciprocal causality. Unlike family disease models, however, CRAFT does not regard CSOs as helpless or powerless to effect change in the IP or in the family system. Rather than recommending that CSOs distance or withdraw themselves from the IP (what is often recommended in Al-Anon), CRAFT is designed to *empower* CSOs to become actively involved in the process of helping the IP initiate change by entering treatment. The primary outcome measured in CRAFT studies is treatment entry by the family member. A review of CRAFT studies conducted over 25 years indicates that 55–86% of treatment-refusing family members enter treatment as a result of their CSO participating in CRAFT (Manuel et al., 2012). The first CRAFT study conducted outside the United States reported a 50% IP treatment entry rate at 12 months after CSOs had completed 12 one-hour weekly CRAFT sessions (Bischof, Iwen, Freyer-Adam, & Rumpf, 2016).

Teaching CSOs to encourage their relative to enter treatment does not mean the CSO uses confrontational skills consistent with the Johnson model of intervention (Johnson Institute, 1987) and depicted on the reality television show *Intervention*. From their review of the first six seasons of this popular television show, Kosovski and Smith (2011, p. 853) concluded that *Intervention* conveys "contradictory and misleading messages" about addiction and family functioning and "grossly exaggerates and misrepresents both treatment approaches and outcomes." They proposed (p. 857) the "exaggerated narratives" featured on the show "have the potential to do harm" by (1) fostering a false sense of optimism about the success of family-based interventions and the availability of desired treatments, (2) creating backlash from viewers and reduced public support for treatment and research because of the overly narrow definition of addiction portrayed, and (3) influencing viewers with addictions to not get treatment because their experiences of addiction may not be consistent with the experiences of addiction among family members on the show. Unlike the confrontational methods shown on *Intervention*, CRAFT uses a motivational style (Smith et al., 2008) and teaches CSOs to engage in positive communication skills with their relative, such as avoiding blaming and name calling, and stating what is wanted rather than what is not wanted. These skills are practiced routinely in CRAFT sessions through role plays. The seven CRAFT guidelines for positive communication are listed in Table 8.1.

From their review of four trials of CRAFT, Roozen and colleagues (2010) found that CRAFT was three times more effective than Al-Anon and 2 times more effective than the Johnson model of intervention in getting the IP to enter treatment (i.e., completing at least one treatment session after assessment). Kirby and colleagues (2017) reported similar findings: IPs of CSOs who participated in CRAFT were three times more likely to enter treatment than IPs whose CSOs participated in Al-Anon or Narcotics Anonymous only. In Roozen and colleagues' study, CSOs also demonstrated improvement (e.g., lower levels of depression and anger, higher levels of relationship happiness), but this was equally true for CRAFT and Al-Anon; there was limited evidence for CSO improvement in the Johnson model.

In one of the early studies of CRAFT (Miller et al., 1999), CSO self-improvement occurred whether or not their relatives entered treatment.

TABLE 8.1. CRAFT Guidelines for Positive Communication Skills

1. Be brief. Avoid lengthy communications with your loved one because they are a "turn-off" and often include irrelevant and emotionally charged information that diverts attention away from the main point.

2. Be positive. Avoid blaming, name calling, and overgeneralizations. Use language that indicates what is wanted rather than what is not wanted (e.g., behavior that needs to stop).

3. Refer to specific behaviors. Do not make vague requests. Rather, describe specific and observable behaviors (not thoughts or feelings) that are desired.

4. Label your feelings. Describe your own feelings in a calm, nonjudgmental, and nonaccusatory manner.

5. Offer an understanding statement. Verbalize understanding and empathy, even though it may be very difficult to do so.

6. Accept partial responsibility (for the *non*-substance-using behavior being addressed). Identify a small piece of the problem situation for which you can accept some responsibility. This reinforces your role in the relationship and conveys your willingness to consider change of your own. (It is very important to note that although CSOs are instrumental in creating positive changes with and for their loved one, they are *not* held accountable for their loved one's substance use or other negative behaviors.)

7. Offer to help. Ask generally, "How can I help?" in a manner that is genuine and supportive.

Note. From Smith and Meyers (2004). Copyright 2004 by The Guilford Press. Adapted by permission.

This was also reported in a study of parent CSOs who attended an average of 10 CRAFT sessions to encourage their adolescent to enter treatment (71% of whom *did* enter treatment; Waldron, Kern-Jones, Turner, Peterson, & Ozechowski, 2007). Although CSOs did not report self-improvement in Manuel and colleagues' (2012) study of CRAFT, they did report significantly improved family functioning at both 3- and 6-month follow-up. In this same study, CRAFT was delivered in a group format (12 weekly sessions with four CSOs per group) and a self-directed format (CSOs received a self-help book only). IP treatment entry rates (within a 6-month window) were 40% for the self-directed format and 60% for the group format, the latter format demonstrating comparable rates to those of individually delivered CRAFT in previous studies. Furthermore, 71% of CSOs who attended only one group session were able to encourage their loved one to enter treatment. Manuel and colleagues' findings suggest that effective CRAFT delivery can be flexible and cost-effective.

Behavioral Couples Therapy

Behavioral couples therapy (BCT; O'Farrell & Fals-Stewart, 2006) is another evidence-based practice designed to help two persons in an intimate and committed relationship (i.e., married or cohabitating) address substance use problems in their relationship. More often than not, BCT is applied when only one person in the relationship is struggling with substance use. Only recently has it been used when both persons misuse substances (Schumm et al., 2012). Unless otherwise noted, we limit our review of BCT in this section to its application when only one member of the couple is misusing substances. We retain Orford and colleagues' (Orford, Copello, et al., 2010; Orford, Velleman, et al., 2010) reference to the person struggling with substance use as the *relative*; the affected family member (AFM) is their *partner*.

BCT seeks to strengthen relationship stability and support abstinence from drinking and drug use. The strategy is based on two assumptions: (1) the partner can reward the relative's abstinence and (2) the likelihood of substance use and relapse are reduced when relational distress is low. The three primary objectives of BCT are to (1) eliminate problematic drinking and drug use, (2) engage the partner's support for their relative's efforts to change, and (3) change couple and family interaction patterns in ways that are conducive to long-term, stable abstinence and a happier and more stable relationship. BCT consists of a minimum of 12 and up to 26 weekly (or twice weekly) couples sessions. In most cases, the relative (as primary client) is also involved in a 12-step program and possibly individual therapy.

The BCT clinician's first aim is to engage the partner in the process of helping his or her relative. This is done after the therapist obtains the relative's permission to contact the partner, so that the partner can be invited to a conjoint interview. In the initial conjoint session, the couple is asked to make a commitment to therapy and to not threaten separation while in BCT (Ruff, McComb, Coker, & Sprenkle, 2010).

Once the relative and his or her partner have committed to BCT, daily sobriety contracts are presented and reviewed by the clinician with the couple. The contracts require the couple to commit to maintain daily sobriety, participate in a 12-step program, and hold trust discussions that facilitate the relative's expression of commitment to abstinence and the partner's offer of emotional support. In addition, BCT clinicians teach effective listening skills and conflict resolution strategies and provide guidance on how to solve problems together. Homework exercises also are assigned. The most common assignment encourages partners to initiate affectionate interactions with their relative. BCT often relies on disulfiram (Antabuse) medication to bolster the relative's daily sobriety. The act of swallowing a disulfiram tablet in the presence of one's partner may be a component of the daily sobriety contract. (Note: Disulfiram produces unpleasant physical effects if taken with alcohol.)

In the continuing recovery stage, the clinician helps the couple create a posttreatment plan that identifies how partners will promote sobriety after their BCT sessions end. The plan is intended to help couples anticipate challenges to maintaining sobriety and avoiding relapse. The plan also provides guidance about actions to take if a relapse occurs. Post-treatment follow-up visits with couples can be scheduled for up to 5 years (Ruff et al., 2010).

Compared to individual- and other couple-based treatments, BCT has produced better outcomes in partner relationships observed at 1- and 2-year follow-up assessments (Kelley & Fals-Stewart, 2008; O'Farrell, Choquette, & Cutter, 1998; Schumm, O'Farrell, Kahler, Murphy, & Muchowski, 2014). When these gains have not been demonstrated at posttreatment, relapse prevention (RP) sessions have been added to BCT. A comparison of the efficacy of BCT-only versus BCT-plus-RP found that the latter intervention produced improvements in marital relations for 2 years following treatment (O'Farrell, Choquette, Cutter, Brown, & McCourt, 1993). The BCT-only intervention improvements had disappeared at the 2-year follow-up. A recent study (O'Farrell, Schumm, Murphy, & Muchowski, 2017) found that BCT combined with the relative's involvement in 12-step-focused individual-based therapy (referred to as BCT + IBT) was superior to BCT-only at 1-year follow-up on three outcomes: reducing substance-related problems, improving relationship satisfaction, and preventing relationship break-up.

In addition to improving relationship satisfaction, BCT has been shown to be effective in reducing drinking problems (Fals-Stewart, Birchler, & Kelley, 2006; Fals-Stewart, Klosterman, Yates, O'Farrell, & Birchler, 2005; Schumm et al., 2014) and other drug use (Fals-Stewart et al., 2000; Fals-Stewart, O'Farrell, & Birchler, 2001; Kelley & Fals-Stewart, 2007), including opiate use (O'Farrell et al., 2017). Furthermore, BCT appears to be more effective in reducing alcohol and drug use compared to other individual and couples treatment programs (Fals-Stewart et al., 2005, 2006; Powers, Vedel, & Emmelkamp, 2008; Schumm et al., 2014). Improvements in alcohol and drug use following completion of BCT, however, have not always been sustained over time (O'Farrell et al., 1998; Winters, Fals-Stewart, O'Farrell, Birchler, & Kelley, 2002). Although BCT-plus-RP may improve alcohol use outcomes (O'Farrell et al., 1998), it seems the positive effects of the added RP sessions start to wane at 2-year follow-up.

The effectiveness of BCT in reducing intimate partner violence (IPV) is more equivocal. O'Farrell and Murphy (1995) found that during the 12 months following BCT, there was a reduction in IPV in couples where alcoholism was present. However, violence remained higher compared to a demographically matched national sample of nonalcoholic married couples. Further inspection determined that the prevalence and frequency of violence following BCT was associated with alcohol use. A subgroup of male alcoholics who had relapsed after BCT accounted for much of the violence. In couples with drug abuse, one study (Fals-Stewart, Kashdan, O'Farrell, & Birchler, 2002) found that BCT reduced IPV at a 12-month follow-up. Compared to those in individual-based treatment, BCT couples reported a significant reduction in male-to-female physical aggression (43% vs. 18%). A subsequent study (Fals-Stewart et al., 2006) showed that BCT reduced IPV in couples with a female relative who misused alcohol and a male partner who did not misuse substances 1 year after treatment ends. A reduction in IPV 1 year following BCT also was found in a more recent study (Schumm et al., 2014), but this reduction was no different than if the relative had participated in individual therapy only.

In the research community, BCT is considered one of the most effective treatments for alcohol and drug addiction (Carroll & Onken, 2005; Morgenstern & McKay, 2007; Rowe, 2012). It also appears to be the treatment of choice for improving relationship functioning in couples with substance abuse (O'Farrell & Clements, 2012).

Family-Based Approaches for Adolescent Substance Abuse

The four family-based approaches briefly discussed in this section have the largest research base of any family-based therapy for adolescent substance abuse (Baldwin, Christian, Berkeljon, & Shadish, 2012). They are brief strategic family therapy, functional family therapy, multidimensional family therapy, and multisystemic therapy. From their meta-analysis of 24 studies investigating the effects of one of these four approaches on measures of substance abuse and delinquency, Baldwin and colleagues (2012) reported significant ($p \leq .05$) combined effect sizes of 0.21 when compared to treatment as usual, and 0.26 when compared to an alternative treatment (e.g., individual therapy, parent groups). When any one of these four approaches was compared to a control group, the combined or average effect size was sizable (0.70) but not significant. Based on the results of this meta-analysis, Bean (cited in Baldwin et al., 2012, p. 301) argues that "there is no clear evidence to favor one program over another, so there is no wrong choice if an educational program or agency was to select a model for implementation." We interpret these comments as an endorsement of all four approaches.

Brief Strategic Family Therapy

As its name suggests, brief strategic family therapy (BSFT) is a brief intervention (delivered in 8–24 sessions) developed from two family systems approaches: structural therapy and strategic therapy (Szapocznik, Hervis, & Schwartz, 2003; Szapocznik, Muir, Duff, Schwartz, & Brown, 2015). It is intended to treat child and adolescent problem behaviors (including drug and alcohol use) in the context of the family system (Briones, Robbins, & Szapocznik, 2008). It originated from research and practice at the University of Miami Center for Family Studies and has been found to be particularly appropriate for, and effective with, cultural groups that emphasize family and interpersonal relationships, such as Hispanics/Latinos (Santisteban et al., 2003). BSFT research represented some of the first systematic efforts to establish an empirical basis of support for adolescent substance abuse treatment (Waldron & Turner, 2008).

The focus of BSFT is on inappropriate family alliances (e.g., a parent–child coalition that challenges another parent, parents "triangulating" a child), excessively rigid or permeable boundaries between family members, and the identification of individual family members (often the adolescent) as the source of familial dysfunction. What is referred to in BFST as the *principle of complementarity* assumes that for every action by a family member, there is a corresponding reaction from the rest of the family (Szapocznik et al., 2003). This means that a substance-using adolescent will improve his or her behavior when the family learns how to behave adaptively. BSFT sessions are often conducted with as many family members as possible, and sessions are held weekly for 1 hour. Although initially delivered only in an office or clinic setting, BSFT has expanded its delivery settings to the home and school.

Strategies used are categorized as joining, tracking and diagnostic enactment, and restructuring (Szapocznik, Hervis, & Schwartz, 2003, 2015). *Joining* involves the BSFT practitioner assuming a position of leadership in the family while supporting the existing family power structure. It is as if the BSFT practitioner has been accepted as a "special temporary member" (p. 26) of the family. Joining is critical to family engagement in treatment. *Tracking and diagnostic enactment* strategies identify and track repeated maladaptive interactional patterns, as well as family strengths. Family problems are diagnosed in such areas as power distribution, boundaries, and conflict resolution. Enactment involves family members speaking to one another in session as they would if the counselor was not present. These observations make it possible for the counselor to diagnose problematic relations as well as strengths. *Restructuring* involves change-producing strategies intended to help family members develop new and more adaptive relational patterns. These include cognitive reframing, role reversals (e.g., coaching a family member to do or say the opposite of what he or she would customarily do or say), and boundary shifting (e.g., rearranging seating in therapy sessions to either loosen or strengthen certain alliances between family members). Consistent with its brief and strategic philosophy, only interventions determined to be practical, problem-focused, and deliberate are delivered in BSFT.

Compared to a group treatment, BSFT was found to significantly reduce marijuana use among Hispanic youth (Santisteban et al., 2003). This finding was criticized, however, because the differences were small and not clinically meaningful (Austin, Macgowan, & Wagner, 2005). Drug use reductions were not found in a more recent multisite trial (Robbins et al., 2011) of multiracial/ethnic adolescents who received either BSFT or treatment as usual (TAU). The one significant difference in this study was that TAU adolescents were 2.5 times more likely to fail to engage in treatment and 1.41 times more likely to fail to remain in treatment compared to adolescents who received BSFT.

Functional Family Therapy

Functional family therapy (FFT) is described as "an integrative ecological model that combines a family systems view of family functioning with behavioral techniques and a multi-systemic emphasis" (Waldron & Turner, 2008, p. 240). It was developed more than 35 years ago by Alexander and Parsons (1982) for youth with disruptive externalizing behaviors ("acting-out," e.g., aggression, oppositional and conduct disorders) involved in the juvenile justice system. It is only in the past 15–20 years, however, that FFT has been recognized as an evidence-based intervention program (Hartnett, Carr, Hamilton, & O'Reilly, 2017).

From its start, FFT has focused on engaging adolescents (typically between the ages of 11 and 18) and their families in therapy (Sexton, 2011; Waldron & Turner, 2008). The rates of successful engagement of adolescents in FFT are reported to be between 78 and 89%, considerably higher than engagement rates for other treatments that service youth (Sexton, 2011). Engagement is done in part by having family members focus on how their interactions with one another function to regulate their relationships. The premise is that relationships serve specific functions; that is, relationships generate interpersonal results or payoffs. According to Alexander and Parsons (1982), family members use "the best means they have available to define their relationships in order to meet their functional needs" (p. 25). Three of the primary functions of relationships and their corresponding payoffs are (1) merging (to increase closeness and contact), (2) separating (to increase distance and independence), and (3) midpointing (a combination of merging and separating functions, as in "Listen to me!" and "Go away!"). The task of the FFT practitioner is to help family members recognize that it is their *relationships* that cause problems, not specific behaviors, feelings, or thoughts. Engagement in treatment takes place when family members are able to "see themselves and each other as recipients rather than malevolent causes and to recognize that there will be benefits for each of them in the change process" (Alexander & Parsons, 1982, p. 48).

FFT is conducted in clinical and home settings, as well as in correctional and mental health settings. It is considered a short-term approach, with an average of 12 family-based sessions provided over a 3- to 6-month period. The three phases of treatment and their corresponding functions are assessment (deciding what to change), therapy (instituting change), and education (maintaining change).

The majority of studies on FFT have examined its effects on criminal behavior alone, even though the vast majority of adolescents (80–85%) in these studies report substance use. Sexton and Turner (2011) reported significant reductions in felony (35%) and violent crimes (30%) at 12 months posttreatment for youth probationers who participated in 12 family-based and high-adherence FFT sessions conducted in the home over 3–6 months, compared to youth who received customary probation services.

In a series of 6 meta-analyses of 14 studies of FFT, Hartnett and colleagues (2017) reported effect sizes favoring FFT over comparison groups (e.g., CBT, individual and group therapy for adolescents) for behavioral *and* substance misuse problems. One of these studies was by Waldron, Slesnick, Brody, Turner, and Peterson (2001). In their study, youth who participated in FFT with their primary caregiver demonstrated significant reductions in their marijuana use (particularly from heavy to minimal use) from pretreatment to posttreatament (after 4 months) compared to youth who participated in a group alcohol and drug skills training. These reductions, however, were comparable to those of youth who participated in either individual CBT or a combination of FFT and CBT, although at 7-month follow-up (3 months after treatment completion) reductions were greater for youth in the combined FFT and CBT program compared to those in individual CBT only.

Multidimensional Family Therapy

Multidimensional family therapy (MDFT) is a family-based outpatient treatment for adolescents with drug and behavioral problems. It has been revised and adapted to numerous settings and for varied concerns, such as high-risk sexual behaviors (see Liddle, 2016, for a review). MDFT is most well known for its use in the Cannabis Youth Project (CYP; Liddle, 2002) sponsored by the Center for Substance Abuse Treatment. For the CYP, services were delivered over 3 months, and the first 2 months were mostly taken up with intense services of two to three weekly 1- to 2-hour sessions with various combinations of family members (e.g., adolescent seen alone in individual counseling and joint adolescent and parent sessions). In most applications of MDFT, the majority of sessions occur in a clinic setting, but face-to-face and frequent telephone contact with family members and extrafamilial systems (e.g., personnel from school and juvenile justice) in natural settings occurs throughout the week.

The theoretical foundation of MDFT is family and developmental psychology. The model presumes that adolescent substance abuse and delinquent behaviors begin and are maintained by a complex set of interrelated and mutually reinforcing risk factors, such as family management difficulties (Rowe & Liddle, 2008). Treatment must therefore be multidimensional, meaning that it operates according to a number of dimensions, such as maintaining an outcome orientation (e.g., focusing on long-term, intermediate, and short-term goals), addressing parent–adolescent relationship development, and understanding the multiple psychosocial ecologies of teens and their families. The 10 principles of MDFT are presented in Table 8.2.

A recent meta-analysis (van der Pol et al., 2017) of 8 studies representing a total sample of 1,488 adolescents (mean age of approximately 16 and approximately 75% male) found that MDFT generated improved outcomes (e.g., lower cannabis use severity) compared to three other therapies: CBT, group therapy, and a combination of CBT and group therapy. In particular, MDFT was found to be most effective for adolescents with severe substance use disorders and more effective for adolescents with disruptive behavior disorder.

One study of ethnic minority youth (Henderson, Dakof, Greenbaum, & Liddle, 2010) found that those who participated in MDFT had reduced high-severity substance-related behaviors compared to a peer-based CBT group. Another study of a 3- to 4-month home-based version of MDFT (Liddle, Rowe, Dakof, Henderson, & Greenbaum, 2009) produced superior results compared to a clinic-based adolescent CBT peer group up to 12 months postintake on measures of treatment completion, abstinence from alcohol and drugs, academic performance, and delinquent behavior. A version of MDFT that began while youth were in juvenile detention and then followed them to postrelease (4–6 months total) also produced outcomes superior to a clinic- and group-based treatment up to 9 months postintake, particularly for youth with more frequent drug use (Henderson et al., 2010). Subsequent analyses of data generated from these studies (specifically for youth with cannabis use disorders) suggest that, compared to CBT, MDFT is conducive for younger adolescents (13- to 16-year-olds) with conduct disorders (Hendriks, van der Schee, & Blanken, 2012). Liddle (2016)

TABLE 8.2. The 10 Principles of Multidimensional Family Therapy

1. Adolescent drug abuse is a multidimensional phenomenon.

2. Problem situations provide information and opportunity.

3. Change is multidetermined and multifaceted.

4. Motivation is malleable.

5. Working relationships are critical.

6. Interventions are individualized.

7. Planning and flexibility are two sides of the same therapeutic coin.

8. Treatment is phasic, and continuity is stressed.

9. The therapist's responsibility is emphasized.

10. The therapist's attitude is fundamental to success.

Note. From Liddle (2002).

reports that MDFT is being adapted to treat Internet gaming disorder and for young adults (ages 18–25).

Multisystemic Therapy

Multisystemic therapy (MST; Henggeler, Schoenwald, Borduin, Rowland, & Cunningham, 2009) is a comprehensive, intensive, and team-based treatment approach for adolescents and their families. It is based on the social ecology theory of Bronfennbrenner (1979) that views human development and functioning from a number of overlapping and nested systems or ecological environments. Unlike traditional family systems theory, the theory of social ecology considers broader and more numerous systemic influences on the individual and his or her family system, including contexts and persons not in direct contact with family members (e.g., school board members, ancestors of indigenous families, members of city council). This theory has been used to explain substance use behavior among Asian American youth (Hong, Huang, Sabri, & Kim, 2011), with consideration given to, among others, chronological systems or contexts affected by the passage of time (e.g., acculturation). The social ecological theory proposes that human development and behavior can be fully understood only from the perspective of the natural settings in which human development and behavior occur. This is known as *ecological validity*. MST practitioners therefore meet and work with clients and their families in their natural environments or real-world settings, such as the home, school, and neighborhood. Services are typically provided over 3–4 months.

MST was developed in the late 1970s for serious juvenile offenders and their families. Today, MST is appropriate for adolescents (typically, 12–17 years old) who struggle with both mental health and substance use concerns and, in the process, have become involved in the legal system. According to the MST Services website (*www.mstservices.com*), there are over 2,500 MST clinicians working in 34 states and in 15 countries. The implicit goal of MST is to restructure the adolescent's overlapping environments to reduce antisocial (including substance use) behavior. Henggeler and Schaeffer (2016) reported an MST evidence base that includes 25 randomized clinical trials on a number of behavioral outcomes: reductions in criminal behavior (including decreased incarceration or residential placement and reduced drug-related arrests), improved family relations, decreased drug use and increased abstinence, decreased psychiatric hospitalizations, and increased school attendance. MST outcomes specific to alcohol and drug use are reviewed by Sheidow and Henggeler (2008). An adaptation of MST specifically targets problem sexual behavior (see Letourneau et al., 2009), and it has been applied to address a range of health concerns such as adolescent diabetes, asthma, obesity, and HIV infection. Of the four family-based approaches for adolescent substance use reviewed in this chapter, MST has the most extensive and perhaps most rigorous evidence base.

The beneficial effects of MST tend to be long-lasting. For example, Sawyer and Borduin (2011) located 176 adults who had received either MST or individual therapy as adolescents 18–24 years earlier (average of 21.9 years earlier). Compared to adolescents who had participated in individual therapy only, MST graduates were significantly less likely to have been (1) arrested for felony or misdemeanor crimes and (2) involved in family-related civil suits during adulthood. Demographic characteristics (e.g., race, gender, social class) did not moderate these effects, lending further support to MST's already established effectiveness with a broad range of cultural groups (e.g., African Americans) from varied geographic settings (e.g., rural). The benefit to caregivers of MST graduates also is enduring. Almost 21 years after they and their adolescents participated in MST services, Johnides, Borduin, Wagner, and Dopp (2017) found that caregivers had 94% fewer felonies and 70% fewer misdemeanors than did caregivers whose adolescent (and not the caregiver) participated in individual therapy only. Family involvement in MST therefore benefits the parent or guardian, not just the adolescent.

Although MST is a multisystem approach (i.e., involving contexts in addition to the family), the family is the primary focus of services. Parents and other caregivers are viewed as full collaborators with MST therapists and as crucial change agents for their adolescents. MST therapists work directly with caregivers to equip them with the necessary skills (e.g., discipline, monitoring, empathy, and validation) to help alter their adolescent's behavior, somewhat similar to the practice of CRAFT. Critical to caregiver empowerment is recognizing and reinforcing family and extrafamilial strengths and resources, such as the adolescent's interest in sports and desire to finish school, and the caregiver's commitment to raising and supporting the adolescent. These strengths are considered the key levers for change.

Henggeler (2011) listed five key components of MST that help explain its effectiveness: (1) providing treatment services in the home, at school, and in other community locations; (2) scheduling appointments at the family's convenience, including evening and weekend hours; (3) offering 24-hour-per-day, 7-day-per-week availability of therapists to address crises that might interfere with the success of treatment; (4) maintaining caseloads of four to six families per therapist on an MST team so that intensive services can be modified to accommodate family needs; and (5) including two to four full-time therapists on each MST team so that there is continuity of treatment (e.g., therapists can rotate an on-call schedule during evening, weekend, and holiday hours). Additional practices integral to MST are continuous tracking of the targeted behavior (e.g., parents administering urine drug screens at home, MST therapists observing parent–adolescent communication at their home, parents evaluating MST therapist behavior) and the sequences of behavior within and between multiple systems that maintain the identified problems (e.g., links between parental practices and school behavior), promoting responsible behavior among family members, and adapting services to fit the cultural context of each family (Henggeler et al., 2009).

O'CONNOR FAMILY CASE FUNCTIONAL ANALYSIS

The O'Connor family case presented on page 225 illustrates several reciprocal, reinforcing, and coping behaviors among the four members mentioned. From a behavioral framework, we offer our own functional analysis of this particular system. Several principles of family systems theory are woven into our analysis, and family roles derived from the family disease models are also included.

Hank has been drinking for what appears to be the entirety of his 35-year marriage to Marge. His drinking seems to have had a stabilizing rather than a destructive influence on the marriage and the family system. He and Marge remain married and living together, and their one daughter, Pam, is a frequent visitor to the house, bringing along her young son, Todd. A certain degree or type of cohesion exists.

Early in their marriage, Marge's behavior seems to have negatively reinforced Hank's heavy drinking: She didn't complain about his drinking, and she kept the house clean. These actions removed or at least minimized stressors for him. She also may have assumed primary responsibility for childrearing, thereby freeing Hank from engaging in certain tasks he may have found distasteful (e.g., helping children with homework, taking them to doctor's appointments). From a family disease perspective, Marge fulfilled the role of family manager. Reciprocally, Hank's drinking may have reinforced Marge's caretaking tendencies, especially prior to the arrival of their children. She may have found her domestic duties rewarding, including those duties that catered specifically to Hank's needs.

Once the children were no longer at home full time and Marge was no longer engaged in childrearing behaviors, the benefits available as part of Hank's employment provided the impetus for Marge to work outside the home—first by attending school and then by securing out-of-home employment. The additional family income appears to have been more reinforcing to the family's stability (including perhaps Hank's drinking) than Marge's absence from the home and the disruption to certain routines (e.g., prepared meals) and conditions (e.g., cleanliness). Now that Marge has been employed for 10 years, a new relational pattern has been established. Her coping style appears to have shifted from tolerant coping ("putting up with it") to withdrawal coping ("withdrawing from it"). There is no evidence that Marge participated in engaged coping ("standing up to it") at any point in their marriage, whereby she attempted to change Hank's drinking. This does not mean, however, that she did not try. Marge's decision to spend more time away from home (as a student and now as an employee) may have been in response to some incident that made her realize she would never be successful in changing Hank. She decided to pursue reinforcements outside of the home and to improve herself whether or not Hank changed his behavior. Marge is now spending more time away from home than she used to and has established positive and rewarding relationships with persons at work.

It is not clear how long Hank has been retired, but it seems Marge's absence from home is reinforcing several behaviors, even though he says he is "bored." It may be that Hank's drinking is a function of his boredom and also an expression of his perceived hierarchical position and decision-making role in the family. He can do what he wants even though he apparently cannot influence Marge to retire as well.

Marge's absence also reinforces Pam's behavior. Pam appears to have assumed the role of family heroine, a role she may have assumed early in her life to maintain some order in the family. Her arrival at her parents' home several days during the week is welcomed by her retired father, particularly because she does not say anything to him about his drinking. Pam's silence on the issue is a negative reinforcement for Hank, supplying him with relief from the frustration or even anger that he possibly has experienced from those who have questioned his drinking in the past (perhaps his other children).

Pam is engaged in tolerant coping with her father's drinking. She puts up with it. The function or payoff of this behavior may be the recognition Pam receives from her father for providing him "the son" he will "never have." This male heir in the form of her son Todd is an achievement for someone who remains in the heroine role.

Although Hank does not drink as much on the days he knows Pam and Todd will stop by, the function of this behavior is unclear. It may be that Todd's behavior relieves Hank's boredom in ways that drinking does when Hank is home alone. Todd therefore serves as a substitute and natural reinforcement for Hank, replacing drinking on those days.

CHAPTER SUMMARY

It is imperative that practitioners be familiar with the principles of systems theory and the three family treatment models in the addictions presented in this chapter: family disease models, family systems models, and behavioral models. As the primary social unit, the family exerts a powerful influence on an individual's drinking or drug use. The emphasis on reciprocal causality is unique among the theories of addictive behavior. It proposes that substance misuse: (1) is functional or purposeful; (2) is a manifestation of other concerns, such as relational conflict; and (3) helps the individual to minimize, distract from, or cope with interpersonal problems.

The emerging body of research on family-based approaches for substance and behavioral addiction we have reviewed in this chapter is encouraging. The six approaches highlighted at the end of this chapter are only a sample of the range of programs and interventions available. It is wise, however, to entertain caution when interpreting results because many of the research studies that have informed these practices vary in terms of methodological rigor, implementation and treatment delivery protocol (e.g., many family members seen together or in unilateral therapy), sample size, and ethnic/racial diversity. In addition, substance use is often only one of many variables measured. Despite this caution, the integration of systems theory and behavioral practices offers much promise for the prevention and treatment of addictive behaviors for individuals and their families. The sequential development of family models of addiction—and their corresponding interventions—mirrors the evolution of the addictions field. It remains an exciting and hopeful time for practitioners, researchers, and family members alike.

REVIEW QUESTIONS

1. What are the four principles of systems theory? Specifically, what is meant by *reciprocal causality*?

2. How can substance misuse in a family unit serve to regulate or to stabilize the functioning of family members? What is the name of this principle in systems theory?

3. For a child or adolescent (adopted or not), what are the intrafamilial influences for later addictive behavior? What are some of the extrafamilial influences?

4. Identify five adverse childhood events or experiences. How are these associated with later addictive behavior?

5. Describe the concept of addiction as a *family disease*. How was this concept helpful to certain family members in the early and mid-1990s? How has it proven less helpful today?

6. What are four criticisms of the concept of *codependency*? What is an alternative characterization or reference?

7. Describe the five family roles that are often associated with the family disease model. How might identifying with one of these roles assist a family member

to understand the patterns of interpersonal relationships over a period time in the family's history?

8. From a family systems model of addiction, describe the types of boundaries that may exist between an adult couple or among two or more family members, such as a parent–child dyad. What about addiction may contribute to rigid and diffuse boundaries?

9. How are subsystems in the family unit affected by substance misuse? What alliances or coalitions may explain the initiation and maintenance of substance misuse, as well as its amelioration (e.g., recovery)?

10. How is addiction in a family understood from a behavioral model? What behaviors serve to negatively reinforce and to positively reinforce substance use?

11. Construct a timeline that includes the three family models of addiction discussed in this chapter. Which developed first in the United States? Which followed? How does their developmental sequence explain the state of addiction prevention, treatment, and research today?

12. What are the principles and distinguishing characteristics of CRAFT? For whom is it appropriate? How does it differ from the potentially harmful practices featured on the popular television show *Intervention*?

13. What are the primary objectives of behavioral couples therapy?

14. Name the four family-based approaches for adolescent substance abuse reviewed in this chapter. What is unique about each one? How are they similar? Which one would you recommend to someone who has an adolescent family member with a substance use problem? Explain your reasons for this recommendation.

15. If you had been able to serve in the role of counselor to the Rowan family while Aiden was still alive (and his biological father, Mike, too), which of the six family-based approaches reviewed in the second half of this chapter would you have used? Explain your selection and how you would have applied this approach with them.

CHAPTER 9

Social and Cultural Foundations

Social and cultural foundations of addictive behaviors cover wide territory. A good bit of this territory is covered in other chapters of this book. In Chapter 4, addiction from a public health perspective necessarily involves a consideration of societal views and practices. Federal legislation (e.g., legal drinking age) and institutional policies (e.g., smoke-free work environments) are the result of social influence at various levels of the political spectrum. In addition, as Albert Bandura's social-cognitive theory illustrates, cognitive processes, such as expectancies described in Chapter 6, are cultivated by social interactions and cultural norms. Furthermore, the family system described in Chapter 8 is by definition a social and cultural dynamic.

This chapter focuses on how substance use and other addictive behaviors are understood and controlled by groups of people. These groups are defined by their social status or context (including their decision-making power or lack thereof) and their cultural identity. The terms *social* and *cultural* are often used synonymously or in combination, as in the term *sociocultural*. A sociocultural understanding of addictive behaviors accounts for the beliefs, values, customs, and other patterned behaviors of groups (and subgroups) of persons with a shared identity or social status. These are influenced by their age, gender identity, race/ethnicity, socioeconomic status, educational level, immigration status, career or vocational status, sexual orientation, religious affiliation or practices, and the intersection of these and other identities or contexts.

A sociocultural theory entails two different positions of perspective: how groups of persons make meaning of and manage their own addictive behaviors (an insider's view) and how groups of persons understand and control the addictive behaviors of others (an outsider's view). An insider's view is accessed through in-depth interviews with group members or observations of group behavior over time. This is the work of social anthropologists and qualitative researchers, such as ethnographers. This information helps explain the purpose of substance use and addiction for those who engage in these behaviors, including self- and group-regulatory practices. An insider's view typically regards drinking and other substance use behaviors as normative and acceptable. "This is what we do," group members might say. "This is who we are."

Most social and behavioral scientists (those who study human behavior) assume an outsider's perspective. They are observers and analysts of human behavior, both collective (as in groups of people) and individual behavior. The information they collect, however, may not necessarily be used to regulate the behaviors of persons observed. Those who assume an outsider's perspective and, by virtue of their social influence and decision-making power, attempt to control the addictive behaviors of others include politicians, helping professionals (e.g., physicians, counselors) and their professional organizations (e.g., American Psychiatric Association), pharmaceutical company executives, and judges. It is the outsider's view that generally regards substance use and addiction as non-normative and unacceptable behavior, although insiders can share this view of their own behavior. This chapter offers both an insider's and outsider's view.

PROFESSIONAL NOMENCLATURE

Names are important; they hold meaning and significance. This is true of the personal names we use for ourselves—names given to us by family members or names we ourselves have selected. Our names may connect us to ancestors, historical events, geographic regions, religious figures, or other cultural influences. They define us in many ways; they assert our identity.

The act of naming another person or groups of persons (e.g., according to personal characteristics, geographic place of residence or origin, and medical condition) clarifies, organizes, and categorizes. This is the practice of nomenclature. It is done routinely in the helping professions to classify persons according to medical conditions, such as substance use disorders. Doing so asserts control. It is the professionals with decision-making power who get to name the conditions and, in the process, get to name the *persons* with these conditions. Professional nomenclature therefore must be handled with great care.

A growing number of addiction professionals contend that using the terms *abuse* and *abuser* to characterize, respectively, a medical condition and a person struggling with addictive behaviors is moralistic and pejorative (Kelly & Westerhoff, 2010; Miller et al., 2011; Richter & Foster,

2014). In their persuasive commentary, White and Kelly (2011) contend that these terms are derived not from science but from religion, being vestiges of colonial American Protestantism, which viewed excessive use of alcohol as sinful, an act of the devil or Satan. White and Kelly offer five reasons why "[t]he terms abuse and abuser should be now and forever abandoned" (p. 320). We discuss four reasons here, however, because we interpret two of these reasons as one and the same.

First, the terms *abuse* and *abuser* are technically inaccurate. Persons "do not abuse alcohol or drugs; they treat these substances with the greatest devotion and respect at the expense of themselves and everyone and everything else of value in their lives" (White & Kelly, 2011, p. 318). As one gentleman in long-term alcohol recovery once quipped to William White: "Mixing Jack Daniels Tennessee Whiskey with Hawaiian Punch: anyone who would commit such an abhorrent act deserves serious punishment" (see White & Kelly, 2011, p. 318). Second, "substance abuse" is not a medical condition; it does not exist in the fifth edition of the *Diagnostic and Statistical Manual of Mental Disorders* (DSM-5; American Psychiatric Association, 2013). Third, the terms *abuse* and *abuser* "contribute to the social and professional stigma attached to substance use disorders and may inhibit help seeking" and promote social rejection and isolation (White & Kelly, 2011, p. 319). A fourth and final reason these terms should not be used is that they attribute substance use problems solely to the individual, specifically to personal characteristics and poor choices. By focusing only on the host and not the agent (i.e., substance) and the environment (as is done in the public health model's tripartite explanatory model of addictive behaviors; see Chapter 3), White and Kelly (2011) argue that "the culpability of corporations whose financial interests are served by promoting high-frequency, high-quantity [chemical] consumption" is dismissed (p. 320).

We wholeheartedly support White and Kelly's (2011) claims and recommendations. We have done our best throughout this volume to use terminology respectful of persons with addictive behaviors. We acknowledge inconsistencies, however. There are occasions in this book when we refer to "abuser(s)" and to addictive behavior as "abuse." This reflects the challenge throughout professional organizations to agree on nomenclature.

DIAGNOSIS AS SOCIAL AND CULTURAL CONTROL

From a sociological perspective, the problems of excessive drinking and drug use have become *medicalized* (Patnode, 2007). As we discussed in Chapter 1, the medical and behavioral health communities have redefined addiction as *illness* or *disease* to benefit their respective interests. Moynihan, Heath, and Henry (2002) describe this process as "disease mongering." This labeling process functions as a means of social control. This indicates that persons in influential positions (e.g., leaders of medical associations) shape and control how addiction is defined and how it is addressed. This is not unlike labeling as diseases ordinary life occurrences or common ailments, such as baldness or irritable bowel syndrome, to profit pharmaceutical companies (Moynihan et al., 2002). These persons hold the proverbial and actual purse strings. They determine the norms and standards for others, including the general public.

Diagnosis is one specialized form of professional nomenclature. It also is considered a sophisticated form of propaganda advanced by medicine and other helping professions (Gambrill, 2010). Medicalization gives credibility to physicians' and behavioral health professionals' efforts to control, manage, and supervise the care of persons with substance use problems. It makes legitimate potentially lucrative endeavors such as hospital admissions, insurance company billings, expansion of the client pool, and consulting fees. It also serves to restrict the number and type of practitioners who are permitted to assist people with these problems. Acceptance of the term *treatment* in the addictions field reflects the dominant influence of medicine and the medical model.

The social process of labeling also functions to restrict substance use in the community. It defines for the average citizen appropriate and inappropriate drinking practices. Stopping for one drink after work and before going home (during "happy hour") is distinguished from public intoxication. Social labeling also alerts persons to smoke-free zones, for example, and provides those with criteria to determine whether to call a helpline for smoking.

A *diagnosis* is the formal name assigned to problem behaviors and psychological disturbances by medicine and the behavioral health professions. It classifies conditions into predetermined categories. In the United States, diagnosis originally served as a means to count the frequency of "idiocy/insanity" among citizens for the first U.S. Census of 1840 (Nathan et al., 2016). Diagnosis subsequently became the means for physicians to record uniform statistics across the country's psychiatric hospitals and to be able to communicate with one another about patients. Today, determining and assigning a diagnosis is now standard practice for medical professionals and most behavioral health practitioners. Without a diagnosis, patients or clients cannot receive formal care or treatment. It is the ticket to professional services.

To justify the diagnostic process, helping professions have created elaborate sets of criteria based mostly on clinical experience. The most prominent example in the behavioral health arena is the DSM-5. Its first edition was issued in 1952 in an effort to name the varied conditions manifested by military veterans who had fought in World War II. Another prominent example of a diagnostic naming system or taxonomy is the *International Classification of Diseases* or *ICD* now in its 10th edition (ICD-10), with revisions for the 11th edition underway. The ICD is the world's primary disease coding system. The forerunner of the ICD was the International

List of Causes of Death, adopted by the International Statistical Institute in 1893. It was in 1948, also after World War II, that the World Health Organization (WHO) was entrusted to oversee the ICD. The purpose of the ICD remains the accounting of causes of hospitalization and morbidity in the general population in all countries, regardless of their level of economic development or nature of health care (Saunders, 2006).

Labeling theorists have described the practice of diagnosis as the *medicalization of deviant behavior* (Conrad, 2007). From a sociological perspective, it represents a longstanding effort by medicine and the behavioral health community to redefine deviance from *badness* to *sickness*. Thus, the control of deviance has shifted from the religious community and the criminal justice system to the medical and addiction treatment systems.

Conrad (2007) argues that the social forces driving the medicalization process have shifted and are no longer directed primarily by the profession of medicine. Although physicians remain the gatekeepers for medical treatment, their role in expanding medicalization has become subordinate to three other forces: the biotechnology industry based on genetic and pharmaceutical research, consumer demands, and managed care pressures. As an example, even before its release, Dr. Allen Francis, the chair of the revision of the fourth edition of DSM, criticized the chairs of DSM-5 for over-diagnosis, facilitated by what he regarded as the undue influence of large pharmaceutical companies (see Nathan et al., 2016). Conrad proposed that the process of medicalization will continue, but the modern engines will be driven by commercial and market interests, particularly those based on new pharmaceutical and genetic treatments.

From a sociocultural perspective, diagnostic criteria for addiction are derived largely from cultural norms. Determining "harmful consequences" of use and "neglecting pleasurable activities" for substance use (two criteria in the DSM and the ICD) depends on a person's social and cultural circumstance. The first two editions of the DSM used the terms *alcoholism* and *drug addiction,* two conditions associated with personality disorders, namely, "sociopathic personality disturbance." According to Nathan and colleagues (2016), "It took 28 years and the appearance of [the third edition of the DSM in 1980] for the nomenclature to move away from this harsh moral judgment on these behaviors" (p. 36). Unfortunately, pejorative language and moralistic views persist among health care professionals specific to mental illness and substance use disorders. For example, mental health professionals ($N = 516$) in Kelly and Westerhoff's (2010) study were significantly more likely to associate someone identified as a "substance abuser" with being a perpetrator who deserved punishment compared to someone identified as having a "substance use disorder" (SUD).

Attitudes such as these, even among behavioral health professionals, exemplify a sociocultural perspective that drinking, drug use, and problem behaviors considered *addictive* are behaviors that deviate from socially acceptable standards. These behaviors are considered forms of social deviance rather than medical problems. Sociologically, *treatment* is seen as an effort to persuade the addicted individual to conform to socially "correct" standards of conduct. We provide further discussion of stigma and the control of the treatment industry in subsequent sections in this chapter.

The cultural foundations of diagnoses were recognized by prominent alcoholism researcher George Vaillant (1990, 1995), a proponent of a disease understanding of addiction. Vaillant (1990) stated: "Normal drinking merges imperceptibly with pathological drinking. Culture and idiosyncratic viewpoints will always determine where the line is drawn" (p. 5). The sociocultural origins of diagnoses force practitioners to consider at least three possibilities. First, a diagnosis, as applied to a particular client, may not be very different from a personal opinion: It may be based not so much on scientific evidence as on the values and beliefs of the addiction practitioner. The practitioner's own history, relative to his or her involvement in addictive behavior, clearly influences the opinion.

Second, time and place play important roles in the sociocultural origins of diagnoses. For example, drinking considered *alcoholic* in one period of time or place may not be viewed similarly in another temporal or geographic context. As noted in Chapter 1, Americans in the early and late 1800s consumed approximately three times more alcohol (per capita) than they consume today. Clearly, the notion of what an alcoholic was then would have differed substantially from the conception today.

Third, cultural factors should sensitize clinicians as to the beneficial and negative consequences of rendering a substance use diagnosis for a particular client. In the best of cases, the diagnosis will motivate the client to change his or her behavior. However, a diagnosis also could lead to overly intrusive treatment, social stigma, estrangement from family members, loss of employment, feelings of worthlessness and humiliation, and worsening of problems in living. Obviously, any diagnosis should be made with caution. One can legitimately question the value of making a diagnosis—even when it is clearly appropriate—if there is reason to believe that it will have an adverse effect on a client. It is important to discuss with clients the reason for assigning a diagnosis, its clinical definition (in words the client can understand), and the meaning of the diagnosis for the client. Although the client may not agree with the outcome of a diagnostic assessment, it is the counselor's professional obligation to explain the process and the role of diagnosis in treatment.

THE SOCIAL AND CULTURAL CONTROL OF THE ADDICTION TREATMENT INDUSTRY

Stanton Peele has long been a critic of the U.S. addiction treatment industry. He has claimed for many years that it is big business by virtue of calling addiction a disease. The title of his book, *Diseasing of America: Addiction Treatment Out of Control* (1989), aptly captures this sentiment. As mentioned earlier in this chapter and in Chapter 1, naming a medical condition a disease affords health care providers the opportunity to treat it, generate income from doing so, and control the treatment process.

Social anthropologist E. S. Carr (2011) contends that the American addiction treatment system is a vastly political system that requires its clients to speak a certain way in order to meet predetermined criteria of improvement and earn recovery status. In her 3½-year immersion study of the daily workings of one treatment facility, Carr discovered that practitioners prescribe certain types of talk to their clients and evaluate their progress based on their use of this type of language. For example, in order for residential clients to be issued weekend passes to see their children, they must first have identified themselves as an "alcoholic" or "addict," confessed their earlier "denial" about their substance use, referred to their substance use in the past tense, and publicly declared they are "working the program."

Clients in substance use treatment are thus at the mercy of health care providers. This is likely true more so for clients with limited income than for those of a higher socioeconomic status who have private insurance. The latter group has more options and can assert their preferences compared to the former group. And it is the limited-income group that accounts for the vast majority of clients in substance use treatment. White (2014) reports that 61% of clients in U.S. addiction treatment facilities did not have health insurance; 28% had public insurance, such as Medicaid; and only 11% of clients had private insurance. A treatment industry in control of impoverished persons with limited education who struggle with substance use and its stigma is therefore susceptible to exploitation.

Another recent critic of the addiction treatment industry is Marc Lewis, a neuroscientist. He writes in a sardonic tone that, by calling addiction a disease, one implies that:

> [t]he only hope to control addiction is to accept a regime imposed from outside, from the halls of medical authority, in order to subdue a problem located on the inside, in the mind itself (an approach to the treatment of mental disorders that has governed psychiatry throughout its history—with some unfortunate consequences). (2017, p. 16)

In light of this characterization, it is therefore startling and ironic that physicians play a very limited role as actual providers of addiction treatment and that they receive very limited training in addictions during medical school. The same is true for psychologists (Dimoff, Sayette, & Norcross, 2017). White (2014) acknowledges that "[m]ost addiction treatment programs use medical metaphors to conceptualize the addiction, treatment, and recovery processes, but most people undergoing addiction treatment in the United States have little contact with physicians, nurses, or other medical personnel during their treatment" (p. 427).

Addiction treatment providers are primarily nonmedical addiction counselors who may or may not have a master's degree. The quality of their training and the rigor of their credentialing requirements are subject to scrutiny. As Humphreys and McLellan (2011) observed, credentialing for substance use providers "has become an entrepreneurial activity, with countless organizations developing and selling certificates and licenses" (p. 2060). Organizations such as these feed off and benefit from the big business that is addiction treatment.

The diversity of substance use providers with respect to discipline (e.g., counseling, social work, addictions specific), extent of training and qualifications (including professional or paraprofessional status), and occupational titles (e.g., "technician," "therapist," "intervention specialist") reflects the hazy picture we have of the treatment industry. Coffey and colleagues (2009) noted that the exact nature of addiction treatment services (including expenditures of addiction treatment facilities) remains relatively unknown. This complicates essential evaluation, oversight, and enhancement practices. A burgeoning industry lacking self-regulatory and quality improvement controls—especially one charged with assisting vulnerable and quite often marginalized populations—is an industry that is subject to ineffectiveness.

This issue is particularly concerning because the implementation of evidence-based practices among addiction treatment providers and their receipt of supervision remains questionable, and their annual turnover rates remain quite high (31–33%; see White, 2014). Furthermore, in the general U.S. population, significant comorbidity rates of mental illness (e.g., major depressive disorder, bipolar disorder) and alcohol use disorder (Grant et al., 2015), as well as drug use disorder (Grant et al., 2016), necessitate a treatment workforce prepared to recognize and respond to co-occurring disorders.

STIGMATIZING ADDICTION

Addictive disorders are stigmatizing conditions. In the United States and in other countries, the public holds very stigmatizing views toward persons with substance use disorders, more so than toward persons with a psychiatric illness such as depression and schizophrenia (Yang, Wong, Grivel, & Hasin, 2017). *Addiction stigma* is the practice of endorsing negative stereotypes of persons struggling with substance use and displaying prejudice and discrimination toward them (Corrigan et al., 2017a; Kulesza et al., 2016). Examples of negative stereotypical beliefs are that persons struggling with substance use are dangerous, repulsive, and unpredictable; are to blame for their use and its consequences; are inherently deceitful and perennial liars; and must be pitied and feared. Beliefs such as these account for discriminatory practices, including not hiring or renting to persons with a known history of substance misuse. The effects of addiction stigma on persons with addictive disorders include self-stigma (e.g., believing "I am disgusting and can't be trusted because I'm an addict"), continued and increased substance use, social isolation, and refusal to seek professional medical or behavioral health care, including substance use treatment.

In the United States, the vast majority (approximately 82%) of persons who meet the criteria for a SUD diagnosis do not seek treatment (Substance Abuse and Mental Health Services Administration, 2017). This includes persons with an opioid use disorder, only 19.44% of whom reported involvement in opioid-specific treatment (Wu, Zhu, & Swartz, 2016). The primary reasons given for not seeking care involve cost and lack of health care coverage, accessibility, and unreadiness to stop using. Additional reasons are stigma-related, such as being perceived negatively by neighbors and the community, and believing that treatment involvement may negatively impact their job status.

These are valid reasons. Although Kulesza and colleagues (2016) reported a general pattern of compassion among members of the public toward persons who inject drugs, they also found evidence of racial/ethnic bias. Specifically, members of the public who participated in an online survey believed that Latinos/Latinas who inject drugs deserve punishment, whereas white persons who inject drugs need help. These and other negative stereotypes can prevent persons from seeking treatment. Professionals themselves can be barriers to care by holding stigmatizing attitudes.

Addiction Stigma among Helping Professionals

Health care professionals are not immune to holding stigmatizing attitudes toward persons who use and misuse substances. Indeed, it is from a position of power that stigma is exercised (Link & Phelan, 2001). Negatively stereotyping and discriminating against those who struggle with substance use is associated with lower job satisfaction and higher turnover among treatment professionals (Kulesza, Hunter, Shearer, & Booth, 2017). Stigmatizing attitudes may be due to lower or limited education (e.g., lack of a graduate degree), lack of specialized training in addictions, work in a stressful environment with low pay and other limited supports (e.g., lack of routine and effective supervision), and lack of exposure to persons who have achieved and maintained sobriety. Compared to primary care physicians and psychiatrists, van Boekel, Brouwers, van Weeghel, and Garretsen (2014) found that addiction treatment providers had less stigmatizing attitudes toward clients presenting with substance use concerns. The researchers attributed this mindset to addiction professionals' specialized training, their routine care for persons with addictive behaviors, and their exposure to clients who may have greater motivation to change than patients who seek care from the other two professional groups.

In a February 2018 letter to the editor of a Midwestern city newspaper (*www.ohio.com*), a "retired advanced practice nurse" blamed "the patient with the addictive personality" for "this opioid crisis," not physicians or drug companies. Even though this retired nurse mentioned that persons in her own family were "caught up in this mess," she stated: "The fault lies squarely in the lap of the addicted person. . . . My relative chose to stick a needle in his arm, not me or the health care profession." Little does this retired nurse realize: There is no such condition as a so-called addictive personality; it is not included in the current editions of either the DSM or the ICD. It is a remnant of early editions (e.g., 1952) of the DSM. Perhaps this retired nurse did not have specialty training in addictions. Her notions exemplify a vastly outdated addiction treatment industry, one that retains a moralistic suasion despite its claims that naming addiction a disease destigmatizes persons with the condition. Her views actually reinforce addiction stigma.

So do the behaviors of addiction professionals on television shows, such as *Celebrity Rehab* and *Intervention*. According to Oksanen (2014), these shows often feature persons with severe forms of addiction, some of whom have subsequently died. The exact details of the treatment process are kept brief, whereas displays of extreme emotion are magnified. Baker (2016) conducted a qualitative content analysis of 117 episodes of these two shows and determined that the treatment providers featured (e.g., Dr. Drew Pinsky) actually contribute to the stigmatization of persons with addictions. They do this in their carefully controlled behaviors that flaunt their privileged status, responding to resistance by asserting their authority, and explaining their views to audience members. In doing so, they encourage the belief that "individuals with addiction are unable to speak authoritatively about their own problems and needs" (Baker, 2016, p. 494).

Kelly and Westerhoff (2010) distributed two versions of the same written client case to mental health care providers attending professional conferences and asked them to respond to questions about the case. One version of the case described the male client as "a substance abuser" (version A); the other described him as having "a substance use disorder" (version B). All other descriptions of the client were the same in both versions. Compared to professionals who received version B, professionals with version A were significantly more in agreement that the client was personally responsible for his condition (e.g., "caused by his reckless behavior") and deserving of punitive measures (e.g., "He should be given some kind of jail sentence to serve as a wake-up call"). Kelly and Westerhoff (p. 205) explain:

Referring to an individual as a "substance abuser" may elicit and perpetuate stigmatizing attitudes that appear to relate to punitive judgments and perceptions that individuals with substance-related conditions are recklessly engaging in willful misconduct. . . . Compared to the [substance use disorder] individual, the "abuser" may elicit greater perceptions of blame because they are perceived as more able to self-regulate behavioral impulses and, consequently, as bringing the problems on themselves, and more deserving of punishment.

As did White and Kelly (2011; discussed earlier), Kelly and Westerhoff (2010) recommend discontinuation of the term *substance abuser* because of its promotion of stigma. They contend that "its nonuse would be unlikely to produce any detrimental results" (p. 206). One of these detrimental results is the prevention of help-seeking behavior among persons who need professional care.

What can helping professionals do to mitigate their own and the addiction stigma of others, including the self-stigma of persons who struggle with substance use? For professionals, targeted educational initiatives involving interaction with recovering individuals is recommended (Crapanzano, Vath, & Fisher, 2014). Flanagan and colleagues (2016) reported that primary care providers exhibited less stigma after hearing firsthand the recovery stories of persons, particularly learning of their strengths, interests, and contributions to their communities. In providing care to persons struggling with substance use, Askew (2016) argues that exploring the reasons for use can minimize stigma. Her interviews with illicit drug users revealed a "functional and controlled" pattern of use, one that did not compromise their long-term health or sociocultural status (e.g., employment, family roles). Askew states: "Recognising the positives of drug use, as well as responding to the risks . . . helps to reduce the social and cultural harm caused by stigma and negative stereotypes" (p. 118).

SOCIOCULTURAL FUNCTIONS OF SUBSTANCE USE AND MISUSE

Many (e.g., Hardon & Hymans, 2014; Meier, Warde, & Holmes, 2018) have argued that science has failed to uncover the social structures that perpetuate or explain substance use. In other words, little is known about what chemicals "do" for those who use them. Still less is known about routine substance use practices and the meaning of these behaviors for those who engage in addictive behaviors. Without these discoveries, effective regulatory mechanisms (e.g., federal policy), prevention efforts, and treatment approaches cannot be developed or implemented. Understanding the role and purpose(s) of certain substances for specific groups of persons in particular contexts allows for targeted and relevant response initiatives. This is similar to the practice in business and industry, and specifically marketing, of conducting a needs analysis. In counseling, learning what is important to the client, what he or she values, and what regulates client behavior is part of the standard practice of case conceptualization. A comprehensive understanding of client situational and cultural factors makes it possible for the counselor to develop an individualized treatment plan. Furthermore, learning the purpose or function of substance use for an individual and for specific sociocultural groups (e.g., men who have sex with men, impoverished persons in rural parts of Appalachia) is humane and humanistic practice. It prioritizes the perspectives and lived experiences of others. It also is consistent with a sociocultural theory of addiction.

From a sociocultural perspective, the use and misuse of substances serves at least five broad functions: (1) social facilitation, (2) release from social obligations, (3) repudiation of social norms, (4) marking boundaries, and (5) crossing boundaries (symbolic mediation). Clearly, these do not capture the wide range of functions, and therefore this list is far from exhaustive. However, these five comprise common functions across cultural groups. They are not distinct functions; they overlap, as depicted in Figure 9.1.

Social Facilitation

Many substances are used to promote social interaction and cohesion; this is true particularly for alcohol. Because its consumption is legal, alcohol is often associated with good times, parties, and fun with others. This may explain the phrase "social drinking" and the reference to being a "social drinker." This function normalizes and legitimizes drinking: "I'm not an alcoholic. I'm a social drinker. I only drink with my friends." Implied in this self-assessment is that one's drinking is not problematic, even if the amount and frequency are above recommended guidelines. The National Institute on Alcohol Abuse and Alcoholism (NIAAA; *www.niaaa.nih.gov*) defines low-risk drinking for women as no more than three standard drinks on a single day and no more than seven standard drinks in one week. For men, low-risk drinking is no more than four standard drinks on a single day and no more than 14 standard drinks in a given week. Drinking rates higher and more frequent than these may not appear problematic to the self-identified "social drinker" if others in one's drinking cohort also are drinking above these guidelines. Because drinking is done with others, heavy alcohol consumption may be legitimized and any negative effects minimized.

The use of alcohol to facilitate social pleasure and interactions with others has been reported for thousands of years among most cultures of the world. For example, the Code of Hammurabi, the earliest known legal

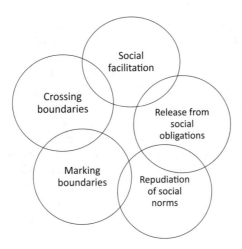

FIGURE 9.1. Five sociocultural functions of substance use and misuse.

code (promulgated circa 1758 B.C.E. in Babylon), contains laws governing the operation and management of drinking establishments (King, 2005). Today, *drinking* has been thoroughly integrated into mainstream U.S. culture. Alcoholic drinks are known simply as a *drink*. If a person invites a friend to "come over for a drink," everyone usually recognizes that alcohol is the planned drink. In Japan, alcohol consumption is socially acceptable, and drinking parties are commonly held to strengthen social and business connections (Yoshimura, Komoto, & Higuchi, 2016).

Alcohol consumption is expected behavior at various social, family, and business gatherings, both formal and informal. Although individuals are not usually directly pressured to drink alcohol in these gatherings, there often is a subtle pressure to do so. A blunt refusal often generates puzzlement, covert speculation, or even suspicion as to one's motives. Frequently, refusing to drink is interpreted as passing on an opportunity to meet and talk in an informal way. This is particularly true in business or other work settings characterized by formal or professional relationships. In such settings, people often desire to escape from the restrictive confines of stiff or rigid professional roles. Drinking together is seen as the way to "loosen up."

Certain illicit substances, such as marijuana and ecstasy, are also used to enhance sociability. "To have a good time with my friends" was the second top reason for smoking among more than 6,500 high school seniors (12th graders) nationwide who reported frequent marijuana use (Palamar, Griffin-Tomas, & Kamboukos, 2015). The number one reason was "To feel good or get high." Dubbed as an "empathy agent," ecstasy reportedly generates feelings of closeness to others. One person interviewed in Hunt and Evans's (2008) study of 300 club drug users in San Francisco described the effects of ecstasy this way: "You like . . . open up to people. . . . Like you don't feel like threatened by anybody, there's no like . . . worrying about trying to be something you're not. Like you can just open up and talk about whatever you want" (p. 339). Another person described the experience as helping to establish new social connections: "There's definitely a lot of . . . meeting new people and talking to new people. And like new people you meet, you're like 'you're my best new friend' " (pp. 339–340).

Some illicit drug use, such as LSD, is associated with motivations unrelated to increased sociability. These include gaining relief from negative mood states (e.g., anxiety) or active psychotic symptoms (e.g., hallucinations), enhancing creativity or concentration, and losing weight.

Release from Social Obligations and Minority Stressors

A second function of substance use is release from normal social role obligations and varied stressors of contemporary life. Drinking or using drugs provides a time-out from the stress associated with certain responsibilities, such as parenting, work, and school. It also is a release from the effects of discrimination and oppression experienced by members of certain cultural groups (e.g., African Americans, women, transgender persons).

As a release from social obligations and the stressors that accompany being a cultural minority, substance use is considered an occasional activity. It is controlled behavior and not dysfunctional. Askew (2016) described this as the "planned celebration" function of drug use, a notion derived from her interviews with 26 drug users. This function reflects the capitalist principle that permits leisure to balance or complement hard work ("work hard, play hard"). "Loosening up," "lounging" or "chilling out," and even experiencing being "out of control" on an occasional and limited basis is a desired and intended function of substance use. Social role obligations remain a priority and take precedence over substance use; drinking or drug use does not compromise the responsibilities important to a person. For some, it may even be a means to promote an enjoyable and productive life. Although intoxication and other forms of substance misuse occur, these are occasional, limited, and manageable repercussions of use.

Time-Out Hypothesis

The time-out hypothesis applies to both alcohol and drug use. It maintains that using substances serves to release individuals temporarily from their ordinary social obligations. By becoming intoxicated or getting high, they are excused from their obligations as parents, spouses, students, employees, and so forth. Prescription drug misuse among young adults has been reported as one way to "turn off" from the stress of work and other responsibilities (LeClair, Kelly, Pawson, Wells, & Parsons, 2015).

Many years ago, MacAndrew and Edgerton (1969) came upon the time-out hypothesis by observing that many cultures exhibit a certain flexibility in norms that allows for suspension of certain role obligations during times of drunkenness. They were careful to point out, however, that the option of *time-out* does not suspend all the rules. In all cultures, certain behavior, even while intoxicated, is considered inexcusable; thus, intoxicated persons are viewed as *less* responsible rather than as *un*responsible (Heath, 1988). According to MacAndrew and Edgerton, "the option of drunken time-out affords people the opportunity to 'get it out of their systems' with a minimum of adverse consequences" (p. 169).

The time-out hypothesis is not limited to alcohol use. Illicit substances, such as marijuana and ecstasy, also can be used on an occasional basis to escape momentarily the burden of school or work responsibilities. This typifies *recreational use*. Askew (2016) describes this use behavior as *planned celebration*. It is behavior intended as release from social role constraints, one often engaged in with other persons for a limited period of time (e.g., weekend). Any negative consequences of use are minimal and contained; the consequences do not "spill over" into the person's workweek or family responsibilities. Feeling "out of control" may be the purpose of substance use: The person seeks relief from the control or regulations of work, family, or other obligations. The person does not feel controlled by the substance or by substance use (as the disease perspective suggests); rather, the person feels *controlled by social roles and obligations,* and substance use thus provides a temporary relief from these burdens.

One person interviewed by Askew (2016) described his planned celebration this way:

> "I had been on holiday for a week . . . it was a friend of mine's wedding, and I was out there with all of my friends and we were dancing around having a really good time and we all took some pills. It was totally premeditated fun, we danced around and made fools of ourselves, and I have got no problem with that. It doesn't happen as much as it should. . . . It's like once a year when I might be in those conditions, when I am neither exhausted nor tired. I am using it partly as a pick me up, when I am not worried about the consequences." (p. 116)

Askew interpreted this person's drug use behavior as a peripheral activity, one that he is able to control and that he believes balances his stressful work. The time-out is not enduring, and there is a return to social role responsibilities.

It is important to note that young people who get intoxicated or repeatedly engage in substance use to avoid or escape from social role expectations may be susceptible to developing more serious drinking or other substance use problems, as well as mental health problems. When use breaches the confines of occasional use, it ceases to be a time-out activity. Thus, the time-out hypothesis does not always explain substance use behavior among youth.

Achievement Anxiety Theory

The time-out hypothesis essentially describes *escapist drinking* or *escapist using*—that is, drinking or drug use to escape role obligations of any sort. Misra (1980) outlined a model that describes substance use as an effort to escape a specific class of role obligations. This model proposes that a person uses substances in an attempt to evade the specific pressures of achievement and productivity. The person is not to blame for substance use; rather, the blame is on U.S. culture and its obsession with materialism, financial success, and personal achievement.

Achievement anxiety theory maintains that drug misuse is a response to a "fear of failure" (Misra, 1980, p. 212). It allows the person to withdraw from the pressures placed on him or her to achieve. At the same time, substance misuse induces and maintains a sense of apathy toward standards of excellence that U.S. culture defines as important. According to Misra (1980), one of the chief characteristics of technologically advanced countries such as the United States is anxiety about achievement. Obtaining or reaching socially prescribed goals can become a compulsion in itself (i.e., *workaholism*). Such competitive conditions cause people to feel anxious, fearful, inadequate, and self-doubting. As a result, many Americans are likely to rely on alcohol and drugs as a way to cope.

This also is true of persons in other countries and cultures where achievement and productivity are not only encouraged but expected. In Indonesia, for example, the stimulant methamphetamine had been sold in pill form in pharmacies beginning in the 1960s as a type of performance-enhancing drug. Cohen (2014) explains that it was commonly referred to as the "diligent drug" (*ya khayan*). Truck drivers and factory workers, for example, used *ya khayan* to work longer hours and to withstand manual labor. As methamphetamine use increased and became widely available on the streets, the Indonesian government implemented strict regulations in what Cohen describes as "a punitive and ruthless three-month 'war on drugs'" (p. 777). Indonesian youth who use methamphetamine today (now referred to as *ya bah*) do so for a variety of reasons, chief among them "to keep up with the demands and expectations of a modern capitalist society" (p. 781).

According to achievement anxiety theory, drugs are initially used to seek relief from the pressures of achievement and productivity. In effect, they provide a quick chemical vacation from the stresses of contemporary life. This conceptualization is quite similar to that of *time-out*. However, Misra (1980) further developed the concept by noting that continued misuse of drugs tends to reduce the difference between work life and leisure-time activities. In essence, the chemical vacations gradually change from being infrequent, temporary respites to full-time pursuits (i.e., addiction).

Minority Stress Theory

Persons who are members of racial and ethnic minority groups and those who identify with any other cultural minority group (e.g., lesbian, gay, bisexual, or transgender [LGBT]) are prone to chronic and high levels of stress simply because of their cultural minority status. Stressors include discriminatory actions (e.g., sexism in the workplace), hostile or micro-aggressive behaviors exhibited by dominant group members, and oppressive governments (e.g., regimes that ban and punish certain religions). Cultural minority stress emanates from direct and vicarious experiences. Persons of minority status experience cultural stress at both first and second hand, the latter by hearing of or having witnessed (e.g., through social media) the victimization of relatives, ancestors, and contemporaries. Cultural stress also can result from acculturation, attempts to assimilate, and efforts to balance two cultural heritages at the same time, referred to as bicultural stress. Alcohol, drugs, and other addictive behaviors can thus serve as an outlet for culturally related stress. As with social roles and achievement anxiety, cultural stress is a burden for which substance use offers temporary relief.

Meyer (2003) described *minority stress* as the excess of physical, mental, or emotional pressure, strain, or tension experienced by members of stigmatized cultural groups because of their minority status. She offered three underlying assumptions of minority stress: it is (1) unique and in addition to general stressors experienced by all persons, (2) chronic, and (3) socially based, stemming from social processes, structures, and institutions beyond the individual. Minority stress involves the experience of stressful events or conditions, the expectation of these events that requires vigilance, and the internalization of negative societal attitudes (e.g., internalized homophobia). In their meta-analysis of 15 studies exploring LGB youth and substance use, Goldbach, Tanner-Smith, Bagwell, and Dunlap (2014) found that general and LGB-specific stress was moderately correlated with substance use in LGB adolescents. The experience of victimization in particular, or threats of violence, was strongly correlated with substance use in this population. What Goldbach and colleagues were unable to detect, however, was the specific role of minority stress unique to being an LGB adolescent, separate from general stress.

Some research has been able to isolate the unique effects of racial discrimination experienced by African Americans on substance use. Thompson, Goodman, and Kwate (2016) sampled 144 black residents recruited from two predominantly African American neighborhoods in New York City. Participants reported experiencing discrimination in four settings or contexts: while getting service in a store or restaurant (69%), on the street or in other public settings (63%), getting hired or getting a job (57%), and from the police or in court (57%). Thompson and colleagues found that for each additional setting in which racial discrimination was reported, the likelihood of using alcohol problematically increased by one-third. They also found a significant association between reports of racial discrimination and currently smoking cigarettes. Their findings support previous studies that substance use among some African Americans is a form of coping to relieve stress from the experiences of racial discrimination.

Repudiation of Norms

A third function of substance use is to repudiate certain societal or other group norms. Think of this as behavior that "goes against the grain," "swims upstream," or "gives the finger" to conventional mores and norms, particularly those related to morality and economic productivity. One example is college students who establish their own weekend, beginning on Thursday and ending on Saturday. In their seven-semester longitudinal study of first-year college student drinking and other leisure behaviors at one large university, Finlay, Ram, Maggs, and Caldwell (2012) found higher rates of alcohol consumption on "social weekend" days (Thursdays–Saturdays) than on weekdays (Sundays–Wednesdays), particularly for women.

By definition, illicit substance use is a repudiation of state and/or federal laws governing substance use. The same is true for underage substance use. Although researchers predicted an increase in marijuana use for college students age 21 and older after recreational marijuana legalization in the state of Oregon, the reverse was true. Kerr, Bae, Phibbs, and Kern (2017) found that underage college students from seven different universities in Oregon increased their marijuana use after its legalization, whereas older students showed lower marijuana use rates. Marijuana use was strongly associated with alcohol use, particularly heavy alcohol use. And it was specifically underage marijuana and heavy alcohol users whose marijuana use exceeded that of their peers in states where marijuana use remains illegal. According to Kerr and colleagues, "given that these Oregon minors had consumed alcohol illegally, perhaps it is not surprising that they were similarly undeterred from underage use of marijuana" (pp. 1997–1998).

Prescription drug misuse is another example of use to repudiate norms. Persons who misuse prescription drugs have obtained the drugs from nonmedical sources or use prescription drugs for nonmedical or recreational reasons. Such use is antilabel, not following instructions, and may be associated with other non-normative behaviors such as theft. Young adults who misuse prescription drugs, however, may regard this behavior as unremarkable

(LeClair et al., 2015). From their 12-month ethnographic qualitative study of young adults who attended one of three music scenes (hip-hop, indie rock, and electronic dance music) in New York, Kelly and colleagues (2015) found that prescription drug misuse promoted certain behaviors (e.g., to enhance the effects of alcohol) and clashed with certain values or subcultural expectations, depending on the music scene. These included perspectives on authenticity, preferences for things perceived as natural, and the view that prescription drugs are not suitable for sharing. Kelly and colleagues concluded: "there are cultural dimensions to many youth cultures that both enable and inhibit particular forms of drug use. Although youth cultures are often portrayed as fomenting drug use, as cultural contexts they provide nuanced and varied influences on drug use" (p. 337). These nuances include establishing and promoting social boundaries.

Marking Boundaries

According to sociologist Michéle Lamont (1992), groups of people draw conceptual or symbolic boundaries to create distinctions between themselves and other people. These boundaries mark differences between outsiders and insiders, and signify commonalities among persons in the same group. Those on the outside do not belong; they are at a distance or estranged from members of the in group. Those on the inside belong; their connections with other members over time shape collective and individual identities. Persons are excluded or included according to criteria such as language, values, socioeconomic status (SES), and racial and ethnic identity. The demarcations established—which can be for generations—serve to define status and identity.

Substance use functions as a boundary marker. This means that alcohol and other drug use establishes group boundaries, defining who *we* are and who *they* are. This is true at macro levels (e.g., among religious groups), as well as at community or meso levels (e.g., neighborhoods, voting precincts) and micro levels (e.g., friend groups, gangs). The use of alcohol or drugs also shapes the images that individuals want or expect others to have of them. It is one source of identity. It solidifies a person's social identity and helps the person define him- or herself in reference to others. It also may earn social capital, such as social status.

Alcohol as a Boundary Marker

Anthropologists have identified numerous examples of how drinking has functioned to separate social and cultural groups and to promote cohesion within themselves. The American Temperance movement (1827–1919), described in Chapter 1, is one such example. During the 19th century, temperance groups were widespread in the United States. Initially, temperance groups sought to reduce the consumption of hard liquor and to promote drinking at home, as opposed to saloon drinking. This emphasis on temperance gradually gave way to a demand for abstinence. This led to quarrelsome disputes between "wets" and "drys," and eventually to Prohibition (1920–1933). However, the dispute actually represented deeper ethnic and social class conflict. According to Hart and Ksir (2018):

> Prohibition was not just a matter of "wets" versus "drys" or a matter of political conviction or health concerns. Intricately interwoven with these factors was a middle-class, rural, Protestant, evangelical concern that the good and true life was being undermined by ethnic groups with a different religion and a lower standard of living and morality. One way to strike back at these groups was through prohibition. (p. 190)

For those involved in the Temperance movement, abstaining (vs. drinking) was a social boundary marker. It served to promote a self-righteous pride within movement workers and was taken as proof that they were morally superior to those who drank alcohol. For the Temperance movement, abstinence was the source of group identification.

Of all cultural groups in the United States today, Native Americans (also referred to as American Indians and Alaska Natives) continue to have the highest rates of alcohol and drug use disorders (Grant et al., 2015). This is true particularly for the diagnosis of severe alcohol use disorder assessed for 12-month ("in the past 12 months") prevalence (7.7%) and lifetime ("ever") prevalence (27.2%). Fish, Osberg, and Syed (2017) found high rates of alcohol use among a sample of 144 Native Americans living on or near a local Indian reservation who endorsed stereotypical beliefs of Native American alcohol use, such as "Drinking is a tradition among Native Americans" and "Getting drunk is a pastime in our culture." This was true particularly of Native Americans who associated more with their cultural heritage (including those who lived on the reservation) than with mainstream or white American beliefs and behaviors. Findings suggest that for some Native Americans alcohol use may signify cultural identity. Among this group, drinking may serve two simultaneous purposes: It preserves a connection among its members, and it separates them from mainstream or white American culture. Fish and colleagues contend that such a belief "could be detrimental to those who are not oriented to the mainstream culture" (p. 241).

Illicit Drugs as Boundary Markers

Illicit drug use also promotes group identity and establishes racial and ethnic boundaries. One disturbing example in the early 1900s was the characterization of "lower class" Southern blacks as cocaine "fiends" who were a "menace" to society—that is, to whites—because they had been "deprived of whiskey" due to Prohibition (see Netherland & Hansen, 2016). Another frequently described example involves Chinese laborers brought to the western United States in the mid- to late 1800s to complete the arduous task of constructing new railroad tracks. They brought with them their practice of opium smoking. Opium dens were created as places to spend nonworking hours.

The practice of opium smoking never spread to other social groups. Local community leaders in many jurisdictions (who, of course, were white) passed legislation to forbid the practice. In general, most Americans viewed the use of opium by the Chinese with distaste and repugnance. Thus, for the white majority, opium smoking served as a significant social boundary. It was useful to them as a means of identifying who *we* (the good people) were and who *they* (the Chinese, the bad people) were. Furthermore, the drug experience (opium smoking) itself made apparent the distinctive value structures of the Chinese versus the white Americans. Opium smoking was consistent with the Chinese emphasis on reflection and introspection. It was at odds with the American orientation toward productivity, action, and settling the West.

Today, heroin use is much more prevalent among white Americans than among other U.S. racial or ethnic groups, including Asian Americans. The dramatic increase in heroin use from 2001 to 2013 is prominent among white individuals and reflects a significant racial gap in lifetime heroin use (Martins et al., 2017). Findings of one national household survey indicate that persons with opioid use disorder are 72% white (Wu et al., 2016). A similar racial divide is noted for prescription drug misuse.

White Americans as a whole have far greater access to health care (including addiction treatment) than do blacks. And blacks are disproportionately represented in the U.S. criminal justice system compared to whites. For middle- and upper-class whites, problematic drug use is considered a medical problem resulting from economic or emotional stress. For persons of color and lower-class citizens (including poor white Appalachians addicted to "hillbilly heroin"), problematic drug use is deemed a moral or even a characterological flaw, justifying their treatment as objects of extreme hostility.

The news media perpetuates these racial divides. From their analysis of 100 popular U.S. press articles from 2001 to 2011 on heroin and prescription opioid users, Netherland and Hansen (2016) unveiled subtle yet startling differences. News stories of suburban drug users (i.e., middle-class whites) garnered front-page headlines; their drug use was depicted as novel, shocking, and tragic, providing an example of squandered or "wasted whiteness." Their addiction was traced back to pain medication prescribed to them for an injury, their struggles with depression or anxiety, and their "falling in with the wrong crowd." The consequences of their drug use were a loss of productivity and potential. In contrast, urban drug users, those from primarily black and impoverished areas, earned only below-the-fold news coverage that was brief (compared to the news stories of whites), symbolic of a ho-hum reaction, as if such news is no news, news that is to be expected. The origins of their drug use and addiction were not considered, in stark contrast to the lengthy personal stories granted whites. The consequence of drug use for urban blacks in these news stories was criminality.

Netherland and Hansen (2016) contend that these media accounts make real "the notion that white and black drug use are different and separate—humanizing white drug users while perpetuating the association between black and Latino drug use, crime and violence" (p. 679). As a result, blacks and Latinos/Latinas regard this type of media coverage as another form of institutionalized racism.

Crossing Boundaries

Substance use not only creates and maintains sociocultural boundaries; it also crosses boundaries. These are demarcations of personal or family identity, social status, time, and states of consciousness. Geographical space—as in dance floors, campgrounds, and sporting sites—also may be a type of boundary. Dilkes-Frayne (2016) makes this argument in her ethnographic study of drug use at music festivals. These and other boundaries are crossed for a variety of reasons, many of which are similar to the functions already noted, such as relief from stress and anxiety, and enhancing social connection. What is distinctive about this fifth broad function of substance use is the transitional process itself: Substances are used to symbolize *departure from* one identity or status and *arrival into* another. Alcohol and drug use marks and facilitates these transitions. In doing so, new connections may be established, or a new state of consciousness may be experienced. This is the case when substances are used to connect with a transcendental or divine being, as in some spiritual and/or religious practices.

Several boundaries and their transitions are worth noting. Alcohol is often used to celebrate personal and family milestones, such as weddings and college graduations. Some new fathers follow a tradition of distributing cigars to family and friends upon the birth of their baby. Members of some amateur and professional sports teams celebrate wins and championships by spraying one another with champagne on the field or in the locker room. Their fans also celebrate with alcohol the end of a losing season and the commencement of a victorious season.

Substances are also used to commemorate passages of time and to assist in the transition of time. Many persons drink coffee or other caffeinated beverages in the morning to help them transition from sleep to wakefulness. Those who smoke cigarettes may do so during breaks from work, and alcohol commemorates the end of a workday and the beginning of leisure time, as in the proverbial "happy hour." Other passages of time are recognized with substance use. The traditional midnight toast of champagne on New Year's Eve is but one example.

Symbolic Mediation and Commoditization

The boundary crossings described thus far generally reflect normative or nonproblematic substance use. The frequency and amount of substance use, such as nicotine and alcohol, determine in part whether a clinical threshold (e.g., DSM criteria for a substance use diagnosis) is met or crossed. When substances are used primarily to cross cultural group boundaries and temporal divides, they are regarded as *symbolic mediators*. They symbolize a transition from one place or social status or cultural group identity to another. They also are vehicles to alter consciousness for the purpose of connecting with a transcendent other. Ecstasy users in Hunt and Evans's (2008) study described a spiritual connection as a result of their use. In the process, substances mediate a divide (e.g., between human and divine) or facilitate the crossing (e.g., connecting with others outside my customary social group).

Social and cultural anthropologist Carlson (2006) depicted psychoactive substances as symbolic mediators "to help humans deal with a fundamental problem: our biological separateness from each other as well as our separateness from other culturally defined domains of reality" (p. 207). From his investigation of "banana beer" use among the Haya tribe in Tanzania, Carlson extrapolated the purposes of three forms of symbolic mediation: (1) to link perceived domains of reality that are culturally defined as separate (e.g., awake vs. dream state); (2) to mark transitions or boundaries with respect to some aspect of life, such as life status (e.g., birth, marriage) or daily or weekly routine (e.g., from work to relaxation), as we described earlier; and (3) to facilitate social bonding, consistent with the first sociocultural function of substance use. From a sociocultural perspective, these three purposes of substance use are acceptable and valid. They reflect social and cultural values and norms.

When substances are used to accomplish something beyond these three purposes, they cease to be symbolic mediators and have become commodities instead. Carlson (2006) defined a *commodity* as a consumable that brings profit and thereby can be misused. Substances that are commodities are owned, possessed, and traded; they are susceptible to increasing consumption and profits. They are not used to mark transitions or to connect with others, for example. They are not used to express cultural identity or social belongingness. Rather, they isolate and lead to self-destructive consequences. Carlson likened commoditized substance use to addiction. Its sole purpose is to reinforce self-pursuit and neurochemical adaptation. Whereas substances as symbolic mediators have beneficial effects (e.g., group cohesion, spiritual connection), substances as commodities are detrimental to self, cultural group, and society.

THE UPSTREAM SOCIOECONOMIC DETERMINANTS OF THE OPIOID EPIDEMIC

The upstream socioeconomic determinants of health are the "fundamental causes that set in motion causal pathways leading to (often temporally and spatially distant) health effects through downstream factors" (Braveman, Egerter, & Williams, 2011, p. 383). The upstream determinants or "drivers" of health outcomes are income inequality, racial discrimination, and other structural features of society (Alston, 2017; Hill & Jorgensen, 2018). Downstream factors are typically those determinants that are close (and apparent) to health outcomes and include behaviors, neighborhood conditions, workplace exposures, and many other variables. Although research has demonstrated the importance of the socioeconomic determinants of health (Braveman & Gottlieb, 2014), the public's understanding of them is quite limited. Most people believe the quality of one's health is the result of their genetic traits and the lifestyle choices they make, such as exercise, diet, smoking, and drinking. Few recognize the influence of macro-level factors on health outcomes.

Today's opioid epidemic is a good example of a health outcome produced by upstream socioeconomic determinants. The epidemic is essentially the consequence of a confluence of upstream determinants that are temporally and often spatially (including globally) removed from the individual user of these drugs. The discussion in the following sections identifies and describes nine of these macro-level drivers of the epidemic.

Skyrocketing Opium Poppy Production in Afghanistan

One upstream determinant is the United States' failed effort to eradicate opium poppy cultivation in Afghanistan (opium is the source of heroin). The United Nations Office on Drugs and Crime (2017) indicates that opium poppy production is skyrocketing in the country. The area of Afghanistan under opium poppy cultivation was estimated to be over 810,000 acres of land in 2017. This was a 63% increase in just 1 year and marked an all-time high in the country. Opium production grew to 9,000 metric tons, an 87% increase from 2016. Despite a 14% decrease in opium price per unit in 2017, the overall monetary value of the country's poppy crop increased by 55% because of the enormous increase in crop volume (United Nations Office on Drugs and Crime, 2017).

The poppy trade is a significant segment of the Afghanistan economy where approximately three million farmers make their living from the crop. The country is extremely poor. Employment opportunities in legal commerce are scarce. All of these factors contribute to the ready availability of inexpensive heroin in the United States; the latest report from the United Nations suggests that the problem is growing ever worse.

Chinese Production and Sale of Illicit Fentanyl for the Americas

Another upstream determinant of the opioid epidemic in the United States is China's production of illicit fentanyl. China is the primary source of the illicit fentanyl that arrives in the United States (U.S. Drug Enforcement Administration [USDEA], 2016a). The Chinese government claims that its use is not a problem in their country, so production of the drug appears to be for export to the United States and the Americas.

Fentanyl and its analogs are a type of opioid drug, that is, pharmacologically similar to morphine and heroin. However, fentanyl is 50 to 100 times more potent than morphine (USDEA, 2017b), and thus the risk of fatal overdose is very real. Like heroin, fentanyl ingestion is followed by intense euphoria, making it highly addictive. Nausea, fainting, and respiratory failure (or death) are the adverse effects of fentanyl use. In addition to the risks faced by users, fentanyl also presents a serious threat to first responders and law enforcement officials. In handling confiscated fentanyl, these officials must wear protective gear to avoid inhalation of the drug or direct exposure with the skin because it is possible for lethal doses to be accidentally ingested (USDEA, 2017b).

Prior to 2014, fentanyl powder was usually mixed into and sold as heroin. Frequently, the purchaser had no knowledge of the contents of the product. Beginning in 2014, law enforcement agencies in the United States began to discover counterfeit prescription opioid pills containing fentanyl. The counterfeit pills were similar in appearance to legally produced opioid medications. The current global supply chain for fentanyl begins in China (USDEA, 2016a). There, clandestine laboratories produce fentanyl powder and fentanyl precursors, and ship them via mail services to the United States, Mexico, and Canada. In addition, Chinese counterfeit fentanyl pills are smuggled into the United States from Mexico and Canada. Chinese fentanyl powder is pressed into pills in the United States, Canada, and Mexico, and sold in the country where the pills were manufactured or sold in one of these three countries. Some fentanyl powder from China continues to be mixed with heroin and sold as that drug in all three countries. Although U.S. laws require the DEA to be informed of pill presses being imported into the country, overseas vendors of pill presses frequently misidentify their products or ship them unassembled to evade detection by law enforcement.

The USDEA (2016a) reported that counterfeit fentanyl pills cost between $10 and $20 per pill in illegal drug markets in the United States. Bulk quantities of counterfeit pills with fentanyl can be bought for $6.50. The agency estimates that a kilogram of fentanyl processed into counterfeit pills could generate between $5 and $20 million in profit on the street, depending on fentanyl pill dosage.

The outlook of the USDEA (2016a, 2017b) for the fentanyl crisis is quite grim. The flow of illicit fentanyl into the United States is expected to continue to increase, and with it there will be more overdose deaths. The powder form of fentanyl is easy to obtain, the cost of manufacturing counterfeit pills is low, and the potential profits from sales are high. The agency is also concerned that fentanyl will begin to appear in a variety of nonopiate counterfeit pills, as producers look for ways to expand their profits.

The Great Recession and Widespread Unemployment

Another upstream determinant of the opioid epidemic appears to be the Great Recession of 2007–2009 during which the national unemployment rate in the United States reached 10.0% (U.S. Bureau of Labor Statistics, 2012). Recent cross-national research has documented the relationship between diminishing economic opportunity in some segments of the population, particularly middle-aged white men with a high school education or less and increasing mortality (Case & Deaton, 2015, 2017b). This phenomenon has been described as "deaths of despair," including deaths related to opioid and other drug use (see the subsequent discussion in this chapter). This association has been observed only in the United States and not other developed nations of the world.

Hollingsworth, Ruhm, and Simon (2017) examined these conditions in the United States more closely by analyzing data on deaths and emergency department visits due to opioid medication usage and their associations with macroeconomic conditions in the years 1999–2014. They found that as county-level unemployment rates increased by 1.0%, the opioid death rate (per 100,000 persons) rose 3.6% and emergency room visits for opioid overdose (per 100,000 persons) increased 7.0%. Local unemployment rates also increased the death rate for all drugs, but opioid deaths were the primary source. The relationship between adverse opioid events and unemployment was concentrated among whites. Hollingsworth and colleagues also conducted analyses at the state level and reported similar findings. The investigators concluded that during periods of economic decline, such as unemployment, some populations are more likely to cope with anguish and despair by using readily available opiate prescription medication. A question that remains unanswered is: Why has this relationship been found to disproportionately afflict middle-age whites in the United States?

The Politicization of Opioid Medication Production

By law, the USDEA (2016b) establishes aggregate production quotas (APQs) for Schedule I and II controlled substances on an annual basis. These quotas determine the total amount of controlled substances, including opioid medications, which are needed in the United States each year, including a reserve stock. After the DEA determines the aggregate quota for the nation, it then negotiates with pharmaceutical firms to determine their individual allocations. The DEA has authority to change a firm's quota at any time during the year if needed.

In 2015, members of Congress severely criticized the USDEA for poor management of their APQ process. The criticism centered around claims made by some members of Congress that the DEA was creating shortages of Schedule II substances and thereby leaving patients untreated for their pain. As a senior DEA official acknowledged in a 2014 letter to the U.S. General Accountability Office (GAO), establishing APQs "is a delicate balance" (Rannazzisi, 2014, p. 2). A GAO report (2015) contended that the number of drug shortages increased substantially after 2007, and it called for the DEA to better coordinate their efforts with the Food and Drug Administration to address the medication shortages. In turn, the DEA challenged the GAO assertions by finding fault with their analyses and claiming that the medication shortages were not severe and represented a grossly exaggerated narrative of the pharmaceutical industry.

Within a year, the political pressures applied to the USDEA came from the opposite direction; that is, they were allowing the pharmaceutical industry to flood the market with opioid painkillers. According to the *Washington Post*, Senator Richard Durbin stated in a Senate Judiciary Committee hearing with the DEA director at the time that oxycodone production jumped from 3.5 tons to 150 tons between 1993 and 2015 (Davidson, 2016). In this same time period, hydrocodone production increased 12-fold and fentanyl production 25-fold. The USDEA director did not dispute Durbin's figures and acknowledged, "I think we are part of the problem" (i.e., the problem of opioid addiction and overdose) (Davidson, 2016). Three months later, the agency announced that it was reducing the amount of almost every Schedule II opiate and opioid medication that might be produced in the United States in 2017 by 25% or more (USDEA, 2016b). As this review of the political pressures placed on the USDEA reveals, the federal government's erratic regulation of opioid medication production is an upstream determinant of the opioid crisis.

Industry Attempts to Change the Opioid Prescription Practices of Physicians

Prior to the 1990s, the risks associated with heroin use and opioid prescription medication were readily accepted in medical education and practice. However, this view began to change following the results of a handful of peer-reviewed studies conducted in the 1980s (e.g., Portenoy & Foley, 1986). In the 1990s, a national debate emerged about whether patient pain was being undertreated. Some argued that not treating chronic pain adequately was cruel and amounted to inhumane care. Responding to this narrative, in 1994 Purdue Pharma began developing OxyContin as a painkiller designed for long-term use. The giant pharmaceutical manufacturer introduced the new opioid painkiller to the market in 1996 amid an aggressive promotion campaign aimed not only at physicians, but pharmacists and nurses as well (Van Zee, 2009).

The primary aim of Purdue Pharma's campaign was to change the prescription practices of physicians—yet another upstream determinant of the opioid crisis (Keefe, 2017). From 1996 to 2002, Purdue Pharma directly sponsored or provided grant funds to carry out more than 20,000 educational programs on the clinical management of chronic noncancer pain using opioid pain relievers (Kolodny et al., 2015). As a result, between 1996 and 2002, OxyContin sales increased from $45 million to more than $1.5 billion (U.S. General Accounting Office, 2003a). As perceptions of opioid risk decreased among the public and the health care professions, the number of prescriptions written for opioid painkillers began to rise rapidly each year, leading many patients to develop addictions (Van Zee, 2009). In 2007, three Purdue Pharma executives pleaded guilty in U.S. federal court to criminal charges that they had deceived government officials, physicians, and their patients about OxyContin's risk of producing opioid addiction (Meier, 2007). The company agreed to pay $600 million in fines and other payments to resolve the case.

In 2010, when the Affordable Care Act was enacted in the United States, the law established the Open Payments Program (Centers for Medicare and Medicaid Services, 2017). One of the primary aims of this program is to collect information about the payments pharmaceutical firms and medical device companies make to physicians and teaching hospitals for travel, research, gifts, speaking fees, food and beverages, consulting, gifts, entertainment, space rental, and facility fees. Essentially, the Open Payments Program was created to monitor the potential influence of pharmaceutical payments on physician prescription practices.

Using data from the Open Payments Program, Hadland, Krieger, and Marshall (2017) determined the extent to which the pharmaceutical industry made opioid-related payments to physicians in the United States.

The investigators found that between August 2013 and December 2015, 375,266 opioid-related payments were made to 68,177 physicians (about one in 12 physicians in the United States). The total value of the payments was $46,158,388. In contrast, during the same time period, physician payments related to nonsteroidal anti-inflammatory drugs (NSAIDs or nonopioid painkillers) amounted to only $13,758. Payments related to abuse-deterrent opioids made up 20.3% of the dollars flowing to physicians, whereas 9.9% were associated with buprenorphine used in addiction treatment. A majority of the physician payments were for food and beverages. Hadland and colleagues concluded that the marketing of opioids to physicians needs further evaluation and continued monitoring.

Overprescription of Opiate Pain Relievers by Physicians

To overcome physician reluctance to prescribe opioid painkillers in the 1990s, Purdue Pharma and other pharmaceutical companies employed physician–representatives who delivered presentations at medical conferences where they claimed that the field of medicine had a mistaken understanding of addiction (Kolodny et al., 2015). In the latter half of the 1990s and the first decade of the 2000s, physician speakers declared that patients diagnosed with chronic pain did not possess the drug-seeking characteristics of drug addicts and thus would only rarely develop addictions. Furthermore, they downplayed withdrawal symptoms as "clinically unimportant" (see Portenoy, 1996, p. 300), and they overstated the benefits of long-term opioid use (Kolodny et al., 2015).

Today, the Centers for Disease Control and Prevention (2017a) advises physicians not to prescribe opioid pain relievers for chronic pain conditions. Unfortunately, recent research suggests that the prescription practices of some physicians has not changed despite the growing opioid epidemic. Barnett, Olenski, and Jena (2017) conducted a retrospective study examining data from a national sample of 215,678 patients treated by low-intensity opioid prescribers and 161,951 patients treated by high-intensity opioid prescribers in hospital emergency departments between 2008 and 2011. Patients in the study had not received prescription opioids in the prior 6-month period. The investigators compared patient rates of long-term opioid use during the 12-month period following their visits. There was a great deal of variation in physician opioid prescribing rates. Most important, long-term opioid use was about 30% higher among patients treated by high-intensity prescribers compared to patients treated by low-intensity prescribers. Barnett and colleagues concluded that prescription opioid addiction is often not the result of a random or chance exposure to an opioid prescription, but instead is at least in part determined by the habitual prescription practices of a subset of physicians.

Purdue Pharma Took No Action to Stop OxyContin Diversion to Drug Dealers

Under U.S. federal law, pharmaceutical firms are required to notify the DEA when customers submit suspicious orders of controlled substances to them (USDEA, 2017a). In addition, the DEA interprets federal law to mean that pharmaceutical firms have a duty to reject any order of controlled substances if they believe the customer is diverting prescription drugs to the black market. According to an intensive investigation by the *Los Angeles Times*, Purdue Pharma had 10 years of data indicating suspicion of illegal OxyContin trafficking and did not share this information with the DEA or other law enforcement officials (Ryan, Girion, & Glover, 2016). The *Los Angeles Times* reported that in regard to distributing OxyContin in the 2000s: "A former Purdue executive, who monitored pharmacies for criminal activity, acknowledged that even when the company had evidence pharmacies were colluding with drug dealers, it did not stop supplying distributors selling to those stores" (Ryan et al., 2016).

Political Influence of the Pharmaceutical Industry

Another upstream determinant of the opioid epidemic is the political influence of the pharmaceutical industry. The amount of money the pharmaceutical industry spends on political lobbying and campaign contributions is staggering. According to the Center for Responsive Politics (2017), the pharmaceutical industry has led all industries in political spending for many years. Over the past decade, the industry spent almost $2.5 billion on lobbying and campaign donations to members of the U.S. Congress (McGreal, 2017). In 2017 alone, the industry spent $132 million in political contributions to members of Congress. In the same year, 90% of the members of House of Representatives and 97 of 100 senators accepted campaign contributions from the pharmaceutical industry (McGreal, 2017). Much of this money was used to block laws that seek to regulate the distribution and prescription of opioid medications. The Center for Public Integrity notes that the industry spent $740 million over a decade lobbying Congress and a number of state legislatures in an effort to block regulation of their business practices and physician prescription practices (Perrone & Weider, 2016).

President Obama and Congress Tie the Hands of the DEA

In April 2016, President Barrack Obama quietly, and with no fanfare, signed into federal law the Ensuring Patient Access and Effective Drug Enforcement Act of 2016 (Public Law 114–145). Despite the human devastation produced by the opioid epidemic, the aim of the legislation was to weaken the authority of the DEA to block opioid prescription shipments in the U.S. drug distribution system. Prior to passage of the current law, the DEA could freeze shipments based on a legal standard of posing an "imminent danger" to the community, which provided DEA broad authority. Under the current law, the legal bar is much higher; that is, the DEA must demonstrate that a pharmaceutical manufacturer's action represents "a substantial likelihood of an immediate threat." Former DEA administrators have indicated that the agency will rarely be able to meet the current legal bar (Higham & Bernstein, 2017).

The Ensuring Patient Access and Effective Drug Enforcement Act was passed by unanimous consent of Congress, a parliamentary procedure that does not require individual Senate and House members to record a vote. According to a *Washington Post*/CBS *60 Minutes* investigation, President Obama and very few lawmakers understood the contents of the bill—with the exception of a handful of bill sponsors and co-sponsors (Higham & Bernstein, 2017). The investigation could not determine why the U.S. Justice Department supported the legislation. Justice officials would not speak to the press. Higham and Bernstein (2017) speculated that members of Congress believed that the DEA had been too aggressive in their enforcement efforts and that it needed to be reined in and develop a more collaborative approach in working with pharmaceutical manufacturers as partners.

DEATHS OF DESPAIR IN A POSTINDUSTRIAL ECONOMY

In an influential paper, Princeton economists Case and Deaton (2015) identified a striking increase in the all-cause mortality of middle-aged (ages 45–54) white men and women (non-Hispanic) in the United States for the period of 1999–2013. This mortality increase stood in contrast to decades of death rate decreases in this subpopulation. Case and Deaton found that this increase in middle-aged white mortality was found in the United States and no other developed nation. Moreover, in the United States, this mortality increase was not observed in middle-aged African Americans and Hispanics or in persons 65 years of age and older regardless of racial and ethnic status. Case and Deaton found that the mortality increase for middle-aged whites was explained mostly by elevated death rates associated with substance use and suicide. Among middle-aged whites, those with a high school education or less experienced the steepest increase in death rate. Middle-aged whites also reported diminished physical health, mental health, and ability to carry out daily living activity; chronic pain increases; and inability to work. In a subsequent paper on this problem, Case and Deaton (2017ab) found that these same trends continued to worsen through 2015; they referred to the phenomenon as "deaths of despair" (p. 398).

What is behind deaths of despair in the United States? Although the opioid epidemic plays a role, deaths of despair among those with lower levels of education are likely the consequences of structural changes in the economy (Case & Deaton, 2017b). Manufacturing output in the United States has grown over the past 30 years. However, the number of well-paying manufacturing jobs not requiring advanced education and training has plummeted. This is the result of labor moving overseas and computer and robotic technology replacing skilled labor in production processes (Desilver, 2017). In this postindustrial economy, there has been no growth in workers' wages (adjusted for inflation) for the last several decades, and the number of well-paying jobs for those without a college degree has fallen sharply (Case & Deaton, 2017a). The result is widespread under-employment and unemployment, rising poverty, depression, and hopeless-ness. The less-educated tend to blame themselves for their plight and turn to substance misuse, including opioids, to cope with their circumstances (Scutchfield & Keck, 2017). In the current political environment in the United States, it is not clear that sound national policy solutions will emerge to address the socioeconomic conditions that underlie substance misuse and suicide.

PRACTICING FROM A SOCIAL AND CULTURAL FOUNDATION

A sociocultural theory of addictive behavior lacks the distinctiveness and specificity of other theories and models covered in this volume. Unlike cognitive and behavioral or conditioning theories, for example, there are no codified or agreed-upon principles that explain addictive behavior and guide its practice to address addiction. As mentioned at the beginning of this chapter, sociocultural theory shares territory with other theories and is not readily discernible as its own standalone model. Nonetheless, enter-taining sociocultural perspectives to inform practice is essential for health care providers. Taking action encompasses a range of advocacy efforts (e.g., correcting misrepresentations in the news media and entertainment indus-try), comprehensive assessment practices (e.g., conducting a cultural inven-tory), and policy restructuring.

Corrigan and colleagues (2017b) identify several strategies to address addiction stigma, including self-stigma. Among these strategies are educa-tion and contact. The primary aim of education is awareness raising, which offers alternative perspectives for clients, students, family members, and the public to make reasoned decisions and take appropriate action. Disput-ing the erroneous belief that there is a medical condition known as "addic-tive personality" and noting the tendency of physicians (who typically have very little training in addictive medicine) to overprescribe opioids are two educational approaches. Contact involves taking the initiative to interact with and learn from persons who struggle with substance use. This can be in the form of attending in-person support groups, such as AA and Al-Anon, as well as groups that focus on managing mental illness, such as those sponsored by the National Alliance on Mental Illness (NAMI; *www.nami.org*).

For direct care providers, such as counselors, nurses, and intervention specialists, socioculturally informed practice entails assessing clients' and students' cultural identity, including their values and belief systems. Asking in a genuinely curious and neutral tone the reasons for their substance use can access these beliefs. We recommend beginning by asking: "What do you *like* about [a particular substance or behavior]? What do you *get* from using? What does using *do* for you?" Responses to one or all three of these questions generally capture what is important and valuable to the person, as well as the purpose or function of their behavior.

It also is important for direct care providers to assess the sociostructural or environmental influences that are and have been part of a person's life, such as experiences of racism and other forms of discrimination. As reviewed in this chapter, substance use can be a means of coping with and surviving societal and other institutional oppressive forces. Learning that substance use is a means to an end and not an end in itself can enhance empathy and decrease self-stigma and open the door to pursuing alternative and feasible health-promoting behaviors. These behaviors include those taken not only by the recipients of care, but also by the providers themselves. One such action is consulting with advocacy groups, such as NAMI and the Legal Action Center (LAC; *https://lac.org*). The LAC provides free resources and support for criminal justice, substance use, and HIV/AIDS concerns. Specific to substance use, the LAC has successfully litigated cases involving employment discrimination and breaches to the longstanding U.S. federal law concerning the confidentiality of drug and alcohol client records.

A final socioculturally informed practice is worth noting. It is not a practice imposed on others by health care professionals, industry executives, or politicians. Rather, it is the proactive practice of members of sociocultural groups themselves, such as injection drug users (IDUs). This "insider" practice is a collection of strategies known as *intraventions*. Friedman and colleagues (2004) coined the term *intravention* to characterize the harm-reduction activities developed and implemented by group members to nurture the health of their fellow group members. From interviews conducted with 120 primarily Latino/Latina (78%) IDUs in Brooklyn, New York, Friedman and colleagues found that 83% had engaged in at least one other-directed prevention activity in the past 3 months. These activities included urging others not to use drugs, urging fellow IDUs to use needle exchanges, and urging condom use for those who had begun a new relationship. The authors concluded that "the common image of IDUs as being little more than sources of social and medical problems is inaccurate." A majority of

IDUs, Friedman and colleagues reported, "had actively urged other persons to take actions that can protect themselves and others against blood-borne or sexually transmissible infections" (p. 258). They encouraged professionals to include IDUs as active participants in their own care planning.

CHAPTER SUMMARY

Sociocultural perspectives suggest that health care providers must be aware of basic human values in working with individuals and communities. Sociocultural analyses do not pass judgment on the "correctness" of the values of persons engaged in addictive behaviors; instead, they serve as relatively impartial analyses of the social phenomena under scrutiny. If sociologists describe a drug subculture as placing a low priority on economic productivity, they are not insisting that such persons are "lazy." They are simply pointing out that the value structure of those who misuse substances emphasizes other pursuits and that this structure deviates from that of the larger culture.

Those who struggle with substance use may balk at attempts to encourage serious introspection and self-assessment of their behavior. This response may reflect a value structure that elevates social relations, fun, and amusement over rational self-control and serious self-understanding. These conflicts are crucial issues to be uncovered, clarified, and discussed when attempting to help a person with a substance use problem. Many, perhaps most, clients are unaware of their value priorities and of how these priorities relate to their substance use. Although it may be painful, practitioners should help clients bring these issues to the foreground of consciousness while maintaining an objective attitude toward the clients' value structure. This also is true for educators who work with students in a school setting.

As a basis for prevention programming or treatment planning, there are two major limitations to sociocultural concepts. First, many of these concepts do not seem salient to the practice guidelines of medical and human services professions. This may be particularly true of the concepts *social boundary markers, subcultures, conduct norms,* and *time-out.* Critics have occasionally charged that sociocultural theorists are the sideline observers of the drug scene. Their concepts provide intellectual insight but are not helpful in enhancing the direct delivery of treatment services.

The second limitation pertains to the relative inability of prevention and treatment practitioners to significantly alter the social, cultural, and environmental factors that contribute to substance use and misuse. This is apparent in reviewing contributions to the "deaths of despair" discussed earlier. In this vein, sociocultural perspectives may be viewed as intellectual curiosities that provide fodder for stimulating conversations among academics but are of little practical value because these social variables cannot be readily addressed. This lack of practicality is likely to prevent sociocultural perspectives from gaining more prominent status among theories on addictive behavior. It is the challenge of professionals who are both scholars and clinicians to do so—those with graduate degrees who have clinical and/or administrative responsibilities for one or more systems of care, such as schools and treatment facilities.

REVIEW QUESTIONS

1. What is meant by the *medicalization of addiction?*

2. What are the five basic sociological functions of substance use? How do they explain substance use and substance misuse?

3. What explains the recommendation not to use the term *substance abuse* or to refer persons who misuse substances as *substance abusers?*

4. What are the effects of *addiction stigma* for persons struggling with substance use? What can be done to reduce addiction stigma among health care professionals?

5. What are the upstream socioeconomic determinants of the opioid epidemic, and how do they contribute to the crisis?

6. What is meant by "deaths of despair" and what conditions created it?

7. How might the resources provided by advocacy groups such as NAMI (*www. nami.org*) and LAC (*https://lac.org*) be incorporated into prevention and treatment services?

8. What are *intraventions,* and how might professionals and community members promote their practice?

9. What are the limitations of applying sociocultural concepts to addiction prevention and treatment?

CHAPTER 10

The Controversial Science
of Behavioral Addiction

History teaches us that the concept of addiction is in a continual state of flux. In the last decade or so, one of the most important changes to the concept has been the diminishing role assigned to tolerance and withdrawal symptoms. In traditional definitions of addiction, these neurobiological features were centrally positioned, with great emphasis placed on the need of the brain to adjust to chronic, repeated exposure to high doses of alcohol and/or other drugs. This emphasis waned as more attention was directed to drug self-administration as conditioned behavior—that is, a class of activities maintained by the pharmacological rewards provided by drugs. Understandably, as focus shifted to reinforcement mechanisms and the brain's reward circuitry, questions began to be raised about whether addiction can be defined apart from drug taking, *and* how far the concept should be expanded to encompass other pathologies associated with excessive reward seeking, including gambling, eating, having sex, and shopping (Billieux, Schimmenti, Khazaal, Maurage, & Heeren, 2015). This fundamental shift in scientific and clinical perspective ushered in the notion of *behavioral addiction*.

Behavioral addiction, also referred to as *process* or *non-substance-related* addiction, can be defined as a pathological involvement in a drug-free activity that exposes persons to mood-altering stimuli that produce pleasure or relieve pain. More simply, these are activities that have potential for producing excessive reward seeking without drug ingestion. According to Shaffer's (2015) conceptualization, behavioral addiction can be thought to have three primary features:

1. Presence of aberrant psychophysiological responses when exposed to specific environmental cues.
2. Continued involvement in the behavior despite experiencing negative consequences.
3. A perceived inability to reduce engagement in the activity (perceived loss of control).

DSM NOMENCLATURE
AND DIAGNOSTIC CRITERIA FOR ADDICTION

The *Diagnostic and Statistical Manual of Mental Disorders* (DSM) is the most widely used nomenclature for classifying mental disorders in the United States. All disorders recognized by the American Psychiatric Association have specific diagnostic criteria identified in the manual. In addition to use in clinical settings, researchers rely on the diagnostic criteria to study the etiology and treatment of mental disorders, and to document the prevalence and incidence of these disorders in the population.

A major aim of the American Psychiatric Association's (2013) current edition, DSM-5, was to establish a stronger scientific basis for the diagnosis and classification of psychiatric disorders. Substance use and addiction nomenclature underwent substantive revisions in DSM-5. The name of the major category *Substance-Related Disorders* found in DSM-IV-TR was changed to *Substance-Related and Addictive Disorders* in DSM-5 (American Psychiatric Association, 2013). A second revision involved the terms *abuse* and *dependence*. These terms were omitted in DSM-5, and in their place the term *substance use disorder* was used for separate classes of drugs. These disorders are rated on a severity continuum ranging from *mild* to *severe*. In addition, DSM-5 does not use the term *addiction* because of the ambiguities and negative connotations associated with it. A fourth DSM-5 revision was that *Substance-Related and Addictive Disorders* included one behavioral or *non-substance-related disorder*: gambling. This represented a significant change in that DSM-IV-TR classified pathological gambling as one of the *Impulse-Control Disorders Not Elsewhere Classified*. In DSM-5, *gambling disorder* was grouped with Substance-Related and Addictive Disorders, and other non-substance-related disorders were considered future candidates for inclusion in DSM's Substance-Related and Addictive Disorders category as justified by an expanding research base.

It is also important to point out the distinction between behavioral addiction and impulse-control disorders (ICDs; Fauth-Bühler, Mann, & Potenza, 2017). This distinction can be confusing because some disorders, such as pathological gambling, have been referred to as both addictions and ICDs in different versions of the DSM. How are they different? Going forward, behavioral addictions such as gambling will be considered to be similar to substance addictions in that they both involve actions that generate pleasure. In contrast, ICDs will be thought to involve repetitious actions intended to reduce distress. However, the line separating the hedonic features of behavioral addiction from the stress reduction features of ICDs may become blurred as the addictive activity becomes less pleasurable over time and motivated increasingly by a desire to escape from dysphoria (Fauth-Bühler et al., 2017). Therefore, it may be difficult to distinguish the two types of disorders in some cases.

Evolution and Addiction

The theory of evolution has been used primarily to explain biological changes in species. However, in the past decade or so, scientists who study the neurobiological basis of addiction have relied on it not only to explain alcohol and drug dependence, but addiction to non-substance-related behavioral processes as well. The key concept in the theory of evolution is that through a process of natural selection, species evolve by adapting to environmental challenges. Organisms that develop advantageous traits will be more likely to survive and therefore transmit their genetic information to offspring, compared to those failing to develop such traits. Thus, over time, fewer and fewer member organisms with nonadvantageous traits will survive, and their genetic contribution to the species will gradually diminish and disappear.

In the primitive human brain, neural networks are thought to have evolved to adapt to short-term survival and to increase the likelihood of reproduction. Life expectancy in the human ancestral environment (Pleistocene epoch) was relatively short, and many adaptations are thought to have centered on reproduction, which led to increases in the size of the human population (Wall & Przeworski, 2000). Brain functions that today we consider beneficial for modern life, such as long-term planning functions and attention to long-term consequences, were much less relevant to survival in the Pleistocene Age. Thus, the forces of natural selection are thought to have fostered development of pleasure centers in the mesolimbic dopamine pathway of the brain to reinforce those behaviors most necessary for survival, such as eating food and having sex (see Figure 2.3 in Chapter 2). It is by evolutionary design, then, that these behaviors provide immediate rewards in the form of pleasure. The design also helps us understand why humans find it so difficult to resist the ubiquitous opportunities for immediate pleasure in the contemporary world.

In support of this evolutionary view of brain development, provocative research in the last decade suggests that gambling, eating, and having sex activate the same reward circuitry in the brain as do commonly used drugs (Gola et al., 2017; Volkow, Wise, & Baler, 2017). Unfortunately, in the contemporary world where opportunities for food, sex, drugs, and any number of other rewarding substances and behaviors are ever-present, the presence of these pleasure centers serve us less well than they did our early ancestors. Intended to promote human survival, the original design of the brain has been coopted or "hijacked" by the easy availability of modern pleasures. Moreover, the relentless introduction of Internet-based activities exacerbate addiction risk. Online gambling, gaming, shopping, pornography, instant messaging, and overuse of social media use are among the behaviors that can be problematic (Ioannidis et al., 2018).

One way to think of addiction (of any type) is that it represents a modern-day malfunction of an adaptation that once served our ancestors well in a harsh environment. Unfortunately, there is little hope that the neural networks of our brains will adapt fast enough to keep pace with the developing technologies we find so attractive today. Thus, from an evolutionary point of view, we are all vulnerable—not only to alcohol and drug abuse, but to any number of activities, games, foods, and the like, that evoke neural signals in the brain's pleasure centers. For proponents of the behavioral addiction concept, this evolutionary perspective is a critical lynchpin in the argument for expanding the concept of addiction to non-substance-related activities (Linden, 2011). Believing that natural selection is responsible for the presence of brain pleasure centers unlocks them from viewing addiction as exclusively a problem of alcohol and other drug abuse.

Narrow, reductionist explanations deeply rooted in neuroscience alone also raise challenging questions about the brain circuitry–behavioral addiction connection. For example, why are behavioral addictions not more widespread among humans? Why are they not the cross-cultural norm? How do people who regularly engage in hedonic pursuits manage to avoid developing problems? Questions such as these challenge the proposition that the evolution-designed brain is a sufficient basis for expanding the concept of addiction to include non-substance-related activities. This chapter critically examines controversies surrounding the concept of behavioral addiction.

MANAGEMENT OF NEGATIVE PUBLICITY
BY PUBLIC FIGURES

If the concept of behavioral addiction becomes widely accepted in society, from time to time public figures will likely turn to it as a strategy for minimizing media ridicule and securing public forgiveness following disclosure of inappropriate or scandalous behavior. This function is akin to the notion of *time-out* (Heath, 1988); that is, a socially unacceptable action is excused because the actor was intoxicated by alcohol (see Chapter 9). In recent decades, a number of American public figures, primarily men involved in gambling and sex scandals, have put forth claims of behavioral addiction.

Described here are brief stories of five well-known persons from the sports and entertainment industries, as well as the pastoral community, who have made public claims of behavioral addiction.

• *Wade Boggs, baseball player.* Wade Anthony Boggs was born on June 15, 1958 (National Baseball Hall of Fame, 2018). His 18-year Major League Baseball career was spent primarily with the Boston Red Sox. He was inducted into the Baseball Hall of Fame in 2005. *Sporting News* (1998) ranked him 95th on their list of 100 greatest players in baseball history.

In 1989, Boggs was at the center of a media-driven scandal involving his off-field activity (Swift, 1989). A female mortgage broker from California disclosed to the media that she'd had a 4-year extramarital affair with Boggs (who was married). After he broke off their relationship in 1988, the woman filed a $12 million lawsuit against Boggs for emotional distress and breach of oral contract. The woman claimed that Boggs had verbally agreed to compensate her for lost income and "services performed" while accompanying him on Red Sox out-of-town road trips during the baseball season. Boggs did not deny the affair, but mounted his own media campaign to defend his actions and to refute many of the woman's claims about their relationship. At one widely reported meeting with the press, Boggs claimed that he was in recovery from the disease of sex addiction. His comments set off a media frenzy, and they remain a stain on his reputation today.

• *David Duchovny, actor and director.* David William Duchovny was born on August 7, 1960. He has appeared in a number of television shows and feature films during his acting career. He won Golden Globe awards for his television roles in *The X-Files* and *Californication*. In the latter television series, Duchovny played a journalist beset with conflicts often involving sex, alcohol, and drugs.

In 2008, he entered a program for the treatment of sex addiction. There was considerable speculation in the entertainment world that Duchovny's personal life and his role in *Californication* could not be easily distinguished from each other (Fisher, 2008; Marikar, 2011). Duchovny is believed to be the first celebrity from the entertainment world to specifically cite *sex addiction* as his motivation for seeking treatment.

• *Ted Haggard, evangelist pastor.* Ted Arthur Haggard was born on June 27, 1956. He was founder and former pastor of a 14,000-member evangelical church in Colorado Springs, Colorado, and from 2003 to 2006 he was leader of the National Association of Evangelicals. The latter position provided him with a national platform for promoting conservative Christian views on social issues, such as gay marriage and homosexuality.

After being accused of participating in a 3-year cash-for-sex relationship with a male prostitute from Denver, Colorado, Haggard was forced to leave his church position. The Denver man was apparently motivated to expose Haggard because the pastor had made public comments condemning homosexuality that the male prostitute believed to be hypocritical (Associated Press, 2006). At the time, Haggard acknowledged being in contact with the man, admitted to sexual "immorality" and to purchasing methamphetamine, but claimed he'd never used the drug. He subsequently entered a 12-step program for the treatment of sex addiction and later stated that, although he is a recovering sex addict, he is not homosexual. According to Haggard's website (*http://tedhaggard.com*; accessed September 1, 2012), he now leads a second church in Colorado Springs.

• *Pete Rose, baseball player.* Peter Edward Rose was born on April 14, 1941 (National Baseball Hall of Fame, 2018). He played Major League Baseball from 1963 to 1986, and managed professional teams from 1984 to 1989. He holds several Major League Baseball records, most notably as the all-time leader in career hits (4,256). Rose was named Rookie of the Year; played on three World Series Champion teams; won three league batting titles; once was named league Most Valuable Player; won two Gold Glove awards; and appeared in 17 Major League All-Star Games.

Three years after he retired in 1989, Rose agreed to a permanent separation from Major League Baseball in an attempt to address accusations that he had violated league rules by gambling on baseball games as a player and as a manager of the Cincinnati Reds, including betting on games played by his own team. After many years of denying that he had bet on baseball, Rose (2004) confessed in a *Sports Illustrated* interview that he had indeed bet on baseball games as a player and manager. In the article, Rose claimed that he suffered from an addiction to gambling and reported receiving treatment for the problem. At the time, some speculated that Rose might have confessed in an attempt to sway public opinion about his ban from the Baseball of Hall of Fame, which continues to block his induction today, despite his outstanding baseball records. His ban from the Baseball Hall of Fame remains a controversial issue among sportswriters and fans (Heller, 2011).

• *Art Schlichter, football player.* Arthur Ernest Schlichter was born on April 25, 1960. He is a former college and professional quarterback well known for his troubled life resulting from his persistent involvement in theft and embezzling schemes to secure funding for his gambling activity. Schlichter was arguably the most celebrated high school quarterback in Ohio football history (MacGregor, 2000). He subsequently played at Ohio State University (1978–1981), where he was the last quarterback to play for legendary Coach Woody Hayes. He then joined the Baltimore/Indianapolis Colts in 1982 as the overall number-four selection in the National Football League rookie draft. As a result of his serious gambling and legal problems, Schlichter never lived up to his potential on the football field. He appeared in just one preseason game in 1986, in what would be his last year in the

National Football League. The NFL Network (2011) rated Schlichter as the number-four "draft bust" in league history.

Schlichter has identified himself as a gambling addict for many years (Wagner, 2011). To finance his gambling activity, Schlichter estimated that he had stolen at least $1.5 million from friends and strangers by 2007. He was convicted of more than 20 felonies, mostly fraud and forgery convictions. From 1995 to 2006, he served 10 years in 44 jails and prisons across the Midwest. After prison, he may have owed as much as $500,000 in restitution to various parties. In 2009, Schlichter and his mother appeared on television in Ohio delivering political announcements in opposition to a statewide casino ballot issue. In March 2011, he was once again jailed on felony charges alleging that he had swindled a Columbus-area widow out of more than $1 million to support his gambling habit (Wagner, 2011).

POPULAR CLAIMS AND THE RESEARCH EVIDENCE

Today, gambling and sexual activities are not the only problems being defined as addictions. In popular culture as well as in some segments of the mental health treatment and self-help communities, a large number of behaviors that produce harm for self and/or others are now claimed to be addictions. The Internet is populated by websites that define and describe these problems in living and offer help, sometimes including 12-step recovery programs. However, these popular notions may be based more on pseudoscience than on evidence-based science.

We employed Shaffer's (2015) three key diagnostic symptoms (noted previously) to evaluate involvement in harmful non-substance-related activities of abuse as possible behavioral addictions. In this diagnostic scheme, individuals experiencing problem behavior must possess attentional biases for craving-related stimuli (Smeets, Roefs, & Jansen, 2009). This means that they must experience cravings when exposed to specific stimuli associated with the behavior, or the stimuli must trigger speeded detection, heightened engagement, greater sustained attention, or slower disengagement from the stimuli. The second criterion is that the person with a potential behavioral addiction persists in maintaining the harmful activity even though he or she is penalized in some way for these actions. The third criterion is that the person believes that he or she is unable to refrain from future involvement in the activity.

Our review of the existing literature review found scientific support for no more than five possible behavioral addictions, based on Shaffer's (2015) criteria. At this time, the strongest scientific support probably exists for gambling, followed by growing, but not yet compelling, support for Internet use (including social networking), video gaming, overeating, and skin tanning.

Our observations are consistent with past literature reviews on behavioral addiction (e.g., Grant, Potenza, Weinstein, & Gorelick, 2010). The existing literature also indicates that the activities identified as behavioral addictions appear to frequently co-occur with other problems such as depression, anxiety, and substance abuse. Prevention and treatment strategies need to anticipate the clustering of these problems within affected individuals.

Free-Market Drivers of Excessive Consumption and Hedonic Pursuits

Our contemporary society has been negatively characterized as a consumption-based culture focused on immediate gratification (Alter, 2017; Bryant-Jeffries, 2001). All manner of products and services are marketed to consumers who have available to them a large number of hedonic attachments and activities, which are often affordable, that can facilitate adoption of maladaptive behavior. Although it may be simplistic to claim that a toxic social environment is the cause of excessive consumption, we certainly must recognize that our free-market economy supports and accentuates myriad problems that may be defined as *behavioral addiction*. In his analysis of the social consequences of globalization, Alexander (2001) goes even further to say that "addiction is mass produced in free market society" (p. 2). In this section, we provide an overview of the contemporary free-market, technological, and social conditions that support five putative behavioral addictions. Internet access is a significant support for two of these activities: gambling and Internet use (including social networking).

Gambling

Legal gambling is a big business today. In the United States, the state-regulated gambling (gaming) industry is composed of nearly 1,000 casinos in 39 states and state-sponsored lotteries in 44 states and the District of Columbia. According to a gaming industry trade report, casinos alone generate about $81 billion in revenue each year (Oxford Economics, 2014). This same report claims that in 2013 commercial casinos paid $38 billion in local, state, and federal taxes, and supported employment for 1.7 million people. Offering some perspective on entertainment preferences, one should note that Americans spent almost 3.5 times more money at casinos than at movie theaters! In 2013, Americans lost $119 billion through gambling, an amount that far exceeded amounts in other developed countries of the world (Brandt, 2014). The top five states for casino-generated consumer spending in 2012 were Nevada ($10.9 billion), New Jersey ($3.1 billion), Pennsylvania ($3.2 billion), Indiana ($2.6 billion), and Louisiana ($2.4 billion).

Internet Use

Internet access is an expectation of most Americans and part of their daily routine. In 2015, 77% of Americans reported that they had Internet access in their home (Ryan & Lewis, 2017). Broken down by age, 85% of 35- to 44-year-olds indicated that they had home Internet access, followed by 15- to 34-year-olds (81%), 45- to 64-year-olds (81%), and those 65 years of age and older (63%). Racial/ethnic differences are relatively small, though African Americans and Hispanics are somewhat behind Asians and whites. Educational attainment and income disparities do appear to persist in home Internet access. For example, in 2015, 91% of persons with at least a bachelor's degree indicated that they had home Internet access versus only 49% of persons with less than a high school degree (Ryan & Lewis, 2017). Americans with annual incomes of at least $150,000 were more likely to report home Internet access (96%), than those who earned less than $25,000 (52%). Overall, home Internet access appears to be highest on the east and west coasts of the United States and lowest in the Southeast and much of Appalachia (Ryan & Lewis, 2017).

In January of 2018, the Pew Research Center found that YouTube was used by 73% of American adults, compared to 68% using Facebook (Smith & Anderson, 2018). However, among those ages 18 to 24, platform use varied a great deal, with 78% using SnapChat and a large majority of these users (71%) visiting the platform many times a day. The Pew report found that the average American uses three of the eight major social media platforms (Smith & Anderson, 2018). Pinterest is much more popular among women (41%) than among men (16%). LinkedIn is much more widely used by college graduates and in high-income households. Among American Hispanics (49%), the messaging service WhatsApp is popular, but this appeal does not extend to whites (14%) or to blacks (21%). Although a majority of Americans now use one or more platforms, 59% do not believe they would have difficulty giving up social media (Smith & Anderson, 2018).

Overeating: Binge-Eating Disorder and Food Addiction

Among Americans 20 years of age and older, 38% of women and 34% of men were estimated to be obese in 2011–2014 (Ogden, Carroll, Fryar, & Flegal, (2015). These U.S. prevalence rates represent a 7 percentage point increase over the level of obesity that had existed during the period 1999–2000. This trend is a major public health concern because obesity is a risk factor for chronic medical problems such as diabetes, hypertension, elevated cholesterol, stroke, heart disease, arthritis, and some cancers (Maffetone, Rivera-Dominguez, & Laursen, 2017). Equally alarming are the health care costs attributable to obesity. These costs increase each year, and they are shared by all citizens whether obese or not. For example, in the United States in 2015, total medical expenses of obese adults were estimated to be about $500 billion compared to about $420 billion among normal-weight adults (Biener & Decker, 2018). Extremely obese adults incurred an average of $7,800 in yearly medical expenses, which was about 76% more than that experienced by normal-weight adults. In addition, prescription drug use, across a number of different therapeutic classes, was significantly higher among obese adults than among normal-weight adults (Biener & Decker, 2018).

In their explanations of the modern obesity epidemic, policy researchers have come to describe developed countries as *obesogenic* environments (Ananthapavan, Peterson, & Sacks, 2018; Townshend & Lake, 2017). *Obesogenic* refers to social conditions that have made overeating and obesity normal biological conditions. The major alterations in societal work conditions, daily transportation, and the production, distribution, and sale of food have made obvious the human biological tendency to gain weight under sedentary living conditions. Through natural selection, our metabolic systems evolved to allow us to engage in sustained vigorous physical activity needed to survive in the human ancestral environment. In this view, individuals are not particularly gluttonous or lazy today, but rather have a biological system for weight maintenance that is no longer in step with modern lifestyles.

The global obesogenic environment is thought to have become pervasive during the past 40 years or so (Swinburn et al., 2011). The primary drivers of this environment are within the food production and distribution system, including the increased supply of inexpensive, palatable, and energy-dense foods; greatly improved food distribution systems that make it easy to obtain foods; and industry marketing practices that have been persuasive in leading people to increase their energy intake beyond energy needs (Butland et al., 2007). Additional drivers include modern jobs that do not require vigorous physical activity; heavy reliance on motor vehicle transportation rather than walking and other forms of transport that require physical effort; leisure and recreational activities devoted to television watching, computer use, video games, and other sedentary pursuits; and government failure to recognize and address these basic societal changes (Townshend & Lake, 2017).

Skin Tanning

American consumers spend a large amount of money on indoor tanning services, on products to reduce skin cancer risks related to outdoor sun exposure, and on products to treat skin damage caused by sun exposure. The *indoor tanning industry* provides services to consumers at on-premise salons. The *sun care products industry* sells three types of over-the-counter products from retail outlets: sun protection, self-tanning, and after-sun skin repair. These services and products are used to expose consumers to, and protect them against, ultraviolet (UV) radiation from both the sun and artificial sources, such as tanning beds and sun lamps. There is no question that UV radiation, from any source, including indoor tanning facilities, increases risk for cancer (U.S. Preventive Services Task Force et al., 2018).

In 2017, it was estimated that the U.S. indoor tanning industry generated $2 billion in revenue from 13,586 salons that employed 35,570 persons (IBIS World, 2017). Fortunately, these numbers represent a steep decline in the use of retail tanning services since 2010. Among non-Hispanic, white women, ages 18 to 29, indoor tanning dropped by about 30% from 2010 to 2015 (Guy et al., 2017). Growing public concern about skin cancer seems to be the driving force behind the decline of the indoor tanning industry. However, outdoor tanning does not seem to be in decline. Market research companies expect the sale of sun care and sun protection products to continue to increase through at least 2024 (e.g., Transparency Market Research, 2016).

Challenges to Redefining Pleasurable Activities as Behavioral Addiction

Obviously, the market conditions described here exist because of our inborn drive for pleasure. This is a universal human experience. Motivation, learning, and even survival are based, at least in part, on the experience of pleasure. Various forms of pleasure motivate us to engage in a wide range of behavior, including eating, drinking, having sex, gambling, working, engaging in recreation, and serving others (Linden, 2011). Different forms of learning—ranging from academic to social—are shaped by rewards involving pleasure. Of course, sexual pleasure is integral to human reproduction, ensuring that our species produces future generations.

However, individuals and societies have long been conflicted about the experience of pleasure, producing a fear of succumbing to hedonistic pursuits perhaps because they are an ever-present distraction from the often mundane or tedious routine of daily existence (Shaw, 1996). Thus, through the centuries all cultures have developed legal codes, religious doctrine, and social customs to restrict access to and regulate pleasurable activity deemed immoral conduct. Interested readers should acquaint themselves with St. Augustine's Christian treatise "On the Good of Marriage" (Kearney, 1999), as well as passages in Chapter Four of the *Holy Qur'an* (An-Nisaa, Verse 15) for notable historical examples of doctrine warning against sexual pleasure. In the modern era, societal concerns about pleasurable activities have focused heavily on restricting youth access to them. Zimring (1998) noted that those pleasures about which adults are most ambivalent or conflicted are those we tend to quickly prohibit our teenage children from partaking in (e.g., smoking, alcohol use, gambling). The cross-cultural ambivalence about pleasure has been recognized by Linden (2011), who notes that the following ideas and conventions exist in all societies:

1. Pleasure should be sought in moderation.
2. It is important to earn pleasure.
3. Naturally achieved pleasures are more acceptable.
4. Pleasurable activities should be transitory.
5. Spiritual growth can be aided by the denial of pleasure. (p. 3)

Despite findings from a growing number of neurobiological studies suggesting that substance addictions and behavioral addictions arise from a common neurobiological substrate (Volkow et al., 2017), their interpretation does not necessarily lead to the conclusion that so-called *behavioral addiction* represents a mental disorder (Frances, 2017). In their argument, neurobiological researchers contend that in the contemporary world, there has been a commandeering or overriding of the pleasure circuitry in the brain; that is, addiction is simply a malfunction of a specific neural network originally designed for our ancestral environment. Such an explanation can be considered a classic example of *methodological reduction* in science (Bechtel & Richardson, 1993). This is the idea that biological systems are best studied at the lowest possible scientific domain and that the benefits of science are maximized by discovering causes at the molecular and chemical level. The longstanding argument against this exclusively reductionist approach to science is that by setting aside multilevel analyses, which may include higher-level environmental, social, and psychological factors, the risk of systematic bias in research is increased. This bias may obscure our understanding of phenomena under study. As applied to behavioral addictions, the basic question is whether these problems in living can be adequately explained as well as treated by concepts, explanations, and methods derived almost exclusively from neurobiological research.

As noted in Chapter 3, there is often a collision of views about how to improve the health of human populations (see Figure 3.1). On one side is the traditional biomedical approach, which often favors biological reductionism and focuses on the characteristics of individuals and access to medical treatment as the primary determinants of health status. On the other side is the approach of the progressive public health movement, which arises from a collectivist social philosophy that is more holistic and ecological, focusing on multilevel determinants and interventions (Galea, Riddle, & Kaplan, 2010; Huang, Drewnowski, Kumanyika, & Glass, 2009; McKinlay & Marceau, 2000). Progressive public health proponents are skeptical of using evidence, limited largely to molecular biology research, to reduce problems in living to mental disorders by describing them in new psychiatric nomenclature as *behavioral addictions*. The concern is that by medicalizing such problems, we fail to recognize the larger system of contributing causal factors that are "upstream" from a manifest case of behavioral addiction. For instance, many of the activities now being considered for classification as behavioral addictions are mediated by rapidly developing computer software applications (gambling, video gaming, texting, pornography, etc.). Such diverse forces as engineering advances in integrated circuits, business marketing strategies, and social diffusion of innovations, which influence the introduction, adoption, and impact of computer "apps," would be among the many upstream, indirect determinants of these behavioral problems from a multilevel, systems perspective.

In addition, serious questions can be raised about the less obvious social functions of promoting the behavioral addiction concept. A useful framework for analyzing the social consequences of an expanded definition of addiction is to apply the notions of manifest and latent functions, as described by distinguished American sociologist Robert K. Merton (1910–2003). In regard to the aims of social actions, Merton (1968) believed that there were two types of distinctive forces in operation in society. *Manifest* functions are those consequences of social action that people expect to occur and are communicated by those participating in the same action. In contrast, *latent* functions are those social consequences that are not intended or recognized by the parties involved in introducing, implementing, and carrying out the action. The intention of manifest functions is obvious and explicitly stated by proponents, whereas latent functions require interpretation that goes beyond the motives recognized and expressed by its proponents. In many cases, manifest functions are supported by propaganda; that is, a set of justifications for action are employed that perhaps may be ahead of compelling evidence, or as Gambrill (2010) defines it, are "encouraging beliefs and actions with the least thought possible" (p. 302). In her analysis of helping professions, Gambrill contends that the propaganda of the movement to expand the application of psychiatric diagnoses (including behavioral addiction) to an ever-greater range of human activity serves to reduce the challenges and complexities faced by practitioners. For example, critical thinking about the problems presented by a client becomes unnecessary, and uncertainties about prospects for insurance reimbursement (for services rendered) are diminished. Furthermore, the introduction of new psychiatric nomenclature offers practitioners "ready-made opinions for the unthinking. . . . It decreases anxiety and prevents confusion about 'what to think.' . . . It allows us to identify with the heroes of society. It provides group belonging" (Gambrill, 2010, p. 307). The seductive and dangerous aspect of helping profession propaganda is that it can create a world view in which practitioners believe their toolkit is adequate for addressing the problems they face, or, as Ellul (1965) observed, "It permits him [or her] to participate in the world around him [or her] without being in conflict with it" (p. 159).

Now, it is obvious that in expanding the concept of addiction, the manifest purpose of helping professions, such as the American Psychiatric

Association, is to extend and improve care for groups of sufferers who are underserved in the current health care system. Indeed, a past president of the American Psychiatric Association noted that DSM-5 would assist clinicians with making more useful diagnoses (Bernstein, 2011). Of course, this is a commendable aim. However, another distinguished psychiatrist, in commenting on the prospect of DSM-5 including behavioral addiction as a psychiatric disorder, argued: "In a statistical sense, it is completely 'normal' for people to repeat doing fun things that are dumb and cause them trouble. This is who we are. It is not mental disorder or 'addiction'—however loosely these much freighted terms are used" (Frances, 2010).

We should not ignore the social consequences of redefining addiction, and we should not be naïve about claims made by helping professions (Conrad, 2007; Gambrill, 2010). Analysis of the larger societal context suggests that a number of latent or unintended functions are associated with officially recognizing the diagnosis of behavioral addiction. First, the culture of psychiatry and mental health treatment will be further infused into everyday life. Questions can be raised about whether this infusion operates to reduce the influence of other value and belief systems informed by different ethical, philosophical, or religious principles. Are the so-called *behavioral addictions* medical/psychiatric conditions or simply foolish indulgences? Does redefining a problem in living as a behavioral addiction help persons avoid the moral dilemmas arising from their problem behaviors? If so, is it a benevolent goal in service of the person labeled an *addict*?

Second, expanding the definition of addiction will significantly extend the authority of mental health professions to determine the boundary between normal and abnormal human behavior (Horgan, 2011). Is it wise to leave the boundary line to a relatively small group of experts? Will these experts shrink the range of normality? Will they become promoters of social conformity? How will they apply the notion of personal responsibility in arriving at their clinical judgments?

Third, official recognition of the behavioral addiction concept will inevitably lead to the demand for funds to support research to investigate the problem. Given that these funds are a finite resource, is behavioral addiction an important future direction for research investment? Will it become a research priority with potential for draining money away from other critical lines of inquiry? Skeptics argue that many of the putative behavioral addictions are trivial in their consequences, as compared to alcohol and drug dependence, and thus have potential to divert attention from higher-priority substance abuse problems. On the opposite side of the debate, proponents of the concept argue that enhancing research into behavioral addiction has the promising prospect of discovering new "crossover" medications that can effectively treat both substance addictions and non-substance-related addictions (Frascella, Potenza, Brown, & Childress, 2010).

Legal and Health Care Implications of Defining Behavioral Addictions as Medical Conditions

The legal system in the United States has been built largely on the doctrine that the conduct of individuals is freely chosen (Colasurdo, 2010). *Mens rea,* or the intent to commit a prohibited act, is a major component of individual responsibility in this system (Mack et al., 2005). With the introduction of problematic gambling as a behavioral addiction in DSM-5, a host of contentious questions will likely arise about the legal and social implications of redefining compulsive, non-drug-related, problem behaviors as medical conditions (Frances, 2010). The central issues in this debate will focus on colliding beliefs about the legal doctrine of intent. Arguments will divide persons on matters of personal responsibility for which blame can be assigned and on whether intense cravings and perceived loss of control truly represent medical conditions (Shaffer, 2015). At issue: Under what conditions, and to what extent, will conditions referred to as *behavioral addiction* mitigate personal responsibility? Clearly, an expanded definition of addiction offers the prospect of extending help to many persons who need assistance. However, new social problems may be created by recognizing these new disorders (Gambrill, 2010).

One concern of critics is that expanding the definition of addiction has potential to create "false epidemics" (Miller & Holden, 2010, p. 771). This concern is not based on conjecture. The front-page news story of *Newsweek* magazine (December 5, 2011) read: "The sex addiction epidemic. It wrecks marriages, destroys careers, and saps self-worth. Yet Americans are being diagnosed as sex addicts in record numbers. Inside an epidemic." Frances (2010), a distinguished psychiatrist who chaired the American Psychiatric Task Force that developed DSM-IV, worried that

> during its history, psychiatry has gradually, but consistently, spread its purview. In the first official diagnostic system for the United States, developed in the mid nineteenth century, there were six diagnoses intended to be used mostly for inpatients. Now we have close to three hundred mental disorder diagnoses covering all sorts of problems that straddle the boundary of normal. The "behavioral addictions" would be another great leap forward pushing mental disorder into the shrinking realm of normality. Eventually having one, or several, mental disorders would become the new normal. (p. 2)

Colasurdo (2010) asserts that, if the legal system were to recognize behavioral addiction as a medical disorder, the impact would be greatest in three areas: employment and disability law, family law, and criminal sentencing. The Americans with Disabilities Act (1990) prohibits employer discrimination against qualified individuals "on the basis of disability in regard to job application procedures, the hiring, advancement, or discharge of employees, employee compensation, job training, and other terms, conditions, and privileges of employment" (Section 12112). Although the Americans with Disabilities Act expressly excludes compulsive gambling, substance abuse disorders, and a number of other mental health problems as disabilities, there appears to be little in the law that prohibits broadening the category of qualified disability. Thus, successful claims of workplace discrimination based on behavioral addiction could possibly occur in the future. In family law, acceptance of behavioral addiction as a medical disorder could affect divorce and child custody decisions (Colasurdo, 2010). Claims by one spouse against another spouse could allege that a behavioral addiction impaired the partner's ability to be a suitable mate or impaired his or her ability to function as a parent. In criminal sentencing, defendants could be given reduced sentences if they were found to be suffering from a reduced mental capacity because of a behavioral addiction (Colasurdo, 2010). For instance, might a person charged with soliciting prostitution or rape claim he or she suffers from sex addiction? Or might a person faced with theft charges contend that he or she is disabled by an addiction to shopping?

Other concerns about expanding the definition of addiction to non-drug-related behaviors focus on the health care system and the possibility that it would increase costs. A major fear is overidentification of "addicted" patients needing treatment. What proportion of overweight patients would be diagnosed by their physicians as food addicts? Would the large number of persons who work long hours need treatment for workaholism? Some psychologists are not alarmed by the prospect of recognizing behavioral addiction, contending that its prevalence is probably underestimated in society. They actually speculate that "addiction is a natural state of affairs as a human being" (Sussman, Lisha, & Griffiths, 2011, p. 46).

Concerns also focus on the enterprising nature of pharmaceutical companies and the likely scenario that they would turn their attention to developing and marketing new medications to aid physicians in treating these "medical conditions" (Horgan, 2011). This advertising practice has for some time been known as *disease mongering* (Moynihan et al., 2002; Payer, 1992). It is not difficult to imagine the pharmaceutical industry pitching new medications for hypersexuality or binge eating. Of course, the net effect of directing resources to these newly discovered addictions would be to add costs to our society's already overly expensive health care system.

CHAPTER SUMMARY

Recognition of behavioral addiction in DSM-5 by the American Psychiatric Association will not resolve the controversy about expanding the concept of addiction to include non-substance-related problem behaviors (Yau &

Potenza, 2015). Adoption of the concept of behavioral addiction will elicit new debates about where to draw boundaries between normal and abnormal behavior, and about how far we should go in applying the medical model to the classification of human behavior. Of course, the controversy will also invite new clashes between law and psychiatry over matters of personal responsibility and who gets to make decisions about blameworthiness and culpability. Concept expansion would seem to have potential for adding to the costs of health care and open new markets for the pharmaceutical industry that some will argue are more exploitative than curative.

Considerable scrutiny will likely be given to the standards of evidence used by the American Psychiatric Association in any future consideration of adding candidate behaviors to the behavioral addiction category. Neither should we expect that multidisciplinary interpretation of the research evidence will produce incontrovertible conclusions that resolve the controversy. Opposition to extending the concept beyond substance (alcohol and drug) addictions will continue, as will opposition to extending it beyond pathological gambling (the problem behavior with the most support in the neurobiological literature). Many critics, including quite a number within the mental health professions, will contend that defining non-substance-related activities as addiction amounts to trivializing the serious problems of alcohol and drug dependence. At the same time, there will likely be mental health professionals and groups and a self-help community that will lobby in different ways for a continually expanding concept of behavioral addiction. They will contend that the science is adequate for expanding the concept; that a knowledge base in support of it will only grow further with time; and that many additional needy persons will seek treatment as a result of recognizing behavioral addiction. Indeed, the history of the DSM suggests that, with the passage of time, the general psychiatric nomenclature will expand rather than contract.

REVIEW QUESTIONS

1. In the past decade or so, which features of addiction have been given more emphasis and which have been deemphasized?

2. According to Shaffer (2015), what are the three primary features of behavioral addiction?

3. What substance abuse and addiction-related changes are included in DSM-5?

4. Why did the human brain evolve in such a way that it includes pleasure centers?

5. Which non-substance-related behaviors, claimed to be addictive, have at least some scientific evidence to back them?

6. What are the free-market drivers of gambling, Internet use, overeating, skin tanning, and video gaming?

7. When evaluating the scientific evidence supporting behavioral addiction, why might it be a problem to rely exclusively on neurobiological research?

8. What are important challenges to the concept of behavioral addiction?

9. What are the negative legal and health care implications of adopting the concept of behavioral addiction?

10. Does the current scientific evidence support the behavioral addiction concept? Or is it largely a view based on propaganda as defined by Gambrill (2010)?

CHAPTER II

Promoting Motivation and Autonomy for Personal Change

There are clear distinctions among the theories of addiction reviewed in this book. Explanations differ with respect to the etiology, maintenance, and prevention and treatment of addiction. What is common across these theories is the role of motivation. This underscores Baumeister's (2016) contention that motivation is a primary human process, explaining all human behavior.

Heather (2005) characterizes addiction as a disorder of motivation. More specifically, addictive behaviors are manifestations of abnormalities in the motivational system (West & Brown, 2013). West and Brown describe this system as "a set of brain processes that energise and direct our actions" (p. 8) specifically in the present moment (see *www.primetheory. com*). These processes encompass internal influences (e.g., physiological and affective states, cognitive constructions such as values) and external influences (e.g., environmental factors, including people). It follows that a disorder, abnormality, or disruption in the motivational system due to the effects of addiction is incapacitating; it prevents the person from responding in the moment and autonomously to internal and external influences in healthy ways. It curtails living a meaningful life (see Heintzelman & King, 2014).

THEORIES OF MOTIVATION

Human motivation has been studied scientifically for over 100 years (Bernard, Mills, Swenson, & Walsh, 2005; Ryan & Deci, 2017). The earliest theories of motivation focused on the biological aspects of human behavior. These comprised largely unconscious mechanisms, such as needs, drives, and instinct. The next generation of theories defined motivation in strictly behavioral terms, as an automatic process shaped by environmental influences and satisfying basic organismic requirements such as hunger and sleep. Chief among the environmental influences is social context and interaction. From this perspective, motivation is behavior that satisfies the need for belongingness, cohesion, and approval from others. Around the time of behavioral explanations for human motivation was the advent of cognitive theories of motivation that replaced earlier drive theories. These cognitive explanations included considerations of expectancy and psychological values. Consistent in these versions of motivation through the last century is that motivation is a unitary construct and thus is only or primarily understood in terms of quantity, as in how much motivation a person has. Only recently has motivation been studied with respect to type, quality, and orientation.

Current theories of human motivation attribute behavior to specific cognitive processes such as expectancies, values, self-concepts of ability (e.g., self-efficacy), and future-time orientation (e.g., goal theory). One of these theories, self-determination theory (SDT; Ryan & Deci, 2017), assumes that humans are growth-oriented organisms whose behavior is pursued to satisfy three basic and universal needs: autonomy, competence, and relatedness or belonging. SDT distinguishes between autonomous motivation and controlled motivation. Autonomous motivation is defined as self-governing and intrinsically regulated behavior that expresses and is consistent with one's values. Controlled motivation, by contrast, is contrived behavior that often is regulated by extrinsic forces such as laws and rules, social approval, and economic security. According to SDT, psychological well-being is the product of intrinsically motivated and autonomous behavior. We return to this theory later in the chapter.

According to Ainslie (1992), none of the major theories of motivation explains addictive behaviors in an adequate fashion. A multidimensional concept of motivation therefore is indicated, one that can account for, or explain, the broad reach of addictive behaviors, including biology and physiology (e.g., genetics, craving states), specific observable behaviors (e.g., self-administration of a drug), cognitive processes (e.g., expectancies), and emotion. Bernard and colleagues' (2005) evolutionary theory of human motivation is multidimensional and incorporates many of the constructs that pertain to addictive behaviors. It defines human behavior as purposeful and ultimately oriented to the survival of one's genes, what Bernard and colleagues refer to as *inclusive fitness*. This evolutionary perspective, distinctive among the theories of motivation, specifies 15 purposeful behaviors that may be useful in understanding addictions (e.g., curiosity, safety, play, meaning). However, Bernard and colleagues' evolutionary theory may be too comprehensive to explain the particularities of addictive behaviors.

The PRIME Theory of Motivation

Specific to theories of addiction is the multidimensional or synthetic theory of motivation that West first proposed in 2006 and has since revised (West & Brown, 2013). It is referred to as the *PRIME theory of motivation*. PRIME is the acronym for its five primary components. This theory assumes that the human motivational system operates at the levels of Plans (intentions or conscious mental representations of future actions, including commitment), Responses (starting, stopping, or modifying actions), Impulses and inhibitory forces (e.g., urges, drives, emotional states), Motives (experienced as desires, wants, and needs), and Evaluations (beliefs about what is good or bad). All five components interact with one another in a dynamic fashion to explain human motivation; they are not sequential, and one component is not primary.

Below, we apply the PRIME theory of motivation to the case of Gary. Notice how each of the PRIME theory components explains Gary's motivation to continue to smoke cigarettes. The first letter of each PRIME component is underlined, as they are in the preceding paragraph.

> Gary is a maintenance worker on the campus of a large university that recently instituted a tobacco-free policy. He has been employed there for many years, plans to retire in 2–3 years, has been a smoker since he was 16 years old, and believes the new policy is "another form of discrimination against those of us who smoke" (his evaluation). He does not intend (or plan) to stop smoking. From the lens of the PRIME theory, Gary's deliberate intention (or plan) to walk alone and take an alternate route from one building to another on campus on a particular work day (and stop in a cluster of trees near the border of campus) can be understood as a response to an impulse or urge to smoke, generated by a desire or need (motive) for decreased anxiety and calm that he believes (or evaluates) as favorable. The impulse to smoke on that particular morning is also in response to an argument Gary had earlier with a coworker about smoking that raised his level of distress (an emotional state or motive).

Redvers (2007) praised the first draft of the PRIME theory of motivation (West, 2006) for its common sense. However, the PRIME theory may be too simplistic; it also may be too broad or inclusive to account for the vicissitudes of addictive behaviors. Nevertheless, it is useful in its description of a motivational system applicable to addictions, and it does centralize the role of motivation in understanding addictions. To learn more about the PRIME theory of motivation (and view a diagram of the five components), go to *www.primetheory.com*.

A Preview of Other Theories and Models of Motivation

The evolution and integration of theories of human motivation have contributed to the development of approaches to the prevention and treatment of substance use problems that target motivational processes, including more autonomous or self-governing behaviors. These include the transtheoretical model (TTM) and its stages of change dimension, motivational interviewing (MI), and, as mentioned, SDT. We describe each of these three approaches in the remainder of this chapter, along with three others that facilitate motivation for change and promote autonomy: harm-reduction approaches, mindfulness-based approaches, and twelve-step facilitation (TSF). The focus is clinical in nature; that is, the emphasis is on how practitioners can guide students, clients, and other interested persons toward beneficial personal change.

WHAT IS MOTIVATION?

Despite its everyday use and the abundance of motivational theories, the concept of motivation remains little understood. Is it a "thing" a person has or does not have, or has in different quantities or to varying degrees, as in "He just doesn't have enough motivation to stay clean"? Is it something like willpower that somehow can be manufactured, implied in the statement: "I need to get myself motivated"? Is it a condition that develops—or regresses—over time, such as the so-called (and now widely disputed) *amotivational syndrome* associated with chronic marijuana use? Or is it a personality trait that is relatively stable over time and, as a result, defines an individual and explains his or her general behavior? This version is implied when the reason given for a person's failure to enter treatment is that he or she simply is not motivated and the person is then told: "Come back when you're ready."

The conclusion of a vast amount of motivational research in the behavioral sciences, including addiction, is that motivation is none of these entities. It is not a "thing" or a condition that people have in their possession, nor is it a stable and permanent trait that defines an individual. It is a complex interplay of internal and external forces that stimulate and direct behavior. It is, as Bernard and colleagues (2005) explain, "what animates us, what prompts our initiation, choice, and persistence in particular behaviors in particular environments" (p. 137). As such, motivation is expressed in behavior; it implies behavior. Indeed, the two are inseparable. This is evident in the etymology of the word *motivation,* which originates from the Latin words *motus,* meaning "to move," and *motivus,* or "of motion." According to Draycott (2007), what prompts or influences a particular behavior (i.e., motivation) cannot be separated from the behavior itself, further complicating efforts to define motivation.

Motivation as Purposeful Behavior

Human motivation is best understood as *purposeful behavior*. It is "the *why* that causes an organism to initiate and persist in certain behaviors as opposed to others" (Bernard et al., 2005, p. 134, original emphasis). West and Brown (2013) argue that motives "[lie] at the heart of purposeful behavior" (p. 200). Although purposeful behavior takes place only in the present moment, its focus is (unconsciously or consciously) on the future. Current behavior is therefore always in service of, or a function of, an imagined or anticipated goal or outcome. According to Bernard and colleagues (2005), motivation or purposeful behavior involves "if–then" thinking, where *if* is the mental image of desired or intended behavior (e.g., drinking) and *then* is the mental image of the result of engaging in that desired behavior (e.g., relaxation). This cognitive process is consistent with expectancy theory and goal theory, but it is only one aspect of motivated behavior, as seen in the theories of motivation mentioned earlier—evolutionary theory and PRIME theory.

Understanding motivation as purposeful behavior helps explain addictive behaviors and is useful in devising methods for preventing and treating problematic substance use. Motivation understood as purposeful behavior rejects a generic, all-encompassing explanation of addiction because motives (e.g., values) are plentiful, context- or environment-specific, and often person-specific. Knowing what propels and sustains activity cannot be surmised from observation alone, as is done in animal studies; it only can be understood by asking the person(s) engaged in the behavior. Doing so prevents erroneous assumptions and misguided decision making on the part of prevention and treatment practitioners.

Learning the purpose or function of a behavior requires direct interaction with, and listening to, an individual with substance use problems or persons from a targeted population at risk for developing addiction (e.g., low-income adolescents exposed to repeated trauma). One way to do this is to ask about the benefits of substance use, such as "What do you like about smoking weed? What's the payoff for you?" Simons, Correia, Carey, and Borsari (1998) found that the primary motives for adolescents and young adults to use marijuana were to enhance positive experiences ("It's fun and exciting") and to expand personal qualities and traits ("I want to know myself better, be more creative, and understand things differently"). These motives differed from the primary motives for drinking alcohol, which were to be social ("It improves parties") and to conform ("So others won't kid me about not drinking"). Asking someone about the specific motives or reasons for substance use supplies more personalized and credible information that may prove useful in constructing tailored prevention and intervention strategies.

Viewing motivation as purposeful behavior also rejects the idea of perpetual inertia, "stuckness," or "amotivation" and suggests an amenability to change. Persons are motivated to do something, even if that something is avoidance behavior (e.g., *not* drink, *not* finish school) rather than approach or proactive behavior (e.g., work a recovery program, graduate). Remember that West and Brown (2013) describe motivation as the forces that energize and direct human behavior on a moment-to-moment basis. This implies that forces are always present to incite behavior, and once these motives are brought into awareness and understood and accepted, more self-governing or self-regulated and autonomous behavior can be shaped and exerted.

This implication also applies to impulsive behavior, which Bernard and colleagues (2005) regard as the opposite of self-control. Madden and Johnson (2010) define *impulsivity* as the "tendency to act on a whim and, in so doing, disregard a more rational long-term strategy for success" (p. 11). Impulsive behavior is evident in the phenomenon of delay discounting: the practice of devaluing or discounting the value of an outcome because of the delay in its arrival. The longer one has to wait for something of value (e.g., money), the less valuable it becomes and the more likely the person will not wait for it. Immediate and smaller rewards (e.g., $10 now) are preferred to later or deferred and larger rewards ($50 in 2 weeks). The field of behavioral economics suggests that a range of behaviors, including impulsive behaviors, can be shaped through the use of money and other tangible rewards. (Delay discounting and behavioral economics are described more thoroughly in Chapter 6.) What is important to an individual—what he or she values—is a significant aspect of human motivation that, according to self-determination theory, fuels both intrinsic and extrinsic motivation.

Feather (1987) defined *values* as "a particular class of motives" that has "an oughtness quality about them" (p. 39). He argued that values influence behavior but do not have the character of a goal. Whereas *goals* manifest primarily as cognitive representations that direct behavior toward specific possibilities or outcomes (Elliot, McGregor, & Thrash, 2002), values are guiding principles of life that organize a person's attitudes, emotions, and behaviors (Kasser, 2002). More so than goals, *values* have an enduring quality to them and thus retain some consistency across time and different situations. Learning what is important to a person, what he or she values or wants out of life, is therefore useful in understanding and then shaping his or her purposeful behavior or motivation. One way this is done in motivational interviewing is to ask persons to sort through a stack of cards, each containing a one-word or two-word value statement, such as *simplicity, faithfulness,* and *popularity,* and then to rank the cards according to their level of importance. Known as the *personal values card sort* (accessible at *http://casaa.unm.edu*), this activity helps individuals make sense of and then prioritize what is important to them in order to guide their decision making and to cultivate behaviors that are more consistent with their values. This process can foster more autonomous or self-regulated and authentic behavior.

Motivation as Practice Centerpiece

Only in the past 50 years has the assessment of human motivation become a central feature and an essential function of prevention and treatment practices in the addictions. This is due in part to an expanded view of addiction, namely, that multiple factors contribute to addiction and to its resolution or management. Addiction is no longer viewed in either–or terms. Dated dichotomies have been replaced with dimensions (see Miller et al., 2011). What once was construed as client "denial" or "resistance" is now regarded as a low level of motivation or readiness to change on the motivation dimension. The revision made by the American Society of Addiction Medicine (ASAM) to *The ASAM Criteria* exemplifies this change (see Mee-Lee, Shulman, Fishman, Gastfriend, & Miller, 2013). Compared to earlier versions that used the dichotomous label "treatment acceptance/rejection" for one of the six client dimensions to assess for level of care, the current version of *The ASAM Criteria* labels that dimension as simply "readiness to change."

Motivation has assumed a more prominent role in general psychotherapy as well. According to Ryan, Lynch, Vansteenkiste, and Deci (2011), this change is attributed to a greater focus on eclecticism and integrationism—or combining different theories and approaches—and to the increased emphasis on short-term counseling by funding sources (e.g., private insurance), making the assessment and incorporation of client motivation early on in the treatment process that much more important. Addressing client motivation in counseling and psychotherapy also is important because the majority of clients present with very low or poor motivation to change and a substantial number of them fail to attend the first counseling session after intake (Ryan et al., 2011). To a great extent, client engagement and persistence in counseling depend on the counselor's ability to connect with the client's motivation (see Miller et al., 2011). West and Brown (2013) maintain that this begins with how the counselor poses the first question. For example, rather than asking the client, "Do you want to stop smoking?" counselors should say, "We have quite a few methods available to help persons stop smoking, and I'd encourage you to give one of them a try." The question posed prompts a negative image in the client's mind, whereas the statement prompts a more promising image or outcome. Cultivating positive images of change in clients is one way clinicians can help clients "tie themselves" to their self-regulating capacity or their ability to change, an important type of motivation.

Several models and practices specifically target and prioritize motivational factors and autonomous or self-regulatory processes in their application. The three models we discuss in the following sections were developed in the early to mid-1980s, and two of them originated from the addictions field: the transtheoretical model (TTM) and motivational interviewing

(MI). The third model, self-determination theory (SDT), is a general theory of personality and began as an exploration of what determines intrinsic motivation. SDT has since been applied to the addictions field, whereas the TTM and MI have expanded their applications beyond the addictions field to physical health (e.g., exercise, nutrition), mental health (e.g., depression, anxiety, eating disorders), and public health (e.g., safe drinking water practices), to name a few. Each of these three models and practices has been compared to and integrated with one or the other two, and evidence suggests that any two in combination are compatible and complementary. Kennedy and Gregoire (2009), for example, found that combining the TTM and SDT for the treatment of persons with substance use disorders provided a more comprehensive view of motivation than either model offered independently.

As you read about the TTM, MI, and SDT in the following sections, we encourage you to think of *conditions* (plural) that enhance or diminish client motivation to change, and to refer to helping professionals who *facilitate* (or forestall) motivation to change in people, rather than to professionals who motivate people. These two recommendations are consistent with the four essential aspects of human motivation emphasized in this chapter:

1. Motivation is not the result of one single source. There is no such thing as direct causation or a singular mechanism of action. Believing otherwise perpetuates what DiClemente (2015) calls naïve simplicity.
2. One external source (e.g., clinician) cannot effect change (i.e., motivation) in another person. No one motivates another. Motivation is not made; it is facilitated.
3. One internal source of motivation (e.g., belief, value, intention) does not necessarily effect behavior change. In other words, *knowing* does not automatically translate into *doing*. Galvanizing interpersonal and contextual motivation (or autonomy support systems) therefore is important.
4. A person is not either motivated or unmotivated. Although SDT refers to amotivation, the legitimacy of this concept is disputed in MI.

TRANSTHEORETICAL MODEL OF CHANGE

The TTM is a model of how individuals intend to change their behavior (DiClemente, 2003; Prochaska & DiClemente, 1982; Prochaska, DiClemente, & Norcross, 1992). Originally, it was developed to understand the process of change that took place in persons who were successful in modifying their nicotine use behaviors, whether or not they made use of

formal intervention, such as counseling. Its theoretical structure is integrative, which explains in part its *trans*theoretical name: It "cuts across" and
combines existing theories. It also transcends existing theories by offering
something new: a theory of when and how people change.

The focus of the TTM is on intentional and self-initiated change rather
than on societal, developmental, or imposed change (Prochaska et al., 1992).
It presumes that most change is gradual and ongoing, not instantaneous
and dramatic, as is characteristic of quantum change, or the experience of
sudden, surprising, and permanent personal transformation (Miller, 2004;
Miller & C'de Baca, 2001). There also is no accounting for happenstance
in the TTM. The TTM therefore is concerned with how people intend to
initiate behavior change and the nature of the process of change once it
has commenced. As such, the TTM seeks to understand and to promote a
person's own and self-reported intentions to change. Nuttin (1987) defined
intentions as a cognitive activity that exists at the preperformance stage
of doing (i.e., behavior) and serves as a motivational force for behavioral
action. Expressing an intention to change suggests a self-assessed readiness
and ability to perform a certain task sometime in the future.

The TTM depicts a temporal sequence of change and identifies common processes or activities that propel behavior change from one time
period to another. The model comprises three dimensions: processes, levels,
and stages of change. Processes in the TTM are common activities, tasks,
behaviors, or strategies that correspond to and mobilize change. They help
explain *how* change occurs over time. There are 10 processes of change in
the TTM, equally divided into cognitive–experiential strategies and behavioral strategies. Cognitive–experiential strategies include consciousness
or awareness raising (promoted by education and feedback, e.g., using a
cost–benefit analysis), self-reevaluation (e.g., values clarification), and dramatic relief or emotional arousal (experienced through grieving, role play).
Behavioral strategies include stimulus control, or regulating exposure to
certain places or people; and counterconditioning, or response substitution
(i.e., engaging in a healthy, alternative behavior instead of the conditioned
addictive behavior). Levels of change in the TTM involve prioritizing five
distinct but related problems addressed in prevention or treatment services:
symptom/situational problems, maladaptive cognitions, current interpersonal conflicts, family/systems conflicts, and intrapersonal conflicts.

Stages of Change

The TTM is best known for its third dimension: the outline of five time
periods or stages in the change process, referred to as the *stages of change*.
The five stages of change are sequential and ordinal, as well as recur-
sive and cyclical (DiClemente, 2003, 2015). They represent *when* people
change. They also are purported to be discrete or mutually exclusive,

meaning that persons are assessed to be in only one stage of change at a time. In research studies, stages are determined by responses to standardized measures, such as the University of Rhode Island Change Assessment (URICA; McConnaughy, DiClemente, Prochaska, & Velicer, 1989; accessible at *http://casaa.unm.edu*). Two other measures of readiness to change specific to alcohol or drugs are the Stages of Change Readiness and Treatment Eagerness Scale (SOCRATES; Miller & Tonigan, 1996; also accessible at *http://casaa.unm.edu*) and the Readiness to Change Questionnaire (Rollnick, Heather, Gold, & Hall, 1992). These briefer measures are also used in clinical practice.

Taken together, the stages of change signify various levels of readiness to change. Each stage represents a step toward a new behavior, and certain characteristics are prominent in each stage. Figure 11.1 depicts the stages of change. Each box corresponds to a stage of change (with the exception of relapse and recycling) and includes the primary goal for moving to the next stage of change. For example, to move from preparation into action, commitment and planning are needed. In what follows, we describe each stage and its corresponding characteristics.

Although regarded as a stage of change, *precontemplation,* as its name implies, describes a state that actually precedes the active process of change. Notice in Figure 11.1 on the next page that precontemplation is located outside the stages of change cycle and that movement is one way only: There is no entry back into precontemplation from the change cycle. This positioning aptly depicts this first stage of change. In precontemplation, persons are unaware of, or are oblivious to, a need to change their behavior; are underaware of, or do not fully comprehend, the need to change; or simply do not intend to change their behavior any time soon (e.g., in the next 6 months). They may be resigned to continue living as they have ("I'm a hopeless drunk"), or they are adamant about not sacrificing something that has become too important for them ("No one can tell me to stop smoking"). Either way, they remain committed to maintaining the status quo. When they enter treatment, it is only the result of being mandated or otherwise coerced to do so by someone else because their behavior has become problematic for others.

Once persons have realized that their behavior is problematic and that change is needed, they move into the *contemplation* stage of change. Again, as depicted in Figure 11.1, there is no going back to precontemplation: No one can claim ignorance or revert to oblivion after experiencing an "aha!" or awakening moment—what has been brought into awareness does not evaporate. However, simply realizing that one's behavior needs to change does not mean that actual change in behavior will occur. Knowing is not doing. Persons in the contemplation stage of change are well aware of the costs, burdens, and other negative consequences of their behavior; they also are keenly aware of the benefits of changing their behavior. At

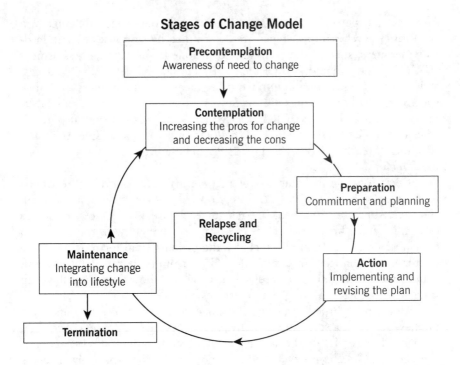

Stages of Change Model

FIGURE 11.1. A cyclical representation of movement through the stages of change. From DiClemente (2003). Copyright 2003 by The Guilford Press. Reprinted by permission.

the same time, they remain attached to the payoffs of their current behavior and realize that change comes at a price. This double-sided awareness or ambivalence is the chief characteristic of persons in the contemplation stage of change. Individuals who are ambivalent are torn between two equally appealing, though opposing, enticements: changing and remaining the same. It is like being perched in the middle of a perpetually fluctuating seesaw; confusion and feeling stuck are common. Persons who are ambivalent know what is good for them (and for others, too), but they are not able to change now (e.g., they lack certain skills or confidence). The benefits of not changing still outweigh the benefits of changing. As a result, contemplation is referred to as prolonged indecision, fluctuating compliance, and behavioral procrastination. Whether or not people are in treatment, they can remain in this stage of change for months or even years.

Persons in contemplation who have weighed the pros and cons of changing and not changing and have tilted their seesaw toward change have entered the *preparation* stage of change. This stage of change characterizes persons who have made a decision to change their behavior in the near future (e.g., next month) because the negative consequences of change are no longer as great as before and because of increased self-efficacy ("I *can* do this"). However, deciding to change does not automatically realize change. Two internal tasks must be accomplished to move forward: creating commitment and planning action (DiClemente, 2003). The first task involves allocating time, energy, and other resources to do the work necessary to realize change; and the second task involves devising a plan of change that is acceptable, accessible, and effective. Preparation may thus be considered the "dress rehearsal" stage of change because persons are trying out their new behavior (e.g., on the third Thursday of November, the American Cancer Society's "Great American Smokeout" day) as one way to convince themselves that they have made the right decision. However, they have yet to "launch" their new behavior. They are still in a trial period of planning, strategizing, and getting ready for their behavioral "debut."

Persons who have followed through on their commitment and plan to change and are deliberately and actively engaged in changing their overt behavior are said to be in the *action* stage of change. Their commitment to making a change is clear and firm, and their efforts are noticeable to others. They have "gone public" with their new behavior and are investing considerable time and energy into making this behavior change routine and permanent (e.g., not smoking since the third Thursday of November). They intend to make this new behavior stick by implementing a relapse prevention plan and revising as needed.

Persons enter the *maintenance* stage of change when they have engaged in their new behavior for more than 6 months and have realized the early benefits of change. New and substitute behaviors have been incorporated into their daily lives, and the "taste" or allure of the problematic behavior is no longer as intense. The "battle" to stay clean, for example, does not require the exertion that it once did. Because of their success, persons in the action stage of change are "sold" on their new behavior and are now invested in "the long haul"; they also want the benefits to "keep on coming." They are intent on consolidating the gains made and living a well-maintained recovery.

Although *termination* is included in Figure 11.1, it typically is not considered a stage of change (as with precontemplation), and rarely is it discussed or mentioned in the TTM literature. It is not measured on any of the three scales mentioned earlier and therefore has not been included in the TTM research. References to termination describe it as the final end state in the TTM, a time when there is little or no activity invested in the change process (DiClemente, 2003).

Because the change process in the TTM is gradual, cyclical, multidimensional, and the product of trial and error, relapse and recycling are built into the stage model (depicted in Figure 11.1 by their location in the center of the change cycle). Persons move through each stage sequentially in their process of change and therefore do not "skip" a stage. They do, however, relapse and thereby revert to earlier stages, such as contemplation. Recycling is a learning process (DiClemente, 2015) that occurs when the change process is reinstated and persons reinvest in a renewed and now altered plan.

Stage–Process Matching and TTM Clinical Application

According to the TTM, movement from one stage to another is facilitated by selecting processes that are appropriate for a particular stage of change. This is known as matching processes to stage of change, a form of individualized care. The cognitive–experiential processes are typically appropriate for persons in earlier stages of change, whereas the behavioral processes are reserved for persons in maintenance and action. Persons in the precontemplation stage, for example, will not benefit from the behavioral task of substituting new activities (e.g., measured breathing to forestall the urge to use) for using behavior (e.g., drinking to calm nerves); they are not ready. Recommending such an activity constitutes a mismatch. What fits for persons who do not want to change or are ambivalent about changing include the cognitive–experiential processes of consciousness raising (e.g., learning about the quantity and frequency of my use) and self-reevaluation (e.g., comparing my use to that of others and to my personal values). Freyer-Adam and colleagues (2014) attributed a significant decrease in alcohol use among adult job-seekers who 15 months earlier presented with problematic alcohol use and low motivation to change to a computer-based intervention tailored to their stage of change.

Norcross, Krebs, and Prochaska (2011) offered nine recommendations for applying the TTM in treatment:

1. Assess the client's stage of change for a specific target or goal behavior. Remember that persons can be at different stages of change for different behaviors. For example, someone can be in maintenance for cocaine use (i.e., abstinent for more than 1 year) while in precontemplation for alcohol use (i.e., "My drinking isn't the problem").
2. Beware of treating all clients as if they are in the action stage of change. This corresponds to Sellman's (2009) adage that "come back when you're ready to change" is no longer acceptable for practitioners to tell a client or a prospective client.
3. Set realistic goals by moving one stage at a time. This fits with the recommendation of AA members to take "one day at a time" in working toward or maintaining sobriety.
4. Treat persons in precontemplation "gingerly," that is, with great care.

5. Tailor the processes to the stages of change; in other words, engage in stage–process matching.
6. Avoid mismatching stages and processes. Meet and work with clients in their stage of change.
7. Prescribe stage-matched relationships of choice as well as treatments of choice. This goes beyond stage–process matching and requires the practitioner to adapt his or her interpersonal style or counseling approach to the client's stage of change. For persons in the maintenance stage, for example, the practitioner is advised to assume a consultation style, not a teacher role.
8. Practice integratively. This means combining prevention and treatment approaches from different theoretical orientations (e.g., experiential, behavioral), as the processes of change represent.
9. Anticipate recycling. Because change is gradual and occurs through trial and error, it is wise to expect persons to move back to earlier stages of change from time to time and not change in a purely linear fashion. Relapse may be considered a sign that an earlier process or approach was a mismatch.

Contributions and Criticisms of the TTM

The TTM and its stages of change dimension have expanded the conceptualization of motivation or readiness to change beyond the longstanding dichotomous understanding of simply *ready* or *not ready*. Indeed, Miller and Rollnick (2009) credited the TTM with "revolutioniz[ing] addiction treatment and more generally how professionals think about facilitating change" (p. 130), characterizing it as "a significant factor in the addiction field's change of heart and mind regarding client motivation" (p. 159). Despite its ongoing criticisms (discussed later in this section), the TTM has become one of the most established and most frequently used theories in health behavior research (Painter, Borba, Hynes, Mays, & Glanz, 2008).

What may explain the popularity of the TTM, specifically its stages of change dimension, is its portrayal of behavior change as something that happens over time. This is its clinical or practical utility—what Littell and Girvin (2004, p. 342) regard as the TTM's "heuristic value"—which has a number of potential benefits. First, it normalizes perceived barriers or complications toward change, such as ambivalence and relapse. Second, it promotes patience and persistence in efforts to change. Rather than expecting or demanding instantaneous or rapid change (and being disappointed and frustrated with the results), persons who view their own or another's behavior change as a process may develop greater self- or other-efficacy, resolve, and endurance. This also may encourage self-compassion and empathy, which are related to a third benefit: that of promoting less pejorative views of persons who are not ready to change or are experiencing difficulty in their change efforts. A final and fourth benefit of accepting change as a gradual process that follows "meaningful segments" (DiClemente, 2003, p. 31) is that specific tasks or activities can be selected to further change or to reinstate the change process following a relapse. This component reflects the "vital implications" that stages of change assessment has for guiding treatment and prevention services and promoting progress (Norcross et al., 2011, p. 151). According to the TTM and its stages of change, when and how behavior change occurs are not a mystery, and established tools and resources (i.e., processes of change) are available for use at specified time periods (i.e., stages of change). These factors, in themselves, can instill hope for recovery to clients and providers alike.

Despite its extensive research base, vast appeal, and seeming entrenchment in the addictions field, the TTM and its stages of change dimension have long been criticized for a number of reasons. Chief among these reasons are that the stages of change are not discrete states or qualitatively different temporal segments (Littell & Girvin, 2002, 2004) but "simply arbitrary lines in the sand" (West, 2005, p. 1037) and therefore not genuine stages. Second, the stages of change do not represent sequential transitions. From their review of the TTM and stages of change research, Littell and Girvin (2002) reported that no study had documented movement through all five stages and that the TTM's claim that progress occurs "one stage at a time" is based on insufficient or flawed evidence (pp. 247–248). What accounts for some people proceeding to behavior change whereas others do not remains unanswered (Urbanoski, 2010). This point relates to a third criticism: that the TTM's processes of change have not been effective in predicting advancement through the change process (Abrams, Herzog, Emmons, & Linnan, 2000; Herzog, Abrams, Emmons, Linnan, & Shadel, 1999). West (2005) voiced further criticisms and argued that the TTM does not account for or explain (1) sudden or "quantum" change; (2) the role of situational determinants in the change process (e.g., recent life events, immediate circumstances, influence of client–counselor conversations); (3) the role of reward and punishment (i.e., principles of learning); (4) intentions about changing, because change from an addictive behavior or other health condition does not necessarily follow a conscious or deliberate process; or (5) readiness to change, because, as Abrams and colleagues (2000) noted, the stages of change are not necessarily "the optimal way by which readiness can be measured."

Hallgren and Moyers (2011) analyzed data from Project MATCH (Matching Alcoholism Treatments to Client Heterogeneity), a multimillion dollar collaborative study of alcoholism treatment in the United States (Project MATCH Research Group, 1997), and were unable to find any consistent associations between client self-reported motivation at the beginning of treatment (based on client URICA responses) and client talk about change in subsequent counseling sessions. Client pretreatment intentions to change their drinking behavior did not match their actual talk about change once they enrolled in treatment. These findings support West's (2005, 2006) contention that motivation to change is not necessarily fueled by early intentions to change and that the TTM (and specifically its stages of change dimension) does not account for situational or in-the-moment influences (e.g., feedback from members in a group counseling session). Although a recommended practice in planning care and prevention services is to assess a client's stage of change first and then select matching or appropriate strategies (see Norcross et al., 2011), Hallgren and Moyers argued against using a pretreatment measure of readiness to change. For care planning purposes, they recommended careful listening to client in-session language about change and selecting services based on how clients talk about change.

Additional criticisms of the TTM include Delinsky and colleagues' (2011) claim that the TTM's conceptualization of motivation is unidimensional rather than multidimensional. In their work with eating disorders (specifically anorexia nervosa), they argue that the TTM does not account for the simultaneous internalization of both the benefits and costs (or burdens) of problematic behavior, and that motivation itself may not be a distinct construct but simply a proxy for illness severity or a positive prognosis. Dare and Derigne (2010) also complain that the TTM adopts a narrow definition of denial (i.e., not capturing its complexity) and that testing other theories of denial has been impeded by the TTM's popularity.

An alternative to the stages of change model is the contemplation ladder (Biener & Abrams, 1991), a measure of readiness to consider stopping a harmful behavior (e.g., smoking). The figure of a ladder with 10 rungs is presented, and persons are then asked: "Each rung on this ladder represents where a person might be in thinking about changing their drinking. Select the number that best represents where you are now." Response options range from "no thought of changing" (0, or ground level) to "taking action to change" (10, or highest rung on ladder). This single-item measure has performed as a modest and reliable predictor of tobacco cessation (Abrams et al., 2000) and intention to quit smoking among chronic pain patients (Unrod et al., 2014). It has been modified for use in an emergency and trauma department (Magill, Apodaca, Barnett, & Monti, 2010) to assess motivation to change drinking behavior. The sparse use of the contemplation ladder may be explained by the popularity of the TTM and its stages of change.

MOTIVATIONAL INTERVIEWING

MI is a particular style of communication intended to strengthen and evoke another person's own reasons and motivation for change (Miller & Rollnick, 2013). It is a way of being with another person, such as a client. Think of MI as the manner in which a clinician interviews a client about his or her motivation—about the internal and external forces energizing and directing the client's behavior. Rather than comprising a set of techniques, MI is a skillful method of helping that employs careful, selective, and responsive listening to gently guide another person toward his or her own self-selected behavior change. It is both a collaborative and a strategic endeavor, and so MI practitioners do not tell clients what to do (not even covertly), and at the same time they do not permit conversations to wander aimlessly. MI gives prominence to what the client wants and believes is necessary for change, and uses that insight to help shape movement toward healthy change.

MI developed from clinical intuition in the early 1980s (see Miller & Moyers, 2017) as an alternative to the direct confrontation methods that were customary in addiction treatment in the United States at that time. Rather than categorizing clients as motivated or unmotivated to change (and equating the latter with being "in denial"), MI proposed a more extensive and sophisticated understanding of motivation. For example, ambivalence is understood in MI as nonpathological and a common occurrence for persons in the change process (e.g., characteristic of persons in the contemplation stage of change according to the TTM). MI also proposes that all people are motivated for something, and therefore no one is "unmotivated" or has "amotivational syndrome." Furthermore, MI views human motivation as malleable and developing in the context of relationships, such as a counseling relationship. MI's proposition that lack of client progress could be attributed, in part, to the counselor and not to the client was quite revolutionary (if not anathema to some). According to Sellman (2009), MI brought about a "seismic shift" in the method of treatment for persons with addictions in the United States, "from noisy confrontation strategies to quiet listening approaches" (p. 9).

MI developed alongside the TTM, and both models still are often used together, especially for persons in early stages of change (i.e., precontemplation and contemplation). Miller and Rollnick (2009, p. 130) acknowledge the "natural fit" between MI and the TTM and characterize them as "kissing cousins who never married." But they insist that MI was never based on the TTM and is not to be confused with the TTM. Whereas the TTM was developed as a comprehensive theory of how and when people change, MI is a specific clinical approach intended to enhance personal motivation for change, and it can be practiced without assessing a person's stage of change.

As with the TTM and its stages of change, MI has become a familiar and strongly endorsed method for delivering prevention and treatment services for addictive behaviors. Heather (2005) referred to MI as a "central plank" (p. 5) in the emergence of a paradigm shift in the addictions field and the "common currency" among many primary health care and other helping professionals, adding that MI is a "truly world-wide phenomenon of our times" (p. 2). In 2007, SAMHSA's National Registry of Evidence-based Practices and Programs (NREPP) recognized MI as an evidence-based practice for the treatment of substance use concerns (see *https://nrepp.samhsa.gov*). Two-thirds of addiction treatment facilities surveyed in the United States report using MI (Rieckmann, Abraham, & Bride, 2016).

Attributes of MI: "Spirit," Skills, and Processes

Miller and Rollnick (2013) define *MI* concisely as "a collaborative conversation style for strengthening a person's own motivation and commitment to change" (p. 12). Notice that this definition makes no reference to counseling or treatment. The focus is on communication. What makes this communication style unique is its integration of relational skills and technical skills applied across four stair-step processes. The relational skills exemplify qualities of the helper. Collectively, they are known as the underlying perspective or "spirit" of MI. Think of them as the core conditions of MI, similar to how person-centered therapy has its core conditions (or qualities and skills of the counselor) of unconditional positive regard, empathy, and genuineness. Applied to client–counselor interactions, the four core conditions that comprise the spirit of MI are: (1) working in *collaboration* and in partnership with a client; (2) *accepting* the client's inherent or absolute worth by expressing accurate empathy, respecting and honoring his or her autonomy or decision-making capabilities, and affirming his or her strengths; (3) demonstrating *compassion* by promoting the client's welfare; and (4) *evoking* or eliciting the client's own ideas and other resources for change. As seen in Figure 11.2 on the next page, these four relational skills overlap as the foundation or essence of MI. Without these four skills in operation, MI is not MI.

The technical components of MI are skills common to many counseling approaches, but they are used strategically in MI. Four fundamental skills or techniques used in MI from start to finish are known by the acronym *OARS*:

- Ask O̲pen-ended questions (questions that often begin with *how* and *what* and open the door to further conversation and exploration).
- A̲ffirm the person's strengths (and do so genuinely, without sarcasm).
- Provide empathic R̲eflections (uttered as statements, not questions that make a guess at the speaker's thoughts or feelings, especially those not yet uttered).
- S̲ummarize content throughout the conversation by collecting and linking material that has been heard, and then transitioning to something new.

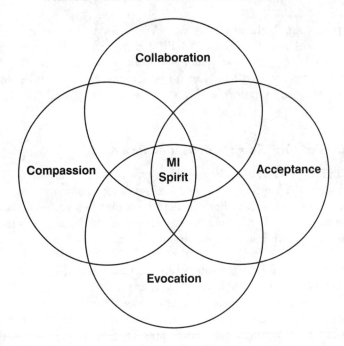

FIGURE 11.2. The underlying spirit of MI. From Miller and Rollnick (2013). Copyright 2013 by The Guilford Press. Reprinted by permission.

In one research study (Moyers, Martin, Houck, Christopher, & Tonigan, 2009), two of these skills prompted more client talk about change (which in turn led to actual behavior change) than the other two skills: questioning the negative and the positive aspects of a target behavior (e.g., drinking) and responding with reflections. A more recent study (Apodaca et al., 2016) also found that reflections and open questions encouraged talk of change (known in MI as "change talk"), but it was offering affirmations that alone generated more change talk and also decreased talk about not changing (known in MI as "sustain talk"). Although many studies of MI do not differentiate between open- and closed-ended questions, Miller and Rollnick (2013) advise that practitioners use twice as many open questions as closed questions. They also recommend that helpers offer two to three reflections for every question asked.

Two additional techniques consistent with the spirit of MI are (1) offering advice or recommendations only with the person's permission and (2) supporting the person's autonomy. The first of these techniques prevents the practitioner from putting words in the speaker's mouth and "plowing through" with prescriptions. This desirable approach is evident in statements such as "I have some ideas about this. Would you care to hear a few?" The second skill further reinforces the humanistic quality of MI that change is always the other person's call and that no one can make anyone do anything. Statements such as "It's your call" and "This is really your decision, not mine" convey this respect. We discuss autonomy more extensively in the section on SDT later in this chapter.

Miller and Rollnick (2013) outline four processes of MI. Consider these as sequential methods for conducting MI, each with a specific purpose that undergirds the work of the succeeding methods. These four processes or stair steps are engaging, focusing, evoking, and planning. *Engaging* refers to establishing a respectful and helpful connection with the speaker (e.g., student, client), and *focusing* involves determining a direction for the conversation, a mutually agreed-upon agenda. Recall that *evoking* is also one of the components of the MI spirit. As a process in MI, evoking deliberately makes use of the person's own momentum toward change; it specifically encourages the person to voice his or her own arguments for change. Although ambivalence is not included in the current definition of MI, it is during the process of evoking that exploring and resolving ambivalence are prominent. The fourth process, *planning,* takes place when it is determined that the person is ready to launch a behavior change, such as reducing alcohol use or no longer playing slot machines. Planning involves cultivating a commitment to change and developing a specific itinerary for making that change happen. As with the TTM stages of change, each of these four MI processes or steps is never entirely accomplished, and all of them often need revisiting as motivation fluctuates.

A surprising finding in Moyers and colleagues' (2009) research was the amount of ambivalence heard throughout MI conversations. They recommend that wise practitioners accept these fluctuations as normal, and they wait patiently and persistently alongside the person (using the relational and technical skills of MI), so that it is this person—the client, for example—who voices self-motivational statements or arguments for change, not the practitioner. MI proposes that change occurs when clients persuade or convince themselves about changing, not when they acquiesce to the coercion of others. Clients may realize beneficial change only when MI practitioners revisit the steps of engaging, focusing, evoking, and planning.

The Language of Motivation in MI

Because MI is a communication style, careful attention is given to the verbal expressions present in conversation. The language of interest in MI is that of change, how people talk about change. It is the talk of change that signals motivation. Motivation also can be detected in the absence of or a reduction in arguments against change or for the status quo (i.e., sustain talk). MI practitioners encourage clients to talk about change, and they reinforce change talk when they hear it. They acknowledge the reasons someone gives for not changing, but they do not cultivate this type of sustain talk; nor do they dispute it. Think of MI practitioners as attentive, empathic, and selective listeners who are highly attuned and ready to promote talk of change. Consistent with West and Brown's (2013) contention that motivation occurs only in the present moment, MI defines motivation according to in-the-moment verbal utterances influenced by another's responses. Motivation in MI thus is assessed according to how people talk about change in the moment and in the context of an interpersonal exchange, such as a counseling session.

There are seven dimensions of motivation in MI, or seven distinct ways people talk about change. These dimensions are known by the acronym *DARN CAT* (Miller & Rollnick, 2013) and are heard when someone talks about his or her:

- Desire, preference, or wish for change.
- Ability or self-efficacy to change (belief that I can effect change, that I can make change happen), as well as confidence in changing.
- Reason for change, or what will be gained by changing.
- Need for change, or the urgency or pressure (internal or external) to change (e.g., what needs to be stopped or relinquished now).
- Commitment to change, or the public declaration of intent to change, signaling a promise to change and a high likelihood of changing one's behavior.
- Activation of change resources or leaning into change ("I'll try," "I'm willing to").
- Taking steps, describing behaviors already and recently accomplished in the direction of change (e.g., "I calmed myself down this morning").

The first four dimensions of verbalized motivation or change talk (DARN) indicate a preparation for change, how people get ready for, or talk themselves into, change. They comprise *preparatory change talk*. Think of this as internal or self-talk language that wrestles with change, a back-and-forth attempt to convince yourself to make a change. In MI counseling sessions, preparatory change talk (DARN language) is often the precursor and harbinger of mobilizing change talk (Amrhein, Miller, Yahne, Palmer, & Fulcher, 2003; Hodgins, Ching, & McEwen, 2009). *Mobilizing change talk* comprises the last three dimensions of verbalized motivation (CAT) and signals an intent to change.

People who talk about wanting and needing to change cite reasons for changing (e.g., getting a driver's license back, regaining custody of children). They are encouraged by an empathic MI clinician's responses to take steps toward change, and they are subsequently likely to promise or vow to change ("I'm gonna get clean," "I'll never pick up again"). MI research has found a compelling link between change talk and actual behavior change (Apodaca & Longabaugh, 2009; Barnett et al., 2014). Moyers and her colleagues (Moyers, Martin, Christopher, Houck, & Tonigan, 2007; Moyers et al., 2009) refer to this link as a *causal chain*. This means that MI interventions lead to an increase in client change talk and/or a reduction in client sustain talk; these in turn lead to overt behavior changes, such as reduced drinking or reduced marijuana use. A similar link was found for persons who received a brief (15- to 20-minute) motivational intervention about their drinking in the hospital's emergency department (Bertholet, Faouzi, Gmel, Gaume, & Daeppen, 2010). Hodgins and colleagues (2009) found that clients who verbalized a commitment to change during MI phone sessions with a therapist later reported positive change in their gambling behavior (e.g., days of gambling, dollars lost, self-efficacy related to gambling abstinence) up to 12 months following the intervention. Voicing motivation to change (preparatory change talk that turns into mobilizing change talk) can thus lead to behavior change.

MI research does not suggest that behavior change occurs by simply uttering the words "I will change." Such a proposition is of course preposterous, as is the contention that knowledge alone effects behavior change (a view still held by many in drug and alcohol prevention and treatment). It is the strength or intensity of change talk (Gaume et al., 2016), as well as its frequency (Moyers et al., 2009) and momentum in session (Houck & Moyers, 2015), that make a difference. Someone who mumbles, "I guess I'll try to stop smoking" is not likely to actually stop smoking. By contrast, someone who verbalizes a genuine desire to stop smoking more than once in a conversation with an MI clinician and does so each time with a sense of urgency, conviction, and confidence is more likely to follow through with the commitment—or to "walk the talk." Gaume, Gmel, and Daeppen (2008) found that, in particular, clients' expressed ability to change (one dimension of preparatory change talk) predicted their report 1 year later of fewer drinks per week.

Findings of recent MI research (Lindqvist, Forsberg, Enebrink, Andersson, & Rosendahl, 2017; Magill et al., 2018) highlight a critical skill for MI clinicians: Acknowledge sustain talk when you hear it, but do not "add fuel to the fire" by spending considerable time exploring it or combatting it. This may be true especially for practitioners who work with adolescents and clients mandated to treatment (Moyers, Houck, Glynn, Hallgren, & Manuel, 2017). Thus, the language of motivation in MI that leads to behavior change is heard in a quieting of sustain talk or decreased arguments against changing. Motivation to change is expressed in sincere, earnest, and confident language that has developed with intensity or conviction over time and through fluctuations. It also is strengthened by a skilled listener who is able to convey empathy, accept the normality of ambivalence heard, not dispute statements opposed to change, and reinforce the person's autonomy or decision-making capacity.

Motivational Enhancement Therapy

Motivational enhancement therapy (MET) is a brief intervention and an adaptation of MI that was developed for Project MATCH, mentioned earlier. MET incorporates the MI spirit and makes use of technical skills associated with MI (e.g., OARS). It is distinct from MI in that MET provides students or clients with personalized and structured feedback (oral and written). Feedback includes comparisons of client or student self-reported alcohol or drug use relative to their peers (e.g., other female freshmen at the same university) and health information (e.g., maximum number of drinks per week recommended), and it is presented in a candid and nonjudgmental manner. In their review of 73 studies, Samson and Tanner-Smith (2015) found that the incorporation of MI into single-session brief interventions to reduce heavy alcohol use among college students was more effective than two other brief interventions, namely, psychoeducation and cognitive-behavioral therapy (CBT).

One example of MET is the Brief Alcohol Screening and Intervention for College Students (BASICS; Dimeff, Baer, Kivlahan, & Marlatt, 1999) conducted in two separate 50-minute one-on-one sessions: an assessment session followed by a feedback session. Maintaining the MI spirit of partnership, acceptance, compassion, and evocation, BASICS is intended to raise awareness of drinking behaviors in older teenagers and young adults. Once awareness has been enhanced and students begin to talk about changing their behavior, they are encouraged in a nonconfrontational manner to develop a personalized plan for healthy change. Amaro and colleagues (2010) adapted the BASICS program to include screening and intervention for alcohol and other drug use and found that it reduced both the quantity and frequency of substance use among college students who sought medical and mental health services at a university health care center.

Feedback is the component that distinguishes MET from MI. Vader, Walters, Prabhu, Houck, and Field (2010) investigated the differences between one-session applications of MI only and MET among college students. They found that student sustain talk (against changing) was lower as a result of receiving feedback (the MET condition) than when no feedback was delivered (the MI-only condition). They also found that how students talked about change during the MET session predicted their 3- and 6-month drinking outcomes (e.g., self-reported drinks/week). Specifically, more change talk predicted less drinking, and more sustain talk predicted more drinking. There was no association between change talk or sustain talk and actual behavior change for students who received only MI. Results suggest that clinician feedback (e.g., provided in BASICS) may serve a distinct and favorable role with respect to how clients talk about change and their eventual behavior change. Compared to MI alone, Vader and colleagues propose that clinician feedback "may tip the balance" toward change talk, which may lead to actual behavior change.

MI Applications and Performance

Although its beginnings are in substance abuse treatment and the vast amount of MI research remains devoted to investigating alcohol and other drug problems, MI has been applied to a wide range of other health-related behaviors such as gambling, HIV/AIDS prevention, eating disorders, diet and exercise, emotional or psychological well-being, and water purification/safety. MI also has been used to address treatment behaviors such as engagement, retention, completion, and intention to change. This model has been found to be particularly useful as a precursor to treatment or program involvement, increasing the likelihood that persons will agree to seek services (e.g., HIV testing), initiate service entry (e.g., go to a clinic for HIV testing and participate in a brief intervention while there), and then engage in prevention or treatment activities (e.g., attend safe-sex programming after learning the results of HIV test; Apodaca & Longabaugh, 2009). In one study (Wain et al., 2011), a significantly greater number of homeless veterans with substance use problems entered a 180-day residential rehabilitation program when they participated in a brief MI intervention (approximately 38 minutes) than veterans who completed a briefer (approximately 27 minutes) standard interview. Although more MI-intervention veterans remained in, completed, and graduated from the program than did standard-interview veterans, these differences were not significant.

From their meta-analysis of 119 studies of MI conducted over 25 years, Lundahl, Kunz, Brownell, Tollefson, and Burke (2010) found that MI exerted a small yet statistically meaningful influence (average effect size = 0.22) across a variety of outcomes (e.g., reduction in risk-taking behaviors, engagement in treatment). Seventy-five percent of participants in these studies improved somewhat from MI, and of those, 50% improved slightly but meaningfully and 25% improved moderately or strongly. Specifically, when compared to "weak" comparison groups (i.e., wait-list/control, nonspecific treatment-as-usual groups), MI performed better, particularly for (1) African American participants, (2) substance-use-related outcomes, (3) gambling, and (4) longer treatment periods. However, when compared to "strong" comparison groups (e.g., specific treatments that included 12-step facilitation and CBT), MI yielded poorer outcomes (i.e., lower effect sizes) for African American participants and when MI studies were of higher methodological rigor. From their meta-analysis of 31 studies of MI for smoking cessation, Hettema and Hendricks (2010) reported an overall modest effect of MI, particularly for adolescents and persons with low tobacco dependence and motivation to quit.

Lundahl and colleagues (2013) conducted a more recent meta-analysis of 48 studies of MI in medical care settings such as hospitals, physician clinics, and dentist offices. Outcomes included decreased alcohol and other drug use (e.g., nicotine), prevention of chronic heart failure, increased fruit and vegetable intake, and prevention of tooth decay. Results for MI were favorable in 63% of the main outcome comparisons (statistically significant differences) and suggested a 55% chance that MI would generate a positive outcome compared to other interventions, such as treatment-as-usual. This meta-analysis also showed that MI increased patient confidence about approaching change when dealing with medical conditions (e.g., smoking) and increased patient treatment or care engagement (e.g., keeping appointments).

One concern about MI is that its benefits do not last. An earlier meta-analysis of 72 studies of MI for a variety of health concerns (Hettema, Steele, & Miller, 2005) revealed a decline in the effect of MI over time. Booster sessions following MI intervention therefore are recommended to sustain its benefits. Lundahl and colleagues (2010), however, reported that lasting and meaningful effects of MI (effect sizes of 0.29 and 0.24) were evident up to 2 years beyond the MI intervention. Similar lasting and significant benefits have been found when MI has been added to another treatment (e.g., CBT), either prior to or throughout treatment (Hettema et al., 2005). For example, combining MI and CBT has been found to increase client retention and active participation in treatment (McKee et al., 2007) and to improve client outcomes, including reduced substance use among persons with psychosis (Barrowclough et al., 2010). In Cleary, Hunt, Matheson, and Walter's (2009) systematic review of 54 studies of treatments for co-occurring disorders (e.g., MI, CBT, contingency management, group therapy, intensive case management), MI was the most effective for substance use reduction, and MI combined with CBT led to the greatest improvements in mental health symptoms as well as reductions in substance use behaviors.

Despite MI's relatively strong performance, especially in changing substance use behaviors (Hettema et al., 2005), little is still known about how MI works. This is the challenge of process research, or the study of how in-session behaviors influence client outcomes. From their review of 19 studies of MI for treating alcohol and other drug use disorders, Apodaca and Longabaugh (2009) found that MI did not increase client readiness to change more so than other treatments (e.g., coping skills training). This finding parallels somewhat Li, Zhu, Tse, Tse, and Wong's (2015) report from their review of 10 studies: They found that MI did not reduce adolescent illicit drug use; MI only was effective in changing adolescent attitudes about drug use. Hunter-Reel and colleagues (2010) contend that no motivation-oriented treatment approach, including MI, should be credited for changing motivation; there is no evidence that these approaches are efficacious because they change motivation. What accounts for increasing motivation to change, they argue, is membership in a social network that does not support drinking, such as AA. Further research on MI must investigate how motivation is influenced by a person's social network. Continued scrutiny of dimensions of client in-session change talk and their link to actual behavior change outside of counseling sessions also is in order.

SELF-DETERMINATION THEORY

SDT (Ryan & Deci, 2017) is a theory of personality, specifically of personal experience, as well as a theory of energy dynamics or how motives determine either vitality or depletion. It developed from exploring what determines intrinsic motivation, or the innate tendency to pursue novelty and challenges, to put into practice one's capacities, as well as to explore and to learn. SDT assumes that people's firsthand subjective experience is the proximal or most authentic determinant of motivation and action. SDT therefore focuses on understanding how people interpret or make sense of internal and external stimuli to explain their motivation and action. According to Williams and colleagues (2002), what distinguishes SDT from other theories of human motivation is its concept of *autonomous motivation*: the belief that perceived autonomy is necessary to maintain behavior change.

Although SDT is a theory and not a practice, through its extensive research base, it supplies empirically informed principles and guidelines for enhancing people's motivation. Motivation enhancement is accomplished by having people reflect on events and experiences to help them make changes in their goals, behaviors, and relationships. SDT has been applied to such varied domains as sport and other forms of physical activity, classroom instruction and student learning, parenting, intimate relationships, pro-environmental behavior (e.g., recycling), politics, video games, mindfulness, and medication maintenance. It also has been applied to counseling and psychotherapy (Ryan et al., 2011). The application of SDT to substance use and addiction is rather limited, even though for some time addiction has been framed as a disorder of motivation (Heather, 2005). In recent years, SDT has been applied to tobacco use and abstinence (Niemiec, Ryan, Patrick, Deci, & Williams, 2010; Pesis-Katz, Williams, Niemiec, & Fiscella, 2011); alcohol consumption among employed adults (Hagger et al., 2012), college students (Chawla, Neighbors, Logan, Lewis, & Fossos, 2009; Hove, Parkhill, Neighbors, McConchie, & Fossos, 2010; Knee & Neighbors, 2002), and high school students (Wormington, Anderson, & Corpus, 2011); and addiction treatment specific to therapeutic communities

(Klag, Creed, & O'Callaghan, 2010) and to methadone maintenance (Zeldman, Ryan, & Fiscella, 2004).

As is true of the TTM and MI, SDT dismisses the notion of a unitary construct of motivation. It identifies different types of motivation that influence different types of behavioral regulation. The types of motivation are conceptualized along a continuum of autonomy ranging from a lack of motivation or volition (amotivation or helplessness) to strong volition or a highly internal influence of self-regulation (e.g., intrinsic motivation). Between these two end points, motivation is regulated according to the different interactions between the person's needs and sources of influence. Unlike the TTM, SDT is not a stage theory, nor does it suggest a developmental sequence (Ryan et al., 2011).

Autonomy

The primary construct of SDT is that of autonomy, which is seen as a natural, inherent, and universal human need (along with competence and relatedness, discussed in the next section) and as a quality of human behavior. It is the lifelong tendency to develop an organized, unified, or integrated sense of self, and it is expressed as volition and congruence. This means that one's actions are self-derived and self-endorsed. Autonomy is experienced as viewing oneself as the locus of causality or the agent of activity—what de Charms (1968) referred to as *personal causation* and described as "being an Origin" (p. 270). It is the feeling of freedom to make one's own choices and then to act on them. Autonomous behavior is therefore self-determined and self-regulated behavior: What a person does originates from within one's self and is consistent with personally endorsed values.

As discussed earlier in the chapter, autonomous motivation is the opposite of controlled motivation. The difference between these two types of motivation is "the most central distinction in SDT" (Deci & Ryan, 2008, p. 182). Whereas *autonomous motivation* implies self-authored volition, choice, and intentionality, *controlled motivation* is the result of pressure or coercion—often external to the self—to fulfill specific outcomes. An example of controlled motivation is attending court-mandated addiction treatment to avoid jail time. Although it is tempting to differentiate autonomous and controlled motivation strictly according to its source of influence— internal (or from within) or external (or from without)—this is not the case in SDT (intrinsic and extrinsic types of motivation are defined later in this chapter). Autonomous motivation can be influenced by external forces (e.g., laws, policies, people) that the person has come to endorse over time. For example, a person who agrees with the sentencing judge's directive to attend addiction treatment because he or she now believes treatment will help achieve desired abstinence, which in turn will help him or her regain child visitation or custody, can be said to be acting autonomously. Again, autonomous motivation involves exerting a choice that by implication is self-derived or self-initiated ("I agree to go to treatment . . . ") *and* reflects self-endorsed values (" . . . because I truly believe it will help me get clean so that I can get my kids back"). This is self-determination in action.

Controlled motivation, in contrast, involves coercion (or seduction) and the eclipse of self-regulation or self-determination. It is experienced as manualization or as operating like a machine in a way that is contrary to one's beliefs. Whereas autonomous motivation feels authentic, controlled motivation feels counterfeit; it is the same as feeling like a pawn and forced to act against one's principles. In this way, independence is differentiated from autonomy in SDT because a person can feel forced by others (e.g., family) to develop less dependence on them. At the same time, autonomous motivation does not imply the dismissal of external sources of influence. A person is acting autonomously when his or her behavior is directed by a value or belief (e.g., abstinence) held by others that he or she has now willfully or voluntarily adopted and integrated. This often takes time and effort. According to Ryan (1992), "Much of the struggle for autonomy . . . concerns gaining regulatory control or management over inner wishes and drives as well as over outer regulations and commands" (p. 13).

Competence and Relatedness

In addition to autonomy, SDT identifies two other basic psychological needs that people innately seek out, whether or not they are aware of these needs. These are the needs for competence and relatedness. All three needs (autonomy, competence, and relatedness) are considered essential for psychological growth, integrity, and wellness and necessary for optimal functioning—which explains why they are referred to as *nutriments*. If any of these nutriments is thwarted or frustrated, the person will exhibit diminished motivation and well-being. These are inherent or natural needs, as opposed to learned desires; they also are universal needs, meaning that they are important to people of all cultures.

Competence is the need to feel effective in one's actions, particularly in one's ongoing interactions with the social environment. It is the experience of opportunities to exercise, expand, and express one's capacities. As with all three psychological needs in SDT, the need for competence is innate and is not the result of experience or learning. It involves the natural urge to have an effect on one's environment, to influence or cause a desired outcome—what has been referred to as *effectance motivation* (Elliot et al., 2002). Although similar to self-efficacy, competence is not an attained skill or capability, but rather "a felt sense of confidence and effectance in action" (Ryan & Deci, 2002, p. 7).

Relatedness is the need to feel a connection to or with other people, or to have a sense of belonging to one's community. It includes caring for others and being cared for by others, and it also entails a sense of being significant or integral to others and accepted by them. An important aspect of relatedness is that a connection with others supplies a sense of security, similar to what is described by the concept of attachment. Although autonomous behavior (and, in general, optimal health) is associated with nourishing or promoting all three psychological needs, Ryan and Deci (2002, p. 14) conceded that relatedness "typically plays a more distal role" in fostering autonomous or intrinsic motivation than do competence and autonomy.

Types of Motivation and Regulation

The two primary and opposing types of motivation in SDT are autonomous and controlled motivation, discussed earlier. Activation of autonomous motivation leads to more self-regulated or self-determined behavior and is associated with health and well-being. Because SDT defines motivation multidimensionally, there are further types of motivation located along the continuum of relative autonomy or self-determination. These additional motivational types are presented in Figure 11.3 and are categorized as either extrinsic or intrinsic motivation.

Intrinsic motivation (on the far right-hand side of the continuum) is expressed as intrinsic regulation, which signifies self-determined behavior. Non-self-determined behavior (far left-hand side of the continuum) is regarded as amotivation or nonregulation. Between these two extremes are four types of extrinsic motivation. Think of these as four regulatory styles, or four ways in which extrinsic motivation is experienced, processed, and expressed. Notice that two types of extrinsic motivation are associated with controlled motivation, whereas the other two types are associated with autonomous motivation. Also notice that extrinsic motivation is not to be confused with external motivation, nor is intrinsic motivation necessarily the same as internal motivation. In SDT, the adjectives *external* and *internal* are used to denote the source of influence or perceived locus of causality, not necessarily a type of motivation. Each of these terms is discussed briefly in this section.

Intrinsic motivation, on the one hand, is defined in SDT as the natural inclination toward personally satisfying behaviors. It is doing something for its own sake—out of curiosity because it is novel or a challenge or both, or for the sheer pleasure of it and not to satisfy anyone or thing external to the self or to receive a reinforcement (Ryan & Deci, 2017). It is associated with spontaneity and is observed in human infancy as exploratory behavior; it is more evident in infants with secure maternal/parental attachments and with a parent who supports autonomy. Intrinsic motivation is autonomous motivation because it is volitional or self-authored, and it involves engaging in self-endorsed rather than controlled behavior. Intrinsic motivation typically diminishes after infancy/childhood, when social pressures to engage

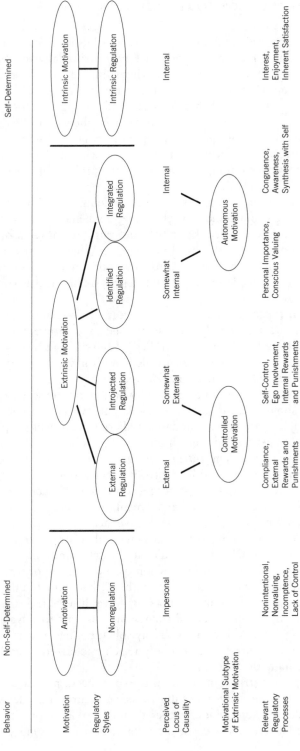

FIGURE 11.3. Types of motivation and regulation in self-determination theory. From Ryan and Deci (2000). Copyright 2000 by the American Psychological Association. Adapted by permission of Richard M. Ryan.

in noninteresting activities and to assume responsibilities become more prominent. Thus, most human behaviors are not intrinsically motivated (Ryan, 1995). These behaviors include initiating substance use (Wormington et al., 2011), limiting alcohol intake (Hagger et al., 2012), and entering treatment for an addictive behavior. Klag and colleagues (2010) did not observe intrinsic or autonomous motivation in clients enrolled in a 2-week therapeutic community program, explaining that "substance users are unlikely to undergo treatment for the mere pleasure and satisfaction they may derive from overcoming their substance use problem and reaching their personal goals" (p. 1118).

Extrinsic motivation, on the other hand, is doing something for its separate consequence or outcome. It is engaging in a behavior to obtain a reward (e.g., drinking to get drunk) or to avoid punishment (e.g., drinking to prevent the onset of withdrawal symptoms). Whereas intrinsically motivated behavior is itself the goal, extrinsically motivated behavior is the means toward a goal—it is doing something to get something else; contingencies are involved.

There are four types of extrinsic motivation in SDT—external, introjected, identified, and integrated—each expressed as a different regulatory style and associated with either controlled or autonomous motivation. *External regulation* is governed by controlled motivation, meaning that the person feels pressured by sources outside and alien to the self to engage in behavior that the person does not like and would not do otherwise; the purpose is to get something tangible or to avoid external contingencies in return. One example is attending mandated addiction treatment simply to avoid jail time and to get one's driver's license back, not because of a belief that one has a drinking problem. *Introjected regulation* is another type of extrinsic motivation also governed by controlled motivation. The purpose of this behavior, however, is to satisfy internal contingencies, such as avoiding the feelings of guilt, shame, or embarrassment. The source of control is also from within, a kind of self-coercion to "save face" or to enhance self-esteem. One example is drinking to assuage perceived peer pressure, which Knee and Neighbors (2002) found predicted greater drinking. Another example is promising the son you love, whom you've hurt before and for whom you now want to finally be a "decent father," that you will take him to the zoo this weekend, which means making yourself not drink the day before or the morning of the promised excursion. It is only to salvage his image in his son's eyes that this father will stay sober, not because he wants to be sober. In this way, introjected regulation is characterized by ambivalence (Wild, Cunningham, & Ryan, 2006).

The third type of extrinsic motivation is experienced, processed, and expressed as *identified regulation.* As illustrated in Figure 11.3, identified regulation is guided by autonomous rather than controlled motivation in that the person endorses or identifies with the value or personal importance of an activity (e.g., abstinence). Although the behavior is still pursued because of its consequences (e.g., preserving one's self-image), the person has claimed ownership of the behavior and takes responsibility for it. The college student who decides to "come clean" to his girlfriend about the extent of his online gambling behavior and to seek help because he realizes it has cost him intangibles more important than money (e.g., her love, his college education) that he now wants restored, can be said to be operating according to identified regulation. In their investigation of clients seeking outpatient treatment for primarily alcohol and cocaine use (the majority of whom reported *not* being mandated to treatment by a legal entity), Wild and colleagues (2006) found that clients' identified motivation (i.e., their personal reasons for seeking treatment) was positively associated with their self-reported substance use severity. They concluded that *clients'* reasons for seeking treatment (e.g., "Things are bad," "I'm in worse shape"—a sign of autonomous motivation) are more influential in predicting client engagement in treatment than controlled motivation or social controls (e.g., treatment mandates, social network pressures).

Integrated regulation is an extension of identified regulation, but the motivation is more autonomous in that the behavior is synchronized and assimilated with other values and goals. It is doing something not just for one outcome or reward, but for several that are interrelated and that satisfy core beliefs and values. The recently retired nurse who stops smoking to prevent her second dog from dying of emphysema and to restore her own health so that she can reconnect with her daughter and get to know her new grandchild exemplifies this type of motivation. Her nicotine-free lifestyle has more than one benefit and is consistent with what is most important to her at this time in her life (e.g., health and family). Clients exhibiting more integrated motivation have been found to demonstrate greater treatment engagement and greater psychological well-being (Klag et al., 2010).

On the one hand, overall research findings associate extrinsic and controlled motivation (specifically, external and introjected regulation) with the negative effects of addictive behavior (e.g., increased drinking, interpersonal violence). Intrinsic and autonomous motivation (primarily integrated regulation), on the other hand, has been found to serve "a clearly protective role" (Wormington et al., 2011, p. 966).

SDT in Practice

The primary purpose of applying SDT to various practice settings is to promote the autonomy and hence the overall well-being of persons seeking services. Its implementation for tobacco cessation also has been found to be cost-effective (Pesis-Katz et al., 2011). Autonomy-supporting environments are characterized by minimal pressure to engage in specific behaviors and the encouragement of individuals to pursue activities based on their own reasons and values (Ryan et al., 2011). In counseling and psychotherapy, creating this environment begins with understanding and validating clients' internal frames of reference, such as what is important and satisfying to them. This does not imply endorsing their values or behavior; rather, it is an effort to grasp how each individual views a particular situation, such as the benefits and the drawbacks of his or her past and current substance use. The autonomy-supporting clinician is not invested in a particular outcome for the client, but instead trusts the client's capacity to engage in integrated regulation. As just described, this is the ability to internalize and assimilate extrinsic motives into one's belief system and then to act accordingly, consistent with that belief system. An example of an autonomy-supporting therapeutic environment is the clinician's commendation of client "Miranda's" decision to engage in substance-free activities because she wants to retain custody of the children she loves and to be able to make decisions for herself and her children, as opposed to others—or a drug—making decisions for her. Discontinuing her substance use and participating in salutary rather than potentially destructive behaviors is congruent with what Miranda values: her children, clear thinking, and the freedom to make her own choices in life.

The importance of an autonomy-supporting environment cannot be overstated. Klag and colleagues (2010) found that clients who felt supported in an autonomous manner by therapeutic community staff saw themselves as more competent and felt more connected to—and understood by—the people around them at the start of treatment. This, in turn, was associated with more autonomous motivation (i.e., integrated motivation) toward treatment. Among clients enrolled in a methadone maintenance program, higher perceived autonomy support predicted low relapse as well as less time to achieve take-home medication status (Zeldman et al., 2004).

Although autonomy support can be thought of as an antidote to controlled motivation, it should not be considered its replacement. Supporting extrinsic motivation by issuing tangible rewards (e.g., vouchers) for achieving targeted behaviors (e.g., abstinence), as is done in contingency management (see Chapter 6), can be used in tandem with autonomy-supporting mechanisms. The two must be balanced carefully. Deci, Koester, and Ryan's (1999) review of more than 125 early SDT studies found that, overall, when tangible rewards (e.g., $3 cash) were given to persons who engaged in tasks they found interesting, intrinsic motivation diminished. However, when positive verbal feedback or praise was provided, intrinsic motivation increased. These findings are consistent with the results of Zeldman and colleagues' (2004) methadone maintenance study. Zeldman and colleagues concluded that unless controlled motivation (e.g., court mandate to be in treatment) is accompanied by high levels of autonomous motivation (e.g., choosing to be free of drug-related negative symptoms in order to be a good parent), treatment may not be successful. However, high levels of controlled motivation may actually aid recovery from addiction when coupled with high levels of autonomous motivation. Zeldman and colleagues explained: "The nature of addiction to either alcohol or drugs may be such that external forces acting or pressuring the individual to engage and remain in treatment are a useful adjunctive when they converge with an inner desire to change" (p. 692). The point, though, is to prioritize autonomy support, to encourage and affirm intrinsic regulation; instituting only mechanisms interpreted as controlling will undermine any inclinations a person has to change problematic behavior and maintain well-being. Self-determined and self-regulated behavior is possible only by promoting autonomy (i.e., one's volition and values) in prevention and treatment services.

INTEGRATING THE TTM, MI, AND SDT

Although they developed separately and each has established its own empirical base and guidelines for practice, the TTM, MI, and SDT are amenable to integration. This makes sense given that all three prevention and treatment approaches target motivational processes by prioritizing autonomous inclinations to change, to varying degrees. The TTM and SDT are both products of theoretical integrations. And the TTM and MI have long been linked, although often mischaracterized as the same approach. Only in recent years have there been efforts to integrate SDT with both the TTM and MI. The developers have welcomed these efforts.

Ryan and Deci (2008, p. 187) described SDT as having "a particular affinity with" MI. They note that MI supports the three basic psychological needs identified in SDT: autonomy (by engaging in nondirective inquiry and reflection), competence (by providing information), and relatedness (by establishing a counseling relationship characterized by unconditional positive regard). Because supporting autonomy is a key principle and skill in MI, Miller and Rollnick (2012) endorse a preliminary integration of SDT and MI, humorously stating, "A marriage may be premature, but the flirtation is not" (p. 2).

Patrick and Williams (2012) noted that SDT and MI draw on the perspectives of Carl Rogers, such as unconditional positive regard, and that both SDT and MI operate according to the same basic assumption: human beings are naturally oriented toward growth, health, and well-being. Patrick and Williams argued that MI provides specific interventions (e.g., empathic listening) to exploit the principles of SDT, namely, autonomous motivation. This is evident in efforts to increase physical activity, such as the web-based physical activity intervention based on SDT and MI and known as *I Move* (Friederichs et al., 2014).

Integrating SDT and MI may improve understanding of the mechanisms of change in MI. For example, one of the findings from Lundahl and colleagues' (2010) meta-analysis of MI studies conducted over a 25-year period was that MI did not significantly enhance client self-reported confidence in changing (one of three variables categorized as reflecting client motivation). In light of this finding, might the effects of MI improve by targeting a more comprehensive and nuanced understanding of confidence, that is, the psychological need of competence, as defined in SDT? Furthermore, Britton, Patrick, Wenzel, and Williams (2011) proposed an integration of SDT and MI with CBT to prevent suicide (and other high-risk behaviors). They speculated that SDT offers a perspective from which to understand how MI-consistent behaviors may improve client retention and outcome.

The integration of SDT and the TTM likewise may enhance understanding of motivational processes at work that explain the movement from one stage of change to the next. Perhaps extrinsic factors (e.g., legal sanctions) influence intent to change for persons who are in early stages of change (e.g., precontemplation) more so than for persons who are further along in the change process. Persons may move from preparation into action, for example, for more intrinsic reasons, such as enhancing the early benefits of mental and emotional well-being. In their study of problem gamblers, Kushnir, Godinho, Hodgins, Hendershot, and Cunningham (2016) found that higher autonomous motivations were predictive of being in the preparation stage of change and intending to quit gambling in the next 30 days, compared to being in the contemplation stage of change. They proposed that early intervention and public health campaigns should promote the positive aspects of quitting gambling, not just the damaging effects.

As mentioned, whereas SDT recognizes amotivation, MI does not. SDT defines amotivation as lacking either intrinsic or extrinsic motivation for certain activities; there is no energy, desire, or intention to act. This description fits persons in the precontemplation stage of change in the TTM. Amotivation occurs because a person does not value an activity, does not feel competent to do it, or does not expect the activity to yield a preferred outcome. By contrast, MI assumes that clients are motivated for something. According to Miller and Rollnick (2013), "No one is unmotivated" (p. 74). The practitioner's task in MI therefore is to elicit and help cultivate the client's proclivity toward change, a proclivity defined in MI as intrinsic motivation for change. In SDT, however, promoting intrinsic motivation is reframed as internalizing extrinsic change intentions. Vansteenkiste and Sheldon (2006) argued that it is unrealistic and perhaps even illogical for practitioners to encourage clients to voluntarily engage in activities that yield only inherent reward or satisfaction (i.e., intrinsic motivation). Just as no person can make another person engage in a behavior for the sake of pure enjoyment, no practitioner can realistically cultivate intrinsic motivation in a client. Rather than enhancing intrinsic motivation, Patrick and Williams (2012) noted, MI facilitates the process of internalizing extrinsic motivations.

The three methods discussed in the following sections are additional and specific approaches for enhancing motivation and promoting autonomy in persons with substance use problems and other addictions. They are neither derived from nor directly linked to the TTM, MI, or SDT. All three approaches, however, share principles common to these three models: Motivation is multidimensional and represents interpersonal, intrapersonal, and contextual influences; change is more often than not developmental and gradual; autonomy is to be respected and promoted; and change occurs in a nonjudgmental, compassionate, supportive, and facilitative environment.

HARM-REDUCTION APPROACHES

Harm reduction is an autonomy-supportive practice that seeks to minimize the risk and extent of harm resulting from addictive and other high-risk behaviors (e.g., unprotected sex, medication noncompliance) and to improve quality of life (Collins et al., 2012). In many ways, harm reduction is similar to moderation-oriented treatment for alcohol abuse and alcoholism (see Chapter 6). It also is a compassionate and pragmatic set of strategies, often formulated at the grassroots level, to reduce harm and increase well-being for individuals, communities, and society. It is particularly appropriate for persons who are not in treatment and are not highly motivated to change their behaviors (see Peavy, Cochran, & Wax, 2010). However, harm-reduction psychotherapy was developed to help persons with problems such as addiction (Tatarsky & Kellogg, 2012). In sum, harm reduction is a belief system and a deliberate plan of action—and it remains highly controversial.

The harm-reduction approach originated outside the United States in the early 20th century as an alternative to legal sanctions for problematic substance use. In countries such as Great Britain, the Netherlands, and Australia, harm reduction remains public policy to varying degrees. Examples of harm-reduction practices specific to substance use are the use of naloxone (or Narcan®, an opioid antagonist) to reverse opioid overdoses; federally funded needle exchange programs for injecting drug users; medication-assisted treatment (i.e., use of medications to reduce cravings) and, specifically, opioid agonist therapy; and supervised consumption sites and "assisted-heroin treatment" (see Collins et al., 2012, for a review).

Harm reduction has never been fully embraced by policymakers in the United States, despite sporadic efforts to do so. Under the Obama administration, for example, a 21-year-old ban on most federally funded needle exchange programs was lifted in December 2009 by the U.S. Congress and the president. However, the ban was reinstated by a new U.S. Congress 2 years later. Nadelmann and LaSalle (2017) characterize this lack of a substantive federal response to harmful and widespread drug injection as a "great shame and tragedy" (p. 1). They note the irony of local, state, and federal jurisdictions refusing to fund needle exchange programs while states increasingly legalize cannabis use. The Comprehensive Addiction and Recovery Act passed by a conservative Congress in 2016 was intended to provide affected citizens with greater access to naloxone and opioid agonist therapies (e.g., methadone). However, the funding approved by Congress in the subsequent 21st Century Cures Act pales in comparison to the great need. Furthermore, in late 2017, the Trump administration refused to call the current opioid epidemic a "national emergency." Doing so would have allocated new funds to address the crisis. Calling it instead a "public health emergency" limits funding to existing funds.

As a form of decriminalization, harm reduction was developed to address the marginalization experienced by many clients informed that abstinence was the only, predetermined, and non-negotiable goal of addiction treatment. Although abstinence is an alternative (and an ideal outcome) in harm reduction approaches, it is not the sole imperative. Using the analogy of traffic lights, Marlatt and Witkiewitz (2010) characterize harm reduction as the yellow light that "signals the driver to slow down, take caution, and notice the potential harms associated with crossing that intersection. . . . [In this way, it] may appeal to many users who are unwilling or unable to completely stop at the red light of abstinence" (p. 592). Harm reduction thus provides persons with choices; more accurately, it honors the right of persons to choose how to live their lives with minimal health risks they and others have incurred. This stance aligns harm reduction with SDT and MI. Indeed, Whiteside, Cronce, Pedersen, and Larimer (2010) claim that "harm reduction strategies based in MI appear to be most effective" (p. 151) when working with adolescents and young adults.

Harm-reduction practitioners typically use the TTM and its stages-of-change dimension (Tatarsky & Kellogg, 2012). One way the two are used in concert is that harm reduction aims to provide some level of protection to those in the precontemplation and contemplation stages of change about their risk behavior, as well as to offer an alternative form of action and maintenance to those who reject abstinence. Harm-reduction approaches are designed to modify addictive behaviors by decreasing the frequency and amount of substance use, for example, and by altering other using practices such as type of substance used and using environment. The *warm turkey* approach (Miller & Page, 1991) and *tapering down* are methods for gradually decreasing substance use (described as *gradualism* and *abstinence eventually*; Kellogg, 2003) and can include *sobriety sampling* whereby the person attempts to abstain for a period of time (e.g., over a weekend) on a trial basis. Substance use is not viewed as inherently immoral, and the user is not regarded as abnormal. The focus is mostly on the *problems* caused by the substance use or other behavior (e.g., hoarding) than the behavior itself. In this way, harm-reduction methods resemble the brief interventions of motivational enhancement therapy.

Other behavioral modifications associated with harm reduction include substituting a safer addictive substance (e.g., methadone, buprenorphine) for another (e.g., heroin, fentanyl) to reduce cravings and prevent withdrawal symptoms, and substituting one type of paraphernalia (e.g., clean syringes for injecting drug users) for another (e.g., used or "dirty" syringes) to reduce the spread of communicable diseases such as HIV and hepatitis. The use of designated drivers, electronic cigarettes, and nicotine replacement therapy are additional harm-reduction practices.

Despite its guiding principle of compassionate pragmatism and its purpose to help persons stay alive, maintain health or get better, and access services (e.g., medical care, education), harm reduction remains highly controversial because it does not forbid ongoing substance use or other high-risk behaviors (e.g., sex). As an example, a condom machine was installed in a San Francisco jail a few years ago, the first of its kind in the United States (Sylla, Harawa, & Reznick, 2010). Preliminary evaluation of this service indicated awareness of condom availability, support of condom use among prisoners, and reports that sexual activity had not increased.

Housing First is another controversial harm-reduction program. It provides shelter for chronically homeless persons with severe alcohol problems and does not restrict on-site drinking. This program was first instituted in New York City in 1992 as an alternative to Treatment First or abstinence-based housing programs that require detoxification, sobriety, and vaguely defined housing readiness before homeless persons can gain access to independent housing (Padgett, Stanhope, Henwood, & Stefancic, 2011). Housing First offers safe housing, meals, and on-site health care services. It is a "safe haven" and a form of palliative care for homeless persons who often have co-occurring mental health and extensive medical conditions. For residents who continue to drink and may die from alcohol-related conditions, Housing First serves as end-of-life care, allowing them to die "at home" in their own bed surrounded by caring staff rather than on the street and alone (McNeil et al., 2012).

Critics of Housing First and other harm-reduction programs often subscribe to a conservative and moralistic ideology and equate harm reduction with permissiveness, or the green traffic light rather than the yellow traffic light. Criminalization is also often championed. The contention is that *permissive* harm-reduction policies and practices *enable* or facilitate continued, harmful substance use and other risk-prone behavior. Findings from several studies on Housing First programs, however, reveal significant reductions in alcohol use when compared to an abstinence-based Treatment First program (Padgett et al., 2011) or other housing programs (Kirst, Zerger, Misir, Hwang, & Stergiopoulos, 2015); significant decreases in days intoxicated (Larimer et al., 2009); and sizeable reductions in alcohol use and alcohol-related problems over 2 years in one program (Collins et al., 2012). Furthermore, Larimer and colleagues (2009) reported significant and substantial cost savings for one Housing First program in Seattle, Washington: Costs to the public prior to Housing First entry (e.g., days in jail, sobering center and emergency department visits, emergency medical services calls and transports) were cut in half (from approximately $8 million to approximately $4 million) for the 95 residents who remained in the program for 12 months. Other harm-reduction programs demonstrate similar results. For example, Wodak and Cooney's (2006) comprehensive review of needle and syringe exchange programs worldwide yielded overwhelming evidence that these programs do not promote negative consequences (e.g., greater injection frequency), are effective in reducing infection (e.g., HIV), and also are cost-effective. They also function as a point of entry or bridge to substance abuse treatment services, which qualifies them as an autonomy-supportive resource.

MINDFULNESS-BASED APPROACHES

Mindfulness can be considered a harm-reduction practice for addictive behaviors. It also is a central component of several counseling and psychotherapeutic approaches. These include dialectical behavior therapy (DBT; Linehan, 2015) and acceptance and commitment therapy (ACT; Hayes, Strosahl, & Wilson, 2012). Both DBT and ACT have been applied effectively to persons who have mental health and substance use disorders. In one study (Harned et al., 2009), DBT significantly outperformed a community-based treatment in remitting substance dependence disorders (i.e., alcohol, cannabis, and cocaine) and increasing drug- and alcohol-abstinent days among persons with borderline personality disorder (BPD) and another mental health condition (primarily major depression). No other additional mental health condition represented in this study sample (e.g., anxiety, eating disorders) demonstrated similar improvement, leading the researchers to herald DBT as particularly well suited for persons with substance use disorders who also have BPD. This endorsement is important because suicidality is common among persons with BPD, and suicidality in this population is often accompanied by substance use. In an earlier study of DBT for opioid-dependent women with BPD (Linehan et al., 2002), DBT was found to reduce opiate use and retain women in treatment significantly more so than a validation-based 12-step treatment program. ACT also has demonstrated positive results for persons with substance use disorders, albeit not as convincingly as DBT. Investigations of ACT include its application for persons with comorbid alcohol use disorders and depression (Petersen & Zettle, 2009), methamphetamine use disorders (Smout et al., 2010), and nicotine dependence (Gifford et al., 2011; Hernandez-Lopez, Luciano, Bricker, Roales-Nieto, & Montesinos, 2009), as well as for problematic Internet pornography viewing (Twohig & Crosby, 2010).

Other therapies have adopted mindfulness as the core skill and have fashioned their practice around it. These include mindfulness-based cognitive therapy (MBCT) and mindfulness-based stress reduction (MBSR). At least three mindfulness-based therapies have been developed for addictive behaviors: (1) mindfulness-based addiction treatment (Vidrine et al., 2016), modeled on MBCT to promote smoking cessation; (2) mindfulness-oriented recovery enhancement (Garland et al., 2017) that uses cognitive–behavior principles and strategies to address chronic pain and opioid addiction; and (3) mindfulness-based relapse prevention (MBRP; Bowen, Chawla, & Marlatt, 2011), modeled on MBSR as a group-based 8-week aftercare program for persons seeking to maintain sobriety from a variety of substances. Of the three, MBRP has an extensive research base, a published training manual, and accessible training and practice-guided resources accessible at *www.mindfulrp.com*. MBRP is described later in this section.

State of Mindfulness

What exactly is mindfulness? *Mindfulness* is heightened awareness of the present moment. It is the deliberate practice of paying attention to, accepting, describing, and not changing or judging one's immediate perceptual experience (Hayes, Follette, & Linehan, 2004; Kabat-Zinn, 1994). It is staying put in the here and now. It is an openness to and an attentional focus on what is taking place in the moment, using as many senses as possible (e.g., sight, sound, smell), including attending to visceral functioning (e.g., breathing). SDT (described earlier in this chapter) speaks of *mindful awareness* (Ryan & Deci, 2017), which is understood as an openness to, and an acceptance of, internal activity, the purpose being to experience freedom from introjects or internal pressures (e.g., judgmental self-commands) and to foster harmony among parts of one's personality. The integration of mindfulness in SDT thus promotes autonomy and healthy self-regulation.

The practice of mindfulness—that is, the concentrated focus on, observation of, and participation in the present moment—eschews any inclinations to think through or make sense of what is taking place. It is not a form of reasoning or the act of interpretation. Rather, mindfulness is an acceptance of the here and now, absorbing the now as it is, for what it is, and not using it to explain past experiences or to strategize (i.e., plan ahead). Its purpose is to soak in the now, letting it be what it is, and not manipulating or otherwise controlling it for another purpose. This is what makes mindfulness a practice—it takes effortful practice!

Mindfulness is inspired by the ancient Buddhist practices of Vipassana and Zen meditation (Chiesa & Malinowski, 2011). Although reference is made to mindfulness meditation, and meditation is one way to develop mindfulness (Marlatt et al., 2004), the two are not entirely the same and can be practiced separately. Rather than focusing on another reality or retreating from the present moment (as can be done in meditation), mindfulness is "a way of living awake, with your eyes wide open" (Dimidjian & Linehan, 2009, p. 425). It is an attentional skill or a way of paying attention on purpose so as to reveal what is occurring internally (e.g., cycle of breath) and externally (e.g., touch). It is therefore not a form of mind-*less*ness (which may be a state achieved in certain forms of meditation). Whereas meditation may have as its goal achieving deep relaxation, spiritual enlightenment, or desensitization to physical pain or anxiety, mindfulness has as its goal only mindfulness (Dimidjian & Linehan).

Mindfulness is the way in which an individual makes direct contact with immediate experience, not with abstractions or concepts. Persons who practice mindfulness are able to control or focus their attention on the present moment. They do not control *what* is being attended to, such as deliberately trying to change internal events (e.g., thoughts, breathing) or external events (e.g., people). Rather, they control *how* they attend to what is happening in and around them in the here and now. Despite the existence of many forms of mindfulness (see Chiesa & Malinowski, 2011), it should not be confused with contemplation or spirituality (Leigh, Bowen, & Marlatt, 2005). It is unlike certain forms of prayer and so should not be confused with prayer. It is not a form of communicating with, or connecting to, a transcendent being (as may be done in certain forms of meditation), nor is it engaging with the specific content of thought or experience. Furthermore, mindfulness does not seek to make something happen, such as "emptying" or ridding oneself of negative thoughts (e.g., urges to use), or to prevent certain kinds of behavior (e.g., gambling). It is, as Chiesa and Malinowski (2011) describe, the process and state of getting used to or "familiarizing yourself" with immediate sensations and experiences.

From a mindfulness perspective, addiction is an attempt either to take hold of or to avoid cognitive, affective, or physical experiences (Witkiewitz, Bowen, Douglas, & Hsu, 2013). A person may continue to use a substance or to gamble to claim ownership of or secure possession of the euphoric high the behavior produces. Addictive behaviors thus are an attempt to manufacture and hoard positive experiences. Addictive behaviors also may be maintained to avoid emotional pain such as shame (Luoma, Kohlenberg, Hayes, & Fletcher, 2012). Either way, addiction, unlike mindfulness, is coerced and nonautonomous behavior that has as its intent the control and manipulation of firsthand experiences.

Mindful behavior is nonpossessive and nonreactive; it holds in abeyance any attempt to change one's immediate circumstance, accepting the here and now (e.g., a craving sensation) as a momentary visitor and remaining alert and open to subsequent immediate experiences. Think of mindfulness as the pause in between a stimulus and a response. Its observant, nonjudgmental, and nonreactive elements make possible the disruption of cyclical or repetitive addictive behaviors. A mindful pause ushers into awareness a menu of response options, including not reacting to an urge or a craving. Mindful behavior thus is in stark contrast to addictive behaviors that are automatic, impulsive, and habitual or compulsive. Adopting a more mindful orientation and practice—implementing a mindful pause—signifies a new form of motivation derived from within and aligned with one's values (i.e., autonomous). Consistent with SDT, mindfulness is self-regulated and authentic behavior.

Mindfulness-Based Interventions for Addictive Behaviors

Mindfulness skills and practices vary widely (see Chiesa & Malinowski, 2011), but they generally include an explicit focus on present-centered awareness, such as paying attention to one's breathing and concentrating on one sense in particular (e.g., hearing) for a short period of time (e.g., 5 minutes). Mindfulness practice is therefore a form of approach coping rather than avoidance coping (Bowen et al., 2014). Because mindfulness has its roots in Buddhist meditation and because meditation can foster mindfulness, guided meditation that "scans" the body (e.g., abdomen, toes, arms) often is used. In MBRP (Bowen et al., 2011), a 20- to 30-minute body scan meditation is conducted at the start of each weekly group session. This type of practice is particularly important for persons with substance use problems and other addictive behaviors because, as Bowen and colleagues (2011) explain:

> Experiences of reactivity, cravings, and urges often manifest physically before the subsequent chain of thoughts or reactions. . . . Thus, coming back to physical sensations is a way of reconnecting the present experience and can be a first step in shifting from habitual, reactive behavior to making more mindful choices. (p. 37)

Overall, MBRP is designed to promote increased awareness of triggers for use, habitual patterns of using, and automatic reactions that appear to control a person's daily living. It integrates mindfulness practice with cognitive–behavioral relapse prevention practices, such as identifying triggers for use. MBRP is an aftercare program for persons who already have completed outpatient or inpatient treatment for substance use disorders. It takes place in 2-hour weekly group sessions over an 8-week period. Sessions provide instruction on and practice of mindfulness skills to implement when urges, cravings, and other triggers to use arise; participants also are encouraged to adopt mindfulness as a recovery lifestyle. In addition to breathing exercises and body scan meditation, skills taught and practiced in MBRP include engaging in mindful movement postures (e.g., yoga) and urge surfing, and exercising SOBER breathing space. Urge surfing (Marlatt & Gordon, 1985) is the intentional practice of staying with an urge to use a substance or engage in an addictive behavior such as gambling by "riding the craving waves," using the "surfboard" of the breath. Focusing on the natural fluctuations of your breathing instead of giving in to an urge or craving to drink or smoke, for example, can result in diminished intensity of urges and cravings. *SOBER* refers to the five sequential tasks of Stopping or slowing down when experiencing a trigger to use, Observing what is happening in the moment, focusing on your Breathing, Expanding your awareness of other sensations (e.g., clammy hands, sweating), and Responding (vs. reacting) with awareness in a healthy, self-compassionate way. Brief audio recordings of guided SOBER breathing practices are available at *www.mindfulrp.com.*

Any of these mindfulness skills can be incorporated into other prevention and treatment practices and adapted for specific populations, substances, and settings. For college students interested in changing their nicotine smoking behavior, for example, Bowen and Marlatt (2009) instructed students to pay attention to their thoughts, sensations, or urges without attempting to change or deflect them when presented with cigarette cues. The urge surfing exercise was described, and students were encouraged to picture their urge as a wave and to imagine riding the wave as it naturally crested and then subsided, rather than fighting the urge or giving in to it (because urges, like waves, gradually decrease in intensity as time goes by). Compared to a control group, students in this study who completed the mindfulness exercises reported 7 days later (1) smoking significantly fewer cigarettes per day and (2) a significantly weaker connection between experiencing a negative affect (e.g., anxiety) and the urge to smoke (i.e., less reactivity). Urge surfing also has demonstrated preliminary positive results for adolescents (ages 14–18) who had completed a school-based alcohol treatment program (Harris, Stewart, & Stanton, 2017). Compared to a wait-list control condition, adolescents who met with an interventionist weekly for four one-on-one sessions to learn about and practice urge surfing reported decreased alcohol quantity and frequency at 4-week follow-up.

MBRP has demonstrated feasibility and efficacy for reducing substance use and craving during and up to 4 months after participating in the program (Bowen et al., 2009; Witkiewitz et al., 2013). Subsequent studies have tested the effects of MBRP up to 12 months posttreatment relative to cognitive–behavioral relapse prevention (CBRP) and treatment as usual (TAU; i.e., process-oriented group based on 12-step programs). Findings from Bowen and colleagues' (2014) study suggest that the beneficial effects of MBRP (i.e., fewer drug use days and a significantly higher probability of not engaging in heavy drinking) are more enduring than those of CBRP. And Roos, Bowen, and Witkiewitz (2017) reported that MBRP was more effective (i.e., involving fewer drug- or alcohol-using days) than either CBRP or TAU, particularly for clients with highly severe substance use symptoms and for those with co-occurring disorders, namely, depression and anxiety.

In describing MBRP, Bowen and colleagues (2011) note that it is not in conflict with the philosophy of 12-step programs, such as AA and NA. Several areas that overlap include the shared emphasis on acceptance ("It is what it is"), relinquishment of personal control, and valuing of prayer and meditation. Areas of divergence, however, are MBRP's nonendorsement of (1) diagnoses or any other labels of people or conditions interpreted as either good or bad (e.g., *addict, disease, alcoholic*) and (2) abstinence as the predetermined and requisite goal for treatment or aftercare.

12-STEP FACILITATION

Unlike AA and other 12-step mutual aid societies (e.g., NA), 12-step facilitation (TSF; Nowinski & Baker, 2003; Ries, Galanter, & Tonigan, 2008) is an intervention delivered by a treatment professional to persons enrolled in a treatment program. It is intended to encourage clients to become active participants in sober social support networks. Specifically, TSF helps clients make use of AA and other mutual aid groups both during and after treatment. This means not only attending AA fellowship meetings, but also becoming actively involved in or "working" the 12-step program by (1) learning and adopting the philosophy of AA (including the 12 steps), (2) securing a sponsor (i.e., enlisting the support of a fellow member of AA with at least 1 year of consecutive sobriety), and (3) identifying oneself as a member of AA or another 12-step program. To accomplish these three components, *facilitating* the process of AA involvement is essential; it is not enough to refer clients to AA meetings. TSF is designed as a time-limited (12–15 sessions) treatment delivered in either individual or group format, and is based on the philosophy of AA, including the 12 steps of recovery. Abstinence is therefore the intended outcome of treatment.

As with MET, TSF was developed in the early 1990s for the Project MATCH study. Since then, TSF has been subjected to extensive research and was recognized by SAMHSA's NREPP in 2008 as an evidence-based practice for the treatment of substance use concerns. Nowinski (2012) outlines its principles and practices to include (1) honoring the locus of change as residing in 12-step fellowships and not in the skills of the counselor, for example; (2) promoting the client's "spiritual awakening" as part of AA fellowship involvement; (3) reinforcing practical methods for achieving and maintaining sobriety; (4) working collaboratively with clients (and not making 12-step meeting attendance a requirement of treatment); and (5) maintaining the focus of treatment on helping clients begin the process of 12-step recovery. Concepts discussed in individual and group TSF treatment are a humble acceptance of one's powerlessness over alcohol and other drugs (consistent with the first step of AA) and the surrender of personal control or willpower to a higher power (consistent with Steps 2 and 3 of AA). Reading material (e.g., AA "Big Book") is provided and reviewed in sessions with clients, and client experiences attending AA and other 12-step meetings are processed.

Since the mid-1990s, considerable and sophisticated research has been conducted on AA and 12-step facilitation, which Kelly and Yeterian (2012) described as an "empirical awakening." Although all three treatments in the Project MATCH study (MET, TSF, and CBT) were associated with improved drinking outcomes, TSF fared better in achieving and maintaining abstinence than did MET or CBT for clients without psychopathology and for those who sought meaning in life (Project MATCH Research Group, 1997). Despite caution about the clinical significance of these and other findings (Ferri, Amato, & Davoli, 2006), the preponderance of evidence suggests beneficial outcomes for persons who attend AA and maintain active involvement while they are in treatment and after completion of treatment (Moos & Timko, 2008).

In their 16-year study of previously untreated individuals with alcohol dependence, Moos and Moos (2006) reported that participation in AA during and after addiction treatment was associated with better alcohol-related outcomes (e.g., abstinence) and improved self-efficacy. The longer these persons remained in AA (even after treatment had ended), the more likely they were to have achieved remission after 16 years. They also were likely to report reductions in anger (Kelly, Stout, Tonigan, Magill, & Pagano, 2010) and in impulsivity and legal problems (Blonigen, Timko, Finney, Moos, & Moos, 2011; Blonigen, Timko, Moos, & Moos, 2009).

What explains the benefit of AA beyond treatment? Moos (2008) offered several explanations, which he categorized as active ingredients: receiving support, having clear goals, participating in structured group activities, having abstinence-oriented norms and role models, being involved in alternative rewarding activities, and focusing on self-efficacy and coping skills. Moos and Moos noted that participation in some form of addiction treatment likely served as motivation for individuals to enter AA. Indeed, 74% of AA members reported that involvement in treatment or some form of counseling (which preceded AA attendance for 59% of AA members) was important in leading them to AA, and 84% reported that their continued involvement in treatment or counseling played an important part in their recovery (Alcoholics Anonymous, 2014). These findings reinforce the beneficial effects of programs such as TSF.

CHAPTER SUMMARY

Human motivation is complex and multidimensional. It comprises intrapersonal, interpersonal, and contextual influences. No one thing or person is responsible for another's purposeful behavior either in the direction of maintaining addictive behaviors or in changing addictive behaviors; many factors contribute. This is true regardless of the theory or model of addiction from which one operates. Among the factors that contribute to behavior change are prevention and treatment methods that honor and promote a person's right to choose what he or she prefers—that is, what a person believes is best for him or her. These are the autonomy-supporting practices of MI and those associated with the TTM and SDT. Additional practices that promote autonomy and enhance motivation to change addictive behaviors, to varying degrees, are harm reduction, mindfulness-based approaches, and TSF. There is compelling evidence, based on well-designed research, to support the continued adoption of these practices.

The evidence is just as clear about what does *not* influence or motivate change in addictive behaviors. These include enlightenment (including fact-based education and scare tactics), confrontation (including coercion), and punishment (Miller, 2006). For example, Apodaca and Longabaugh (2009) found that therapist use of MI-inconsistent behaviors (e.g., engaging in confrontation, offering advice without permission) predicted poorer substance use outcomes. In addition, Pavey and Sparks (2009) reported that among college students, a greater perceived threat to their decision-making freedom (i.e., perception of threat to autonomy) was related to less positive attitudes toward reducing alcohol consumption. And in their study of 672 problem drinkers followed over 11 years (81% of whom maintained their participation), Delucchi and Kaskutas (2010) identified several factors that predicted increased drinking. Four of these factors were (1) experiencing more social consequences of drinking over time, (2) receiving alcohol specialty treatment, (3) receiving suggestions to get help for one's drinking, and (4) taking account of the number of heavy drinkers and drug users in their social network. Factors that predicted *less* drinking over time were the number of contacts across medical, mental health, criminal justice, and welfare systems; and attendance at AA meetings. Attendance at AA reinforces the efforts of TSF.

Nace and colleagues (2007) argued that socially sanctioned mechanisms of coercion (e.g., court-mandated treatment, suspension or threatened loss of licensure for certain professionals, drug testing in sports and other professions) are effective, specifically in initiating treatment for individuals.

However, the arguments for coercion appear to be consistent with their view of addiction as a disease (e.g., "Coercion involves an acceptance of the involuntary aspects of addiction," p. 21) and are subject to hyperbole (e.g., "The swift and predictable punishment and rewards meted out during [drug court] hearings are psychologically powerful," p. 17). In addition, the evidence presented by Nace and colleagues to support coercive methods is not extensive. Furthermore, they appear to equate coercion with treatment and not just as a means to initiate treatment (as in a strategy for treatment). Their assertions run counter to the principles of SDT and harm reduction, as well as the "spirit" of MI.

Given the scientific revolution in the addictions field over the past 35 years, we believe it is time for practitioners to embrace a panoramic view of human motivation rather than the traditional myopic view. The traditional view is quite limiting and inaccurate (i.e., one is neither motivated nor unmotivated), equates the motivation of clients in treatment with their referral source (Wild et al., 2006), and shortchanges prospective and current service recipients of beneficial care. The panoramic view, by contrast, reflects the openness of true scientific inquiry and, we propose, a more humanistic and compassionate stance toward care. A more expansive view of human motivation prioritizes human subjectivity, thereby honoring and promoting autonomy and concomitantly offering options and alternatives to facilitate change. Embracing this evidence-based panoramic view of human motivation and change processes is likely to extend addiction services to a wider range of people who might otherwise scoff at and dismiss efforts to (yet again) control their behavior. What facilitates the motivation of another to change? The evidence is clear: the compassionate and autonomy-supporting approach of the helper.

REVIEW QUESTIONS

1. Motivation is defined as purposeful behavior and, more specifically, as that which energizes and directs action in the present moment. Explain the importance of the present moment to purposeful behavior.

2. How do a person's values influence motivation? How can a prevention specialist or counselor make use of a person's values to facilitate motivation for that person?

3. What are the stages of change in the TTM? How are they useful in understanding and facilitating motivation? What are the criticisms of the stages of change?

4. Referring to its fourfold "spirit," define MI. Identify the four fundamental skills used in MI, referred to by the acronym OARS, and name the seven

dimensions of verbalized motivation (change talk) in MI, referred to by the acronym DARN CAT.

5. How does MET differ from MI?

6. According to SDT, what are the three basic and universal human needs?

7. How does *autonomous motivation* differ from *controlled motivation*? Which one contributes to self-regulated behavior? How does extrinsic reinforcement curtail self-regulated behavior? Does this imply that contingency management is in direct opposition to SDT?

8. If MI and SDT were to "get married" (even though Miller & Rollnick, 2012, said this is "premature"), how would they resolve their differences on the topic of *amotivation*?

9. Define harm reduction and provide five examples of harm-reduction practices. How do these practices promote autonomy?

10. How does the practice of mindfulness facilitate motivation? What are its benefits in the prevention and treatment of addiction?

11. Define TSF. How is it similar to, and different from, attending mutual aid society meetings, such as AA?

12. From your reading of the entire chapter, what specific practices forestall human motivation and squelch autonomous behavior? By contrast, what specific practices facilitate human motivation and promote autonomy?

CHAPTER 12

Linking Theory, Evidence, and Practice

Views of addiction and responses to it are shaped by the political and economic climate of the day. Today's climate remains one of *accountability*. Budget deficits, rising health care costs, and economic instability in the United States explain public health and health care policies that require all practitioners to demonstrate that their work is effective—effective in terms of improved prevention and treatment outcomes, as well as cost savings. When practice is not effective, both the individual and society suffer consequences. The individual continues to have life difficulties, and society pays a high opportunity cost by relying on strategies and services that do not have the highest return on investment (Brownson, Baker, Deshpande, & Gillespie, 2018).

Recognition that ineffective practices need to be replaced led to the introduction of evidence-based practice (EBP) in many health and human services fields in the late 1990s (Brownson et al., 2018). This new principle is based on the expectation that practitioners will use only those practices that have proven track records of effectiveness. More often than not, these track records refer to consistently positive results produced by methodologically sound research investigations. Thus, the new standard calls for only those practices that can be substantiated by evidence to be used in health and human service settings, including programs for problematic substance use prevention and treatment. The delivery of these services is known as EBP.

STANDARDS OF EVIDENCE

When most people hear the word *evidence*, they think of information used in legal proceedings, which may include witness accounts of a crime, testimony from a law enforcement officer or expert, reports from a forensic scientist, and so forth. In the fields that comprise health and human services, evidence is some form of data produced by professional practice, assessment, evaluation, and/or research. These data are often referred to as *outcomes* and are based on behavioral indicators, such as client report of, or biological markers noting, abstinence; court records that reflect no new arrests or charges over a certain period of time; actual costs of conducting a prevention program; and family or staff observation of client medication compliance.

Unfortunately, the quality of evidence is subject to interpretation. Carroll (2012) notes that what constitutes clinically meaningful outcomes remains in dispute in the addiction treatment and research fields. Is simply having a relative who had previously refused to enter treatment now attend an intake session and then one subsequent treatment session sufficient to warrant a family intervention effective? This is the primary outcome used to determine the efficacy of community reinforcement and family training (CRAFT), the family intervention reviewed in Chapter 11. Furthermore, does a client self-report of problem-free substance use at the end of treatment suggest treatment success, or must there be a follow-up period to determine whether or not the effects of treatment have endured? If there is a follow-up period, how long must it be for the effects of treatment to be considered lasting?

The standards used for judging evidence vary tremendously, and frequently are influenced by professional training or stakeholder status. For example, an epidemiologist may employ extremely high standards of evidence, whereas a consumer or client may accept low standards for judging information as credible.

Chambers and Kerner (as cited in Brownson et al., 2018) placed different types of health data on a continuum ranging from *subjective,* representing low credibility, to *objective,* representing high credibility. On this continuum, information in the form of personal experiences, testimonials, and marketing data (subjective sources) were identified as representing low standards of evidence. In contrast, the highest standards of evidence (objective sources) were provided by systematic reviews of scientific literature. In between these two extremes were isolated studies from the scientific literature, program evaluations, and studies relying solely on qualitative methods. Because there are no absolute criteria for determining what type of information constitutes *evidence,* practitioners, stakeholders, and consumers need to be cautious about accepting claims that a practice is evidence-based.

Concerns about practices claiming to be "evidence-based" partially explain the recent decision of the Substance Abuse and Mental Health Services Administration (SAMHSA) to suspend updates to the online registry it has operated since 1997, the NREPP. In a public statement, an assistant secretary at SAMHSA (2018) acknowledged there are NREPP entries "based on review of as few as a single publication that might be quite old and, too often, evidence review from someone's dissertation." Gorman (2017) observed that NREPP-registered interventions include those tested on "a very small, self-selected sample, and in which the findings of the evaluation have appeared only in an internal report or an unpublished manuscript or a pay-to publish online journal" (p. 41). Further criticism is that "NREPP has mainly reviewed submissions from 'developers' in the field. By definition, these are not EBPs because they are limited to the work of a single person or group. This is a biased, self-selected series of interventions" (SAMHSA, 2018). This echoes the potential bias criticism raised by Wright, Zhang, and Farabee (2012). They found that 52% of NREPP entries were evaluated by the developers of those programs, persons eager to claim their program as "NREPP-registered" and "evidence-based." These criticisms support claims that the term *evidence-based practice* represents a form of propaganda (Gambrill, 2010).

THE RELATIONSHIP BETWEEN
THEORY, EVIDENCE, AND PRACTICE

Under ideal circumstances, theory, evidence, and practice should inform one another in a continual process that builds a body of knowledge. The translation of theory and evidence into EBP should always be in flux. As Figure 12.1 depicts, theory comprises constructs that should be tested, and when supported by data, they should be adopted and implemented into routine practice. However, if the evidence does not support the theory under scrutiny, then the theory needs revision (notice the two-way arrow involving theory and evidence in Figure 12.1). Consistent with the attributes of a good theory mentioned in Chapter 1, West and Brown (2013) stipulate that theories must be tested to determine, in part, whether there is "a genuine counter-example that conflicts with the theory" (p. 22). If one exists, the theory should be modified.

The newer concept of *practice-based evidence* that originated from direct service providers may be extremely useful for revising theory and improving practice, primarily because of its relevance to representative community and clinical settings (Barkham & Mellor-Clark, 2003). Practice-based evidence is a "bottom-up" or "grassroots" effort that enlists practitioners and clients in effectiveness research of routine practice, including cost–benefit analyses. Thus, theory should be responsive to data generated from (1) research protocols such as randomized control trials *and* (2) program evaluation conducted in representative or conventional practice settings. The former is often characterized as *efficacy research,* the latter as *effectiveness research.*

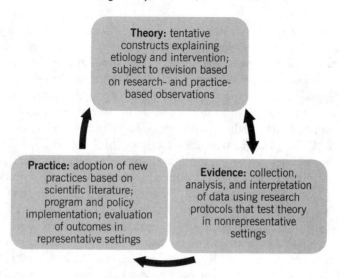

FIGURE 12.1. Ideal relationships between theory, evidence, and practice in substance abuse prevention and treatment.

The Emergence of Evidence-Based Practice

Although the adoption and implementation of EBP in medicine, mental health care, and public health are still relatively new, by comparison, EBP in the addictions field is much more recent. It has taken much longer for addictions professionals to entertain scientific practices. This delay is explained in part by history. As discussed in Chapter 9, addiction remains a stigmatized condition, and the addiction treatment field continues to be heavily influenced by practitioners who themselves are in recovery from the condition. More recently, this includes peer support specialists and recovery coaches. Even though alcoholism and drug addiction are commonly referred to as diseases, their treatment has remained separate from medicine and mental health. Woodworth and McLellan (2016) offer the following explanation for this longstanding separation:

> The prevailing clinical and public perception at the time that the treatment system was being developed was that substance use disorders resulted from a moral failure, and therapy was thus focused on improving the sufferer's spiritual condition. In addition, the financing model for addiction treatment did not comport with the financing of other healthcare, and so the segregation of services was seemingly sensible from a therapeutic, as well as an administrative perspective. The impact of this segregation has been significant, affecting not only the delivery of care, but also shaping public perception and policy-making. (p. 111)

Separate services continue today, despite efforts to achieve integrated health care. The segregation of addiction services is exemplified in the treatment of opioid dependence. Federal law stipulates that methadone (a synthetic opioid agonist medication taken daily to treat the symptoms of opioid dependence, e.g., craving, withdrawal) can be dispensed only in opioid treatment programs, and many private insurance and Medicaid plans remain reluctant to purchase methadone services, instead referring individuals to publicly funded treatment facilities (McCarty et al., 2010).

Developments in the United States over the past 15 years point to increasing reliance on EBP in problematic substance use prevention and treatment. For example, the Paul Wellstone and Pete Domenici Mental Health Parity and Addiction Equity Act (the MHPAEA), passed by the U.S. Congress in 2008, requires health insurance companies to cover mental health and addiction treatment equivalent to physical health coverage. The subsequent passage of the Affordable Care Act (the ACA) by the U.S. Congress in 2010, a law that was upheld by the U.S. Supreme Court in 2012, extended these requirements to Medicaid plans operating through state-based insurance exchanges. Despite the current administration's efforts to stall implementation of specific aspects of the ACA, it remains law. It is intended to address the longstanding health care system fragmentation wherein persons with comorbid disorders are treated in separate service settings and by different service providers. This endeavor—given the long history of separating addiction treatment from primary care and mental health care—is remarkable. As McLellan and Woodworth (2014) noted:

> The implications [of the ACA] are enormous. For the first time, substance use disorders will be treated like other physical illnesses, increasingly by the same providers now practicing general healthcare, and under the same insurance financing conditions. At last, there is the opportunity for consumers to receive care for many of their mental and substance use problems where they receive the rest of their healthcare. This should improve access, choice and quality of care for individuals and society. (p. 541)

Others (e.g., Barry & Huskamp, 2011; Manderscheid, 2014) agree with this assessment, arguing that the ACA has potential to usher in improved coordination of care and the implementation of integrated care models. The ACA considers substance use services one of 10 essential health benefits. Manderscheid (2014) projected that Medicaid expansion will "favor persons with primary substance use conditions" (pp. 88–89); Woodworth and McLellan (2016) project that an approximate 12% increase in persons covered by Medicaid will meet criteria for substance use disorders. The ACA also mandates that new insurance plans cover smoking cessation services (e.g., screening, counseling) without any patient cost sharing or prior authorization, which, if fully implemented, will substantially increase access to care, reduce health care costs, and help end the epidemic of tobacco-related diseases (McAfee, Babb, McNabb, & Fiore, 2015).

These two pieces of federal legislation—the MHPAEA and the ACA— signal further acknowledgment of addiction as a medical condition. They represent a victory for addiction advocacy groups and the recovery movement. They also have significant implications for the addiction treatment field. Specifically, a more sophisticated addictions treatment workforce will be needed to practice effectively in an increasingly regulated and ever-widening treatment industry. As Beutler (2009) noted, no longer can personal experience suffice as the sole or primary standard for justifying treatment decisions. Addictions counselors will be expected to be familiar with a wide range of services and to be able to demonstrate competency in several EBPs, especially those that target co-occurring disorders.

Defining Evidence-Based Practice

According to Brownson and colleagues (2018), there is consensus that EBP needs to be defined within context. This has led professions in the health and human services to define EBP in different ways. For example, the American Psychological Association (APA) has defined EBP as "the integration of the best available research with clinical expertise in the context of patient characteristics, culture, and preferences" (APA Presidential Task Force on Evidence-Based Practice, 2006, p. 273). This is depicted in Figure 12.2 on the next page. Notice that in this definition EBP has three components. Research findings do not constitute the only evidence; rather, clinician and client factors also must be considered (e.g., client cultural diversity). For example, a multisystemic therapy (MST) team (see Chapter 8) must be able to adapt its operations to accommodate adjudicated adolescent sex offenders needing intensive behavioral health services in a specific community. These operations will include consulting recent research on MST for juvenile sex offenders (see Letourneau et al., 2009) and conducting individualized assessment with families to identify their specific characteristics (e.g., gender of adolescent, siblings in the household), culture (e.g., religious beliefs and customs), and preferences (e.g., language).

According to the APA definition of EBP, it is the *integration* of best available research, clinician expertise, and client factors that signifies evidence-based *practice*. One of the three elements on its own—for example, research—does not comprise EBP. It is the coordination and intersection of the three that defines EBP. Evidence-based practice therefore is a program and style of operation that involves routine evaluation of clinical staff performance by a clinical supervisor, clinician self-assessment, consultation of a practice manual that highlights principles of care, and coordination of care with treatment team members, other professionals involved in a case,

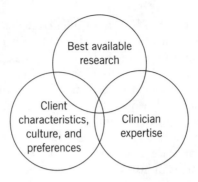

FIGURE 12.2. Evidence-based practice in psychology defined.

and clients and their families. This integrative perspective is in contrast to earlier references to *empirically supported treatments* (ESTs). The distinction between ESTs and EBP is very important. As the name suggests, ESTs, on the one hand, pertain to specific techniques or interventions only, such as conducting a functional analysis or offering empathic reflections. EBP, on the other hand, is inclusive of client and clinician factors, treatment setting and interventions, and research findings. It is a comprehensive package, style, and process of care.

In the field of public health, EBP is defined as "the process of integrating science-based interventions with community preferences to improve the health of populations" (Kohatsu, Robinson, & Torner, 2004, p. 419). This population-level definition attempts to integrate scientific evidence with environmental and organizational considerations, available resources, and perceived needs of communities. These contrasting definitions point out that the translation of science into EBP will take distinct forms in different fields.

EBP is not without controversy. Criticisms include (1) the concern that too much emphasis is placed on science and not on context and resources; (2) lack of clarity as to what constitutes evidence and how to weigh it (e.g., see the criticisms of the NREPP review process noted earlier); and (3) the often cost-prohibitive implementation of many EBPs. Because criteria for determining an EBP originated in clinical medicine and follow guidelines similar to those used to determine safe and effective medications, research studies that provide evidence for a certain practice have been criticized for being unnecessarily rigorous and using nonrepresentative participants or populations. Although these randomized control trials (RCTs) may be the "gold standard" of scientific research, they often produce science that cannot be easily transported to representative settings and populations. This is the argument of proponents of practice-based evidence. Barkham and Mellor-Clark (2003), for example, cite the "high external validity" of practice-based evidence research studies "because they sample therapy as it is in routine practice" (p. 321). One final criticism of EBP is that its implementation is sometimes mandated by funders or policymakers, representing a "top-down" approach and leaving many prevention and treatment practitioners with a distasteful impression of these practices.

Despite these and other controversies about EBP, it is here to stay. A November 2014 Pew-MacArthur Results First Initiative report (a project of the Pew Charitable Trusts and the John D. and Catherine T. MacArthur Foundation; see *www.pewtrusts.org*) noted that from 2004 to 2014, a total of 42 states had passed over 100 state laws supporting the use of evidence-based programs and practices. These laws have been implemented primarily to reduce costs.

Performance-Based Contracting

It is increasingly likely that many states will implement what is referred to as *performance-based contracting* whereby state funding sources, such as Medicaid, will allocate funds to treatment providers only when specified performance measures are met. Performance measures assess meeting goals for program capacity, demonstrating client retention in and completion of treatment, decreased client incarceration, and increased client employment and abstinence (McLellan, Kemp, Brooks, & Carise, 2008). States such as Maine that have enforced these contingencies and for which there are data indicate increased efficiency and effectiveness, but decreased admission of service recipients with severe disorders. Other states (e.g., Delaware) have not demonstrated a decline in admission of clients with severe disorders. On the contrary, Delaware demonstrated an increase in admission of clients with severe disorders, which was likely due to an increase in program capacity (e.g., by extending treatment hours and establishing additional satellites). McLellan (2011) argued that performance-based contracting can only be effective when it operates according to the principles of contingency management (see Chapters 6 and 11), such as linking closely in time the desired (purchased) outcome (e.g., abstinence) to a reward large enough to change the contingent (e.g., addictive) behavior.

Although performance-based contracting and EBP may be thought of as one and the same, they are not. Straus, Glasziou, Richardson, and Haynes (2011) clearly state that evidence-based medicine "is not an effective cost-cutting tool, since providing evidence-based care directed toward maximizing patients' quality of life often *increases* the costs of their care and raises the ire of some health economists" (p. 7, emphasis added). Therefore, adopting and implementing an EBP may not necessarily reflect performance-based contracting and may not always result in reduced costs. The same also may be true for services derived from practice-based evidence. The "evidence" must reflect improved client or consumer outcomes, not necessarily cost savings. Therefore, EBP and practice-based evidence are intended to benefit the recipients of an intervention, not only or primarily the providers of care. According to Carroll (2012), the original aim of disseminating EBPs was to improve client outcome. The challenge is to identify EBPs for prevention and treatment that, in the long run, also reduce costs.

Technology Transfer

The process of connecting practitioners to science is known as *technology transfer* (see Chapter 1). Because EBPs are alternatives to traditional or conventional methods of prevention and treatment, they can be considered innovations. Therefore, technology transfer is also referred to as *adoption of innovation* (as discussed in Chapter 3) and involves three primary steps or phases: training, adoption, and implementation (Flynn & Simpson, 2009). These steps are depicted in Figure 12.3. The process of encouraging the adoption of new practices and investing in them (e.g., EBPs) is often a long-term endeavor. As may be true for most innovations, EBPs often are viewed with suspicion upon first introduction. Training is thus an essential component of this process and must address the preferences and practical needs of practitioners, such as accessibility (including cost), credentialing benefits (if any), and the acquisition of practical knowledge and skills.

Although *adoption* describes the entire process, it also is a specific step of testing and trial learning, and it involves decision making and action taking. According to Flynn and Simpson (2009), these two activities in the adoption phase are enhanced when leadership support is available to facilitate the entire adoption process. It also requires partnerships among various systems (e.g., local and state governments) that may result in the discontinuation of longstanding programs and in the targeting of specific interventions (Schmidt et al., 2012).

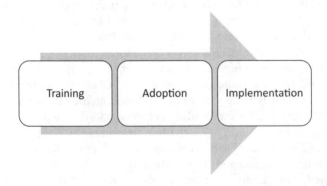

FIGURE 12.3. Three primary steps or stages of technology transfer.

The third step in technology transfer is implementation. This is when a behavioral health treatment facility, for example, puts into routine, everyday practice the program or practice (e.g., motivational interviewing) it adopted following its investment in comprehensive staff training. Implementation is evident in such things as the facility's mission statement, website description of services, consistent in-service training, ongoing staff supervision and fidelity measurement (e.g., periodic audio recording of counseling sessions to determine whether an EBP was delivered as intended), and monitoring of client receptivity to the program or practice.

Carroll and Kiluk (2017) identified a few general barriers to implementing evidence-based behavioral treatments into routine clinical practice. These barriers include a lack of training and certification programs available for clinicians; the cost of training and the high rate of provider turnover in many practice settings; the lack of a feasible means to evaluate and support valid and consistent implementation of an EBP, what is known as fidelity to the model (e.g., providing ongoing clinical supervision); and, as noted earlier, different views on standards of evidence between researchers and practitioners.

Innovations and other EBPs are more likely to be adopted and sustained when practitioners perceive them to have more benefits than shortcomings (including the flexibility or adaptability of an EBP). Furthermore, innovation will occur when resistance and barriers to change are low. During the implementation phase of technology transfer, the adopted innovation or EBP is enforced and conducted on a routine basis. For the EBP to endure and remain viable, the program must be able to sustain it (financially, maintaining a positive work climate), and stakeholders (clients, administration, and practitioners) must view it as effective and feasible. Maintaining strong partnerships among various parties (e.g., funding sources and service providers) also is essential. Although it is a formidable undertaking, the process of implementing EBPs on a wide scale in the addictions field is not impossible (Schmidt et al., 2012).

CHAPTER SUMMARY

Despite investments in technology transfer initiatives, it is our view that insufficient resources are being directed to the implementation of EBP today. Carroll (2012) noted that EBPs "are far from universally available and competently implemented" (p. 1031). Funding sources, leaders in prevention and treatment service provision (e.g., hospital administrators, county mental health and recovery boards), training programs, credentialing bodies, and other professional groups need to invest in a revitalized effort to enhance the quality and consistency of EBP training and delivery in substance use prevention and treatment. The public—current and future consumers of prevention and treatment services—need and deserve such quality care.

This book is intended to address the need for improved prevention and treatment services in the addictions field. It is a mixture of theory, evidence, and practice. It is this kind of mixture—adopted, implemented, and promoted by practitioners and system leaders alike—that is necessary to promote real and lasting change for persons and their families who struggle with addictions.

REVIEW QUESTIONS

1. What societal forces have ushered in evidence-based practice (EBP) in the professions of health and human services?

2. What are the standards for evaluating evidence?

3. What is the ideal relationship between theory, evidence, and practice?

4. How is EBP defined in psychology and in public health? What components comprise the integration in both definitions of EBP?

5. How does EBP differ from (a) empirically supported treatments, (b) practice-based evidence, and (c) performance-based contracting?

6. What conditions impede and facilitate the adoption and implementation of EBP?

References

Abrams, D. B., Herzog, T. A., Emmons, K. M., & Linnan, L. (2000). Stages of change versus addiction: A replication and extension. *Nicotine and Tobacco Research, 2*, 223–229.

Abrams, D. B., & Niaura, R. S. (1987). Social learning theory. In H. T. Blane & K. E. Leonard (Eds.), *Psychological theories of drinking and alcoholism*. New York: Guilford Press.

Adamson, S. J., Heather, N., Morton, V., Raistrick, D., & UKATT Research Team. (2010). Initial preference for drinking goal in the treatment of alcohol problems: II. Treatment outcomes. *Alcohol and Alcoholism, 45*, 136–142.

Administration for Children and Families. (2017). *The AFCARS Report*, No. 24. Retrieved May 23, 2018, from *www.acf.hhs.gov/cb*.

Agrawal, A., Neale, M. C., Prescott, C. A., & Kendler, K. S. (2004). Cannabis and other illicit drugs: Comorbid use and abuse/dependence in males and females. *Behavioral Genetics, 34*(3), 217–228.

Ainslie, G. (1992). *Picoeconomics: The strategic interaction of successive motivational states within the person*. Cambridge, UK: Cambridge University Press.

Ajonijebu, D. C., Abboussi, O., Russell, V. A., Mabandla, M. V., & Daniels, W. M. (2017). Epigenetics: A link between addiction and social environment. *Cellular and Molecular Life Sciences, 74*, 2735–2747.

Alcoholics Anonymous. (1976). *The story of how many thousands of men and women have recovered from alcoholism* [the "Big Book"]. New York: AA World Services.

Alcoholics Anonymous. (1981). *Twelve steps and twelve traditions*. New York: AA World Services.

Alcoholics Anonymous. (2014). Alcoholics Anonymous 2014 membership survey. Retrieved May 24, 2018, from *www.aa.org/assets/en_US/p-48_membershipsurvey.pdf*.

Alexander, B. K. (1988). The disease and adaptive models of addiction: A framework evaluation. In S. Peele (Ed.), *Visions of addiction: Major contemporary perspectives on addiction and alcoholism*. Lexington, MA: D.C. Heath.

Alexander, B. K. (2001, April). The roots of addiction in free market society, Canadian Center for Policy Alternatives. Retrieved February 13, 2018, from *www.cfdp.ca/roots.pdf*.

Alexander, J., & Parsons, B. V. (1982). *Functional family therapy.* Monterey, CA: Brooks/Cole.

Allsop, S. (2018). Advancing alcohol research and treatment: Contentions and debates about treatment intensity, goals and outcomes in the 1970s and 1980s. *Addiction, 113,* 1149–1154.

Alston, P. (2017). Statement on visit to the USA, by Professor Philip Alston, United Nations Special Rapporteur on extreme poverty and human rights (Office of the United Nations High Commissioner for Human Rights). Retrieved February 13, 2018, from *http://ohchr.org/EN/NewsEvents/Pages/DisplayNews. aspx?NewsID=22533&LangID=E.*

Alter, A. (2017). *Irresistible: The rise of addictive technology and the business of keeping us hooked.* New York: Penguin Press.

Amaro, H., Reed, E., Rowe, E., Picci, J., Mantella, P., & Prado, G. (2010). Brief screening and intervention for alcohol and drug use in a college student health clinic: Feasibility, implementation, and outcomes. *Journal of American College Health, 58*(4), 357–364.

American Hospital Association. (1995). *AHA hospital statistics* (1994–1995 ed.). Chicago: Author.

American Psychiatric Association. (1980). *Diagnostic and statistical manual of mental disorders* (3rd ed.). Washington, DC: Author.

American Psychiatric Association. (2000). *Diagnostic and statistical manual of mental disorders* (4th ed., text rev.). Washington, DC: Author.

American Psychiatric Association. (2013). *Diagnostic and statistical manual of mental fisorders* (5th ed). Arlington, VA: Author.

Americans with Disabilities Act. (1990). Public Law No. 101-336, § 2(a), 104 Stat. 327, 328-329 (codified as amended at 42 U.S.C. § 12101(a) (2006).

Amlung, M., Vedelago, L., Acker, J., Balodis, I., & MacKillop, J. (2017). Steep delay discounting and addictive behavior: A meta-analysis of continuous associations. *Addiction, 112,* 51–62.

Amrhein, P. C., Miller, W. R., Yahne, C. E., Palmer, M., & Fulcher, L. (2003). Client commitment language during motivational interviewing predicts drug use outcomes. *Journal of Consulting and Clinical Psychology, 71,* 862–878.

Ananthapavan, J., Peterson, A., & Sacks, G. (2018). Paying people to lose weight: The effectiveness of financial incentives provided by health insurers for the prevention and management of overweight and obesity—a systematic review. *Obesity Reviews, 19,* 605–613.

Anglin, M. D., Brecht, M. L., Woodward, J. A., & Bonett, D. G. (1986). An empirical study of maturing out: Conditional factors. *International Journal of the Addictions, 21*(2), 233–246.

APA Presidential Task Force on Evidence-Based Practice. (2006). Evidence-based practice in psychology. *American Psychologist, 61,* 271–285.

Apodaca, T. R., Jackson, K. M., Borsari, B., Magill, M., Longabaugh, R., Mastroleo, N. R., et al. (2016). Which individual therapist behaviors elicit client change talk and sustain talk in motivational interviewing? *Journal of Substance Abuse Treatment, 61,* 60–65.

Apodaca, T. R., & Longabaugh, R. (2009). Mechanisms of change in motivational interviewing: A review and preliminary evaluation of the evidence. *Addiction, 104,* 705–715.

Artega, I., Chen, C., & Reynolds, A. J. (2010). Childhood predictors of adult substance abuse. *Children and Youth Services Review, 32,* 1108–1120.

Askew, R. (2016). Functional fun: Legitimising adult recreational drug use. *International Journal of Drug Policy, 36,* 112–119.

Austin, A. M., Macgowan, M. J., & Wagner, E. F. (2005). Effective family-based interventions for adolescents with substance use problems: A systematic review. *Research on Social Work Practice, 15,* 67–83.

Azevedo, F. A. C., Carvalho, L. R. B., Grinberg, L. T., Farfel, J. M., Ferretti, R. E. L., Leite, R. E. P., et al. (2009). Equal numbers of neuronal and nonneuronal cells make the human brain an isometrically scaled-up primate brain. *Journal of Comparative Neurology, 513,* 532–541.

Azrin, N. H. (1976). Improvements in the community-reinforcement approach to alcoholism. *Behaviour Research and Therapy, 14,* 339–348.

Bacio, G. A., Mays, V. M., & Lau, A. S. (2013). Drinking initiation and problematic drinking among Latino adolescents: Explanations of the immigrant paradox. *Psychology of Addictive Behaviors, 27,* 14–22.

Baker, K. M. (2016). "I'm going to shut down all of your tricks": Depictions of treatment professionals in addiction entertainment. *Substance Use and Misuse, 51,* 489–497.

Baldwin, S. A., Christian, S., Berkeljon, A., & Shadish, W. R. (2012). The effects of family therapies for adolescent delinquency and substance abuse: A meta-analysis. *Journal of Marital and Family Therapy, 38,* 281–304.

Ball, S. A., Martino, S., Nich, C., Frankforter, T. L., Van Horn, D., Crits-Christoph, P., et al. (2007). Site matters: Multisite randomized trial of motivational enhancement therapy in community drug abuse clinics. *Journal of Consulting and Clinical Psychology, 75,* 556–567.

Bandura, A. (1977). *Social learning theory.* Englewood Cliffs, NJ: Prentice-Hall.

Bandura, A. (1995). Exercise of personal and collective efficacy in changing societies. In A. Bandura (Ed.), *Self-efficacy in changing societies.* New York: Cambridge University Press.

Bandura, A. (1997). *Self-efficacy: The exercise of control.* New York: Freeman.

Bandura, A., Caprara, G. V., Barbaranelli, C., Regalia, C., & Scabini, E. (2011). Impact of family efficacy beliefs on quality of family functioning and satisfaction with family life. *Applied Psychology: An International Review, 60,* 421–448.

Barkham, M., & Mellor-Clark, J. (2003). Bridging evidence-based practice and practice-based evidence: Developing a rigorous and relevant knowledge for the psychological therapies. *Clinical Psychology and Psychotherapy, 10,* 319–327.

Barnett, A. I., Hall, W., Fry, C. L., Dilkes-Frayne, E., & Carter A. (2018). Drug and alcohol treatment providers' views about the disease model of addiction and its impact on clinical practice: A systematic review. *Drug and Alcohol Review, 37,* 697–720.

Barnett, E., Moyers, T. B., Sussman, S., Smith, C., Rohrbach, L. A., Sun, P., et al. (2014). From counselor skill to decreased marijuana use: Does change talk matter? *Journal of Substance Abuse Treatment, 46,* 498–505.

Barnett, M. L., Olenski, A. R., & Jena, A. B. (2018). Opioid-prescribing patterns of emergency physicians and risk of long-term use. *New England Journal of Medicine, 376,* 663–673.

Barrowclough, C., Haddock, G., Wykes, T., Beardmore, R., Conrod, P., Craig, T., et al. (2010). Integrated motivational interviewing and cognitive behavioural therapy for people with psychosis and comorbid substance misuse: Randomised controlled trial. *British Medical Journal, 341,* 6325–6337.

Barry, C. L., & Huskamp, H. A. (2011). Moving beyond parity—Mental health and addiction care under the ACA. *New England Journal of Medicine, 365,* 973–975.

Bartle-Haring, S., Slesnick, N., & Murnan, A. (2018). Benefits to children who participate in family therapy with their substance-using mother. *Journal of Marital and Family Therapy, 44,* 671–686.

Bateson, G., Jackson, D. D., Haley, J., & Weakland, J. (1956). Toward a theory of schizophrenia. *Behavioral Science, 1,* 251–264.

Baumeister, R. F. (2016). Toward a general theory of motivation: Problems, challenges, opportunities, and the big picture. *Motivation and Emotion, 40,* 1–10.

Beattie, M. (1992). *Codependent no more: How to stop controlling others and start caring for yourself.* Center City, MN: Hazelden.

Beauchamp, G. A., Winstanley, E. L., Ryan, S. A., & Lyons, M. S. (2014). Moving beyond misuse and diversion: The urgent need to consider the role of iatrogenic addiction in the current opioid epidemic. *American Journal of Public Health, 104,* 2023–2029.

Bechtel, W., & Richardson, R. (1993). *Discovering complexity: Decomposition and localization asstrategies in scientific research.* Princeton, NJ: Princeton University Press.

Bechtold, J., Hipwell, A., Lewis, D. A., Loeber, R., & Pardini D. (2016). Concurrent and sustained cumulative effects of adolescent marijuana use on subclinical psychotic symptoms. *American Journal of Psychiatry, 173,* 781–789.

Becker, S. J., & Curry, J. F. (2008). Outpatient interventions for adolescent substance abuse: A quality of evidence review. *Journal of Consulting and Clinical Psychology, 76,* 531–543.

Bennett, M. E., Bradshaw, K. R., & Catalano L. T. (2017). Treatment of substance use disorders in schizophrenia. *American Journal of Drug and Alcohol Abuse, 43,* 377–390.

Benowitz, N. L., St. Helen, G., Dempsey, D. A., Jacob, P., & Tyndale, R. F. (2016). Disposition kinetics and metabolism of nicotine and cotinine in African American smokers: Impact of CYP2A6 genetic variation and enzymatic activity. *Pharmacogenetics and Genomics, 26,* 340–350.

Berger, L. M., Slack, K. S., Waldfogel, J., & Bruch, S. K. (2010). Caseworker-perceived caregiver substance abuse and child protective services outcomes. *Child Maltreatment, 15,* 199–210.

Bernard, L. C., Mills, M., Swenson, L., & Walsh, R. P. (2005). An evolutionary theory of human motivation. *Genetic, Social, and General Psychology Monographs, 131*(2), 129–184.

Bernhardt, N., Nebe, S., Pooseh, S., Sebold, M., Sommer, C., Birkenstock, J., et al. (2017). Impulsive decision making in young adult social drinkers and detoxified alcohol-dependent patients: A cross-sectional and longitudinal study. *Alcoholism: Clinical and Experimental Research, 41,* 1794–1807.

Bernstein, C. A. (2011, March 4). Meta-structure in DSM-5 process. *Psychiatric News, 46,* 7.

Berridge, K. C., & Robinson, T. E. (2016). Liking, wanting, and the incentive-sensitization theory of addiction. *American Psychologist, 71,* 670–679.

Bertholet, N., Faouzi, M., Gmel, G., Gaume, J., & Daeppen, J. (2010). Change talk sequence during brief motivational intervention, towards or away from drinking. *Addiction, 105,* 2106–2112.

Besinger, B. A., Garland, A. F., Litrownik, A. J., & Landsverk, J. A. (1999). Caregiver substance abuse among maltreated children placed in out-come-home care. *Child Welfare, 78,* 221–239.

Beutler, L. E. (2009). Making science matter in clinical practice: Redefining psychotherapy. *Clinical Psychology: Science and Practice, 16,* 301–317.

Bickel, W. K., & Marsch, L. A. (2001). Toward a behavioral economic understanding of drug dependence: Delay discounting processes. *Addiction, 96,* 73–86.

Biener, A. I., & Decker, S. L. (2018). Medical care use and expenditures associated with adult obesity in the United States. *Journal of the American Medical Association, 319,* 218.

Biener, L., & Abrams, D. B. (1991). The contemplation ladder: Validation of a measure of readiness to consider smoking cessation. *Health Psychology, 10,* 360–365.

Bigelow, W., & Liebson, J. (1972). Cost factors controlling alcoholic drinking. *Psychological Record, 22,* 305–314.

Billieux, J., Schimmenti, A., Khazaal, Y., Maurage, P., & Heeren, A. (2015). Are we overpathologizing everyday life?: A tenable blueprint for behavioral addiction research. *Journal of Behavioral Addictions, 4,* 119–123.

Bischof, G., Iwen, J., Freyer-Adam, J., & Rumpf, H. (2016). Efficacy of the Community Reinforcement and Training for concerned significant others of treatment-refusing individuals with alcohol dependence: A randomized controlled trial. *Drug and Alcohol Dependence, 163,* 179–185.

Black, C. (1982). *It will never happen to me!* Denver, CO: M.A.C.

Blanco, C., Hasin, D. S., Wall, M. M., Flórez-Salamanca, L., Hoertel, N., Wang, S., et al. (2016). Cannabis use and risk of psychiatric disorders: Prospective evidence from a US national longitudinal study. *JAMA Psychiatry, 73,* 388–395.

Blevins, C. E., Farris, S. G., Brown, R. A., Strong, D. R., & Abrantes, A. M. (2016). The role of self-efficacy, adaptive coping, and smoking urges in long-term cessation outcomes. *Addictive Disorders and Their Treatment, 15,* 183–189.

Blocker, J. S. (2006). Did prohibition really work?: Alcohol prohibition as a public health innovation. *American Journal of Public Health, 96,* 233–243.

Blonigen, D. M., Timko, C., Finney, J. W., Moos, B. S., & Moos, R. H. (2011). Alcoholics Anonymous attendance, decreases in impulsivity and drinking and psychosocial outcomes over 16 years: Moderated-mediation from a developmental perspective. *Addiction, 106,* 2167–2177.

Blonigen, D. M., Timko, C., Moos, B. S., & Moos, R. H. (2009). Treatment, Alcoholics Anonymous, and 16-year changes in impulsivity and legal problems among men and women with alcohol use disorders. *Journal of Studies on Alcohol and Drugs, 70,* 714–725.

Blum, K., Gardner, E., Oscar-Berman, M., & Gold, M. (2012). "Liking" and "wanting" linked to reward deficiency syndrome (RDS): Hypothesizing differential responsivity in brain reward circuitry. *Current Pharmaceutical Design, 18,* 113–118.

Boileau, I., Assaad, J. M., Pihl, R. O., Benkelfat, C., Leyton, M., Diksic, M., et al. (2003). Alcohol promotes dopamine release in the human nucleus accumbens. *Synapse, 49,* 226–231.

Botelho, R., Engle, B., Mora, J. C., & Holder, C. (2011). Brief interventions for alcohol misuse. *Primary Care: Clinics in Office Practice, 38,* 105–123.

Botvin, G. J., Baker, E., Botvin, E. M., Filazzola, A. D., & Millman, R. B. (1984). Prevention of alcohol misuse through the development of personal and social competence: A pilot study. *Journal of Studies on Alcohol, 45,* 550–552.

Botvin, G. J., Baker, E., Dusenbury, L., Botvin, E. M., & Diaz, T. (1995). Long-term follow-up results of a randomized drug abuse prevention trial in a white middle-class population. *Journal of the American Medical Association, 273*(14), 1106–1112.

Botvin, G. J., Baker, E., Dusenbury, L., Tortu, S., & Botvin, E. M. (1990). Preventing adolescent drug abuse through a multimodal cognitive-behavioral approach: Results of a three-year study. *Journal of Consulting and Clinical Psychology, 58,* 437–446.

Botvin, G. J., Dusenbury, L., Baker, E., James-Ortiz, S., Botvin, E. M., & Kerner, J.

(1992). Smoking prevention among urban minority youth: Assessing effects on out-come and mediating variables. *Health Psychology, 11,* 290–299.

Botvin, G. J., & Eng, A. (1982). The efficacy of a multi-component approach to the pre-vention of cigarette smoking. *Preventive Medicine, 11,* 199–211.

Botvin, G. J., Eng, A., & Williams, C. L. (1980). Preventing the onset of cigarette smok-ing through life skills training. *Preventive Medicine, 9,* 135–143.

Botvin, G. J., Griffin, K. W., Diaz, T., & Ifill-Williams, M. (2001). Drug abuse pre-vention among minority adolescents: Posttest and one-year follow-up of a school-based preventive intervention. *Prevention Science, 2,* 1–13.

Botvin, G. J., Griffin, K. W., Paul, E., & Macaulay, A. P. (2003). Preventing tobacco and alcohol use among elementary school students through Life Skills Training. *Jour-nal of Child and Adolescent Substance Abuse, 12,* 1–18.

Botvin, G. J., Renick, N. L., & Baker, E. (1983). The effects of scheduling format and booster sessions on a broad-spectrum psychosocial smoking prevention program. *Journal of Behavioral Medicine, 6,* 359–379.

Bowen, M. (1976). Theory in the practice of psychotherapy. In P. J. Guerin (Ed.), *Family therapy: Theory and practice.* New York: Gardner Press.

Bowen, S., Chawla, N., Collins, S. E., Witkiewitz, K., Hsu, S., Grow, J., et al. (2009). Mindfulness-based relapse prevention for substance use disorders: A pilot efficacy trial. *Substance Abuse, 30,* 295–305.

Bowen, S., Chawla, N., & Marlatt, G. A. (2011). *Mindfulness-based relapse prevention for addictive behaviors: A clinician's guide.* New York: Guilford Press.

Bowen, S., & Marlatt, A. (2009). Surfing the urge: Brief mindfulness-based intervention for college student smokers. *Psychology of Addictive Behaviors, 23,* 666–671.

Bowen, S., Witkiewitz, K., Clifasefi, S. L., Grow, J., Chawla, N., Hsu, S. H., et al. (2014). Relative efficacy of mindfulness-based relapse prevention, standard relapse prevention, and treatment as usual for substance use disorders: A randomized clini-cal trial. *JAMA Psychiatry, 71*(5), 547–556.

Brackenbury, L. M., Ladd, B. O., & Anderson, K. G. (2016). Marijuana use/cessation expectancies and marijuana use in college students. *American Journal of Drug and Alcohol Abuse, 42,* 25–31.

Brandon, T. H., & Baker, T. B. (1991). The Smoking Consequences Questionnaire: The subjective expected utility of smoking in college students. *Psychological Assessment: A Journal of Consulting and Clinical Psychology, 3,* 484–491.

Brandt, M. (2014). Americans lose 119 billion through gambling. Statistica. Retrieved Feb-ruary 23, 2018, from *www.statista.com/chart/1865/gambling-losses-by-country.*

Braveman, P., Egerter, S., & Williams, D. R. (2011). The social determinants of health: Coming of age. *Annual Review of Public Health, 32,* 381–398.

Braveman, P., & Gottlieb, L. (2014). The social determinants of health: It's time to con-sider the causes of the causes. *Public Health Reports, 129*(Suppl. 2), 19–31.

Brecht, M. L., & Anglin, M. D. (1990). Conditional factors of maturing out: Legal super-vision and treatment. *International Journal of the Addictions, 25*(4), 393–407.

Brecht, M. L., Anglin, M. D., Woodward, J. A., & Bonett, D. G. (1987). Conditional factors of maturing out: Personal resources and preaddiction sociopathy. *Interna-tional Journal of the Addictions, 22*(1), 55–69.

Brewer, S., Godley, M. D., & Hulvershorn, L. A. (2017). Treating mental health and substance use disorders in adolescents: What is on the menu? *Current Psychiatry Reports, 19,* 5.

Brick, J. (1990). Learning and motivational factors in alcohol consumption. In W. M. Cox (Ed.), *Why people drink: Parameters of alcohol as a reinforcer.* New York: Gardner Press.

Briones, E., Robbins, M. S., & Szapocznik, J. (2008). Brief strategic family therapy: Engagement and treatment. *Alcoholism Treatment Quarterly, 26,* 81–103.

Britton, P. C., Patrick, H., Wenzel, A., & Williams, G. C. (2011). Integrating motivational interviewing and self-determination theory with cognitive-behavioral therapy to prevent suicide. *Cognitive and Behavioral Practice, 18,* 16–27.

Brodsky, A. (2004). *Benjamin Rush: Patriot and physician.* New York: St. Martin's Press.

Bronfennbrenner, U. (1979). *The ecology of human development: Experiments by design and nature.* Cambridge, MA: Harvard University Press.

Brown, S. A. (1985). Expectancies versus background in the prediction of college drinking patterns. *Journal of Consulting and Clinical Psychology, 53*(1), 123–130.

Brown, S. (1991). Adult children of alcoholics: The history of a social movement and its impact on clinical theory and practice. In M. Galanter (Ed.), *Recent developments in alcoholism: Children of alcoholics* (Vol. 9, pp. 267–285). New York: Plenum Press.

Brown, S. A., Christiansen, B. A., & Goldman, M. S. (1987). The Alcohol Expectancy Questionnaire: An instrument for the assessment of adolescent and adult alcohol expectancies. *Journal of Studies on Alcohol, 48*(5), 483–491.

Brown, S. A., Creamer, V. A., & Stetson, B. A. (1987). Adolescent alcohol expectancies as a function of personal and parental drinking patterns. *Journal of Abnormal Psychology, 96,* 177–121.

Brownson, R. C., Baker, E. A., Deshpande, A. D., & Gillespie, K. N. (2018). *Evidence-based public health* (3rd ed.). New York: Oxford University Press.

Brownson, R. C., Baker, E. A., & Kreuter, M. W. (2001). Prevention research partnerships in community settings: What are we learning? *Journal of Public Health Management and Practice, 7*(2), vii–ix.

Brunette, M. F., Drake, R. E., Woods, M., & Hartnett, T. (2001). A comparison of long-term and short-term residential treatment programs for dual diagnosis patients. *Psychiatric Services, 52,* 526–528.

Brunette, M. F., Mueser, K. T., & Drake, R. E. (2004). A review of research on residential programs for people with severe mental illness and co-occurring substance use disorders. *Drug and Alcohol Review, 23,* 471–481.

Bryant, A. I., Schulenberg, J., Bachman, J. G., O'Malley, P. M., & Johnston, L. D. (2000). Understanding the links among school misbehavior, academic achievement, and cigarette use: A national panel study of adolescents. *Prevention Science, 1,* 71–87.

Bryant-Jeffries, R. (2001). *Counselling the person beyond the alcohol problem.* London: Jessica Kingsley.

Bunker, J. P., Frazier, H. S., & Mosteller, F. (1994). Improving health: Measuring effects of medical care. *Milbank Quarterly, 72,* 225–258.

Burger, K., & Samuel R. (2017). The role of perceived stress and self-efficacy in young people's life satisfaction: A longitudinal study. *Journal of Youth and adolescence, 46,* 78–90.

Burke, D. S. (2016). Forecasting the opioid epidemic. *Science, 354,* 529.

Burns, E. (2004). *The spirits of America: A social history of alcohol.* Philadelphia: Temple University Press.

Bushfield, S. Y., & DeFord, B. (2010). *End-of-life care and addiction: A family systems approach.* New York: Springer.

Butland, B., Jebb, S., Kopelman, P., McPherson, K., Thomas, S., Mardell, J., et al. (2007). Foresight: Tackling obesities: Future choices. United Kingdom Government Office for Science. Retrieved April 22, 2018, from *www.bis.gov.uk/foresight/our-work/projects/published-projects/tackling-obesities.*

Caetano, R., Vaeth, P. A. C., & Canino, G. (2017). Family cohesion and pride, drinking and alcohol use disorder in Puerto Rico. *American Journal of Drug and Alcohol Abuse, 43,* 87–94.

Calabria, B., Clifford, A., Shakeshaft, A. P., & Doran, C. M. (2012). A systematic review of family-based interventions targeting alcohol misuse and their potential to reduce alcohol-related harm in indigenous communities. *Journal of Studies on Alcohol and Drugs, 73,* 477–488.

Calderwood, K. A., & Rajesparam, A. (2014). A critique of the codependency concept considering the best interests of the child. *Families in Society, 95,* 171–178.

Calvey, T. (2017). The extended evolutionary synthesis and addiction: The price we pay for adaptability. *Progress in Brain Research, 235,* 1–18.

Cameron, D., & Spence, M. (1976). Recruitment of problem drinkers. *British Journal of Psychiatry, 11,* 544–546.

Campbell, N. D. (2010). Multiple paths to partial truths: A history of drug use etiology. In L. M. Scheier (Ed.), *Handbook of drug use etiology: Theory, methods, and empirical findings* (pp. 29–50). Washington, DC: American Psychological Association.

Cao, D., Marsh, J. C., Shin, H.-C., & Andrews, C. M. (2011). Improving health and social outcomes with targeted services in comprehensive substance abuse treatment. *American Journal of Drug and Alcohol Abuse, 37,* 250–258.

Caputi, T. L., & McLellan, A. T. (2017). Truth and D.A.R.E.: Is D.A.R.E.'s new keepin' it REAL curriculum suitable for American nationwide implementation? *Drugs: Education, Prevention and Policy, 24,* 49–57.

Carey, T. (2016, October 16). What do Santa Claus and the chemical imbalance have in common? Retrieved May 12, 2018, from *www.madinamerica.com/2016/10/santa-claus-chemical-imbalance-common.*

Carlson, R. G. (2006). Ethnography and applied substance misuse research: Anthropological and cross-cultural factors. In W. R. Miller & K. M. Carroll (Eds.), *Rethinking substance abuse: What the science shows, and what we should do about it* (pp. 201–219). New York: Guilford Press.

Carr, E. S. (2011). *Scripting addiction: The politics of therapeutic talk and American sobriety.* Princeton, NJ: Princeton University Press.

Carr, G. D. (2011). Alcoholism: A modern look at an ancient illness. *Primary Care, 38,* 9–21.

Carroll, K. M. (2012). Dissemination of evidence-based practices: How far we've come, and how much further we've got to go. *Addiction, 107,* 1031–1033.

Carroll, K. M., Ball, S. A., Jackson, R., Martino, S., Petry, N. M., Stitzer, M. L., et al. (2011). Ten take home lessons from the first 10 years of the CTN and 10 recommendations for the future. *American Journal of Drug and Alcohol Abuse, 37,* 275–282.

Carroll, K. M., & Kiluk, B. D. (2017). Cognitive behavioral interventions for alcohol and drug use disorders: Through the stage model and back again. *Psychology of Addictive Behaviors, 31,* 847–861.

Carroll, K. M., & Onken, L. S. (2005). Behavioral therapies for drug abuse. *American Journal of Psychiatry, 162,* 1452–1460.

Case, A., & Deaton, A. (2015). Rising morbidity and mortality in midlife among white non-Hispanic Americans in the 21st century. *Proceedings of the National Academy of Sciences of the USA, 112*(49), 15083. Retrieved December 14, 2017, from *www.pnas.org/content/112/49/15078.full.*

Case, A., & Deaton, A. (2017a). The media gets the opioid crisis wrong. Here is the truth. *Washington Post.* Retrieved December 25, 2017, from *www.washingtonpost.com/*

opinions/the-truth-about-deaths-of-despair/2017/09/12/15aa6212-8459-11e7-902a-2a9f2d808496_story.html?utm_term=.538a63cc3b22.

Case, A., & Deaton, A. (2017b). Mortality and morbidity in the 21st century (Brookings Paper on Economic Activity). Retrieved December 14, 2017, from www.brookings. edu/bpea-articles/mortality-and-morbidity-in-the-21st-century.

Catalano, R. F., Berglund, M. L., Ryan, J. A. M., Lonczak, H. S., & Hawkins, J. D. (1998). Positive youth development in the United States: Research findings on evaluations of positive youth development programs. Paper funded by and submitted to U.S. Department of Health and Human Services, Office of the Assistant Secretary for Planning and Evaluation and National Institute for Child Health and Human Development. Retrieved June 1, 2017, from https://aspe.hhs.gov/execsum/positive-youth-development-united-states-research-findings-evaluations-positive-youth-development-programs.

Catalano, R. F., & Hawkins, J. D. (1996). The social development model: A theory of antisocial behavior. In J. D. Hawkins (Ed.), Delinquency and crime: Current theories. New York: Cambridge University Press.

Catalano, R. F., Kosterman, R., Haggerty, K., Hawkins, J. D., & Spoth, R. L. (1998). A universal intervention for the prevention of substance abuse: Preparing for the drug-free years. In R. S. Ashery, E. B. Robertson, & K. L. Kumpfer (Eds.), Drug abuse prevention through family interventions (NIDA Research Monograph 177, NIH Publication No. 97-4135). Rockville, MD: National Institutes of Health, U.S. Department of Health and Human Services.

Caudill, B. D., & Marlatt, G. A. (1975). Modeling influences in social drinking: An experimental analogue. Journal of Consulting and Clinical Psychology, 43, 405–415.

Caulkins, J. P., Rydell, C. P., Schwabe, W. L., & Chiesa, J. (1997). Mandatory minimum sentences: Throwing away the key or the taxpayers' money? Santa Monica, CA: Rand Drug Policy Research Center.

Center for Behavioral Health Statistics and Quality. (2015). 2014 National Survey on Drug Use and Health: Methodological summary and definitions. Rockville, MD: Substance Abuse and Mental Health Services Administration. Retrieved June 24, 2017, from www.samhsa.gov/data/sites/default/files/NSDUH-MethodSummDefs2014/NSDUHMethodSummDefs2014.htm.

Center for Behavioral Health Statistics and Quality. (2016a). Key substance use and mental health indicators in the United States: Results from the 2015 National Survey on Drug Use and Health (HHS Publication No. SMA 16-4984, NSDUH Series H-51). Retrieved July 29, 2017, from www.samhsa.gov/data.

Center for Behavioral Health Statistics and Quality. (2016b). Results from the 2015 National Survey on Drug Use and Health: Detailed tables. Rockville, MD: Substance Abuse and Mental Health Services Administration. Retrieved August 3, 2017 from www.samhsa.gov/data/sites/default/files/NSDUH-DetTabs-2015/NSDUH-DetTabs-2015/NSDUH-DetTabs-2015.htm.

Center for Responsive Politics. (2017). Pharmaceutical manufacturing. Retrieved December 7, 2017, from www.opensecrets.org/lobby/induscode.php?id=H4300&year=2017.

Center for Substance Abuse Treatment. (2012). Medication-assisted treatment for opioid addiction in opioid treatment programs (Treatment Improvement Protocol (TIP) Series 43, HHS Publication No. (SMA) 12-4214). Rockville, MD: Substance Abuse and Mental Health Services Administration.

Centers for Disease Control and Prevention. (1994). Preventing tobacco use among young people: A report of the Surgeon General. Morbidity and Mortality Weekly Report, 43(RR-4), 1–10.

Centers for Disease Control and Prevention. (1987). Progress in chronic disease prevention cigarette smoking in the United States, 1986, September 11. *Morbidity and Mortality Weekly Report, 36*(12), 581–585.

Centers for Disease Control and Prevention. (1999, April 2). Ten great public health achievements—United States, 1990–1999. *Morbidity and Mortality Weekly Report, 48*(12), 241–243.

Centers for Disease Control and Prevention. (2013). CDC health disparities and inequalities report—United States, 2013. *Morbidity and Mortality Weekly Report, 62*(Suppl. 3), 1–184.

Centers for Disease Control and Prevention. (2016). *Youth Risk Behavior Surveillance System (YRBSS).* Atlanta, GA: Author. Retrieved June 23, 2017, from *www.cdc.gov/healthyyouth/data/yrbs/index.htm.*

Centers for Disease Control and Prevention. (2017a). *Guideline for prescribing opioids for chronic pain.* Atlanta, GA: Author. Retrieved December 23, 2017, from *www.cdc.gov/drugoverdose/pdf/guidelines_factsheet-a.pdf.*

Centers for Disease Control and Prevention. (2017b). *National Notifiable Disease Surveillance System (NNDSS).* Atlanta, GA: Retrieved June 23, 2017, from *www.cdc.gov/nnds/nedss.html.*

Centers for Disease Control and Prevention. (2017c). *Opioid overdose.* Atlanta: Author. Retrieved June 26, 2017, from *www.cdc.gov/drugoverdose/data/index.html.*

Centers for Medicare and Medicaid Services. (2017). Open payments: 2016. Retrieved December 19, 2017, from *www.cms.gov/Openpayments.*

Chang, Y. H., Lee, S. Y., Wang, T. Y., Chen, S. L., Tzeng, N. S., Chen, P. S., et al. (2015). Comorbid alcohol dependence disorder may be related to aldehyde dehydrogenase 2 (ALDH2) and alcohol dehydrogenase 1B (ADH1B) in bipolar II disorder, but only to ALDH2 in bipolar I disorder, in Han Chinese. *Bipolar Disorders, 17,* 536–542.

Channing Bete Company. (2017). Guiding good choices. Retrieved June 28, 2017, from *www.channing-bete.com/prevention-programs/guiding-good-choices/guiding-good-choices.html.*

Charles, V., & Weaver, T. (2010). A qualitative study of illicit and non-prescribed drug use amongst people with psychotic disorders. *Journal of Mental Health, 19,* 99–106.

Chawla, N., Neighbors, C., Logan, D., Lewis, M. A., & Fossos, N. (2009). Perceived approval of friends and parents as mediators of the relationship between self-determination and drinking. *Journal of Studies on Alcohol and Drugs, 70,* 92–100.

Chi, F. W., Sterling, S., Campbell, C. I., & Weisner, C. (2013). 12-step participation and outcomes over 7 years among adolescent substance use patients with and without psychiatric comorbidity. *Substance Abuse, 34,* 33–42.

Chiesa, A., & Malinowski, P. (2011). Mindfulness-based approaches: Are they all the same? *Journal of Clinical Psychology, 67,* 404–424.

Chilkoti, A. (2017, July 15). States keep saying yes to marijuana use: Now come the federal no. *New York Times.* Retrieved August 31, 2017, from *www.nytimes.com/2017/07/15/us/politics/marijuana-laws-state-federal.html?%20rref=collection%2Ftimestopic%2FMarijuana%20and%20Medical%20Marijuana&action=click&contentCollection=timestopics&region=stream&module=stream_unit&version=latest&contentPlacement=5&pgtype=collection.*

Chou, C. P., Montgomery, S., Pentz, M., Rohrbach, L. A., Johnson, C. A., Flay, B. R., et al. (1998). Effects of a community-based prevention program on decreasing drug use in high-risk adolescents. *American Journal of Public Health, 88,* 944–948.

Christiansen, B. A., Roehling, P. V., Smith, G. T., & Goldman, M. S. (1989). Using alcohol expectancies to predict adolescent drinking behavior after one year. *Journal of Consulting and Clinical Psychology, 57,* 93–99.

Christy, S. M., Winger, J. G., & Mosher, C. E. (in press). Does self-efficacy mediate the relationships between social-cognitive factors and intentions to receive HPV vaccination among young women? *Clinical Nursing Research.*

Clark, C. D. (2017). *The recovery revolution: The battle over addiction treatment in the United States.* New York: Columbia University Press.

Clark, H. W., Power, A. K., Le Fauve, C. E., & Lopez, E. I. (2008). Policy and practice implications of epidemiological surveys on co-occurring mental and substance use disorders. *Journal of Substance Abuse Treatment, 34,* 3–13.

Clayton, R. R., Cattarello, A., & Walden, K. P. (1991). Sensation seeking as a potential mediating variable for school-based prevention intervention: A two-year follow-up of DARE. *Health Communication, 3,* 229–239.

Clayton, R. R., Leukefeld, C. G., Harrington, N. G., & Cattarello, A. (1996). DARE (Drug Abuse Resistance Education): Very popular but not very effective. In C. B. McCoy, L. R. Metsch, & J. A. Inciardi (Eds.), *Intervening with drug involved youth* (pp. 101–109). Beverly Hills, CA: SAGE.

Cleary, M., Hunt, G. E., Matheson, S., & Walter, G. (2009). Psychosocial treatments for people with co-occurring sever mental illness and substance misuse: Systemic review. *Journal of Advanced Nursing, 65*(2), 238–258.

Clingan, S. E., & Woodruff, S. I. (2017). Drug-avoidance self-efficacy among exclusive cannabis users vs. other drug users visiting the emergency department. *Substance Use and Misuse, 52,* 1240–1246.

Coffey, R. M., Levit, K. R., Cassed, C. A., McLellan, A. T., Chalk, M., Brady, T. M., et al. (2009). Evidence for substance abuse services and policy research: A systematic review of national databases. *Evaluation Review, 33,* 103–137.

Cohen, A. (2014). Crazy for *Ya Ba*: Methamphetamine use among northern Thai youth. *International Journal of Drug Policy, 25,* 776–782.

Cohen, M., Liebson, J., Fallace, L., & Allen, R. (1971). Moderate drinking by chronic alcoholics: A schedule-dependent phenomenon. *Journal of Nervous and Mental Disease, 153,* 434–444.

Cohen, M., Liebson, J., Fallace, L., & Speers, W. (1971). Alcoholism: Controlled drinking and incentives for abstinence. *Psychological Reports, 28,* 575–580.

Colasurdo, B. S. (2010). Behavioral addictions and the law. *Southern California Law Review, 84*(1), 161–201.

Coleman, J. C., Butcher, J. N., & Carson, R. C. (1980). *Abnormal psychology and modern life* (6th ed.). Glenview, IL: Scott, Foresman.

Collins, F. S., & Mansoura, M. K. (2001). The Human Genome Project: Revealing the shared inheritance of all humankind. *Cancer, 91,* 221–225.

Collins, R. L., Parks, G. A., & Marlatt, G. A. (1985). Social determinants of alcohol consumption: The effects of social interaction and model status on the self-administration of alcohol. *Journal of Consulting and Clinical Psychology, 53,* 189–200.

Collins, S. E., Clifasefi, S. L., Logan, D. E., Samples, L. S., Somers, J. M., & Marlatt, G. A. (2012). Current status, historical highlights, and basic principles of harm reduction. In G. A. Marlatt, M. E. Larimer, & K. Witkiewitz (Eds.), *Harm reduction: Pragmatic strategies for managing high-risk behaviors* (2nd ed., pp. 3–35). New York: Guilford Press.

COMMIT Research Group. (1995a). Community intervention trial for smoking cessation (COMMIT): I. Cohort results from a four-year community intervention. *American Journal of Public Health, 85*(2), 183–192.

COMMIT Research Group. (1995b). Community intervention trial for smoking cessation (COMMIT): II. Changes in adult cigarette smoking prevalence. *American Journal of Public Health, 85*(2), 193–200.

Conrad, K. M., Flay, B. R., & Hill, D. (1992). Why children start smoking: Predictors of onset. *British Journal of Addiction, 87,* 1711–1724.

Conrad, P. (2007). *The medicalization of society: On the transformation of human conditions into medical disorders.* Baltimore: Johns Hopkins University Press.

Conway, K. P., Swendsen, J., Husky, M. M., He, J. P., & Merikangas, K. R. (2016). Association of lifetime mental disorders and subsequent alcohol and illicit drug use: Results from the National Comorbidity Survey–Adolescent Supplement. *Journal of the American Academy of Child and Adolescent Psychiatry, 55,* 280–288.

Conyers, B. (2003). *Addict in the family: Stories of hope, loss, and recovery.* Center City, MN: Hazelden.

Corrigan, P., Schomerus, G., Shuman, V., Kraus, D., Perlick, D., Harnish, A., et al. (2017a). Developing a research agenda for understanding the stigma of addictions: Part I. Lessons from the mental health stigma literature. *American Journal on Addictions, 26,* 59–66.

Corrigan, P., Schomerus, G., Shuman, V., Kraus, D., Perlick, D., Harnish, A., et al. (2017b). Developing a research agenda for understanding the stigma of addictions: Part II. Lessons from the mental health stigma literature. *American Journal on Addictions, 26,* 67–74.

Cottone, R. R. (1992). *Theories and paradigms of counseling and psychotherapy.* Boston: Allyn & Bacon.

Cox, W. M. (1985). Personality correlates of substance abuse. In M. Galizio & S. A. Maisto (Eds.), *Determinants of substance abuse.* New York: Plenum Press.

Crapanzano, K., Vath, R. J., & Fisher, D. (2014). Reducing stigma toward substance users through an educational intervention: Harder than it looks. *Academic Psychiatry, 38,* 420–425.

Crevecoeur, D. A. (2009). Withdrawal. In G. L. Fisher & N. A. Roget (Eds.), *Encyclopedia of substance abuse prevention, treatment, and recovery* (Vol. 2, pp. 1004–1007). Thousand Oaks, CA: SAGE.

Critchlow, B. (1987). Brief report: A utility analysis of drinking. *Addictive Behaviors, 12,* 269–273.

Cummings, K. M., Hyland, A., Saunders-Martin, T., Perla, J., Coppola, P. R., & Pechacek, T. F. (1998). Evaluation of an enforcement program to reduce tobacco sales to minors. *American Journal of Public Health, 88,* 932–936.

Dallery, J., Meredith, S. E., & Budney, A. J. (2012). Contingency management in substance abuse treatment. In S. T. Walters & F. Rotgers (Eds.), *Treating substance abuse: Theory and technique* (3rd ed., pp. 81–112). New York: Guilford Press.

Dalvie, S., Fabbri, C., Ramesar, R., Serretti, A., & Stein, D. J. (2016). Glutamatergic and HPA-axis pathway genes in bipolar disorder comorbid with alcohol- and substance use disorders. *Metabolic Brain Disease, 31,* 183–189.

Dare, P. A. S., & Derigne, L. (2010). Denial in alcohol and other drug use disorders: A critique of theory. *Addiction Research and Theory, 18,* 181–193.

Dart, T. (2016). A mental health template for American jails: Saving lives and money through commonsense reform. Retrieved April 21, 2018, from *http://cookcountysheriff.org/pdf/MentalHealthTemplate_072116.pdf.*

Dattilio, F. M. (2001). Cognitive-behavior family therapy: Contemporary family myths and misconceptions. *Contemporary Family Therapy, 23,* 3–18.

Dattilio, F. M. (2010). *Cognitive-behavioral therapy with couples and families: A comprehensive guide for clinicians.* New York: Guilford Press.

Davidson, J. (2016, June 23). Is DEA a bad guy in opioid addiction fight? *Washington*

Post. Retrieved December 11, 2017, from *www.washingtonpost.com/news/ powerpost/wp/2016/06/23/is-dea-a-bad-guy-in-opioid-addiction-fight/?utm_ term=.0061c4f2bce7.*

De Boeck, K., Wilschanski, M., Castellani, C., Taylor, C., Cuppens, H., Dodge, J., et al. (2006). Cystic fibrosis: Terminology and diagnostic algorithms. *Thorax, 61,* 627–635.

de Charms, R. (1968). *Personal causation: The internal affective determinants of behavior.* New York: Academic Press.

Dear, G. E., Roberts, C. M., & Lange, L. (2005). Defining codependency: A thematic analysis of published definitions. *Advances in Psychology Research, 34,* 189–205.

Deci, E. L., Koester, R., & Ryan, R. M. (1999). A meta-analytic review of experiments examining the effects of extrinsic rewards on intrinsic motivation. *Psychological Bulletin, 125,* 627–668.

Deci, E. L., & Ryan, R. M. (2008). Self-determination theory: A macrotheory of human motivation, development, and health. *Canadian Psychology, 49,* 182–185.

Delinsky, S. S., Thomas, J. J., St. Germain, S. A., Craigen, K. E., Weigel, T. J., Levendusky, P. G., & Becker, A. E. (2011). Motivation to change among residential treatment patients with an eating disorder: Assessment of the multidimensionality of motivation and its relation to treatment outcome. *International Journal of Eating Disorders, 44,* 340–348.

Delucchi, K. L., & Kaskutas, L. A. (2010). Following problem drinkers over eleven years: Understanding changes in alcohol consumption. *Journal of Studies on Alcohol and Drugs, 71,* 831–836.

Dent, C. W., Sussman, S., & Stacy, A. W. (2001). Project Towards No Drug Abuse: Generalizability to a general high school sample. *Preventive Medicine, 32,* 514–520.

Des Jarlais, D. C. (2000). Prospects for a public health perspective on psychoactive drug use. *American Journal of Public Health, 90*(3), 335–337.

Desilver, D. (2017, July 25). Most Americans unaware that as U.S. manufacturing jobs have disappeared, output has grown. Retrieved December 26, 2017, from *www. pewresearch.org/fact-tank/2017/07/25/most-americans-unaware-that-as-u-s-manufacturing-jobs-have-disappeared-output-has-grown.*

Detar, D. T. (2011). Understanding the disease of addiction. *Primary Care, 38,* 1–7.

Deutsch, C. (1982). *Broken bottles, broken dreams: Understanding and helping the children of alcoholics.* New York: Teachers College Press.

Dickey, B., & Azeni, H. (1996). Persons with dual diagnoses of substance abuse and major mental illness: Their excess costs of psychiatric care. *American Journal of Public Health, 86,* 973–977.

DiClemente, C. C. (2003). *Addiction and change: How addictions develop and addicted people recover.* New York: Guilford Press.

DiClemente, C. C. (2015). Change is a process, not a product: Reflections on pieces to the puzzle. *Substance Use and Misuse, 50,* 1225–1228.

Dilkes-Frayne, E. (2016). Drugs at the campsite: Socio-spatial relations and drug use at music festivals. *International Journal of Drug Policy, 33,* 27–35.

Dimeff, L. A., Baer, J. S., Kivlahan, D. R., & Marlatt, G. A. (1999). *Brief alcohol screening and intervention for college students: A harm reduction approach.* New York: Guilford Press.

Dimidjian, S., & Linehan, M. M. (2009). Mindfulness practice. In W. O'Donohue & J. E. Fisher (Eds.), *General principles and empirically supported techniques of cognitive behavior therapy* (pp. 425–434). Hoboken, NJ: Wiley.

Dimoff, J. D., Sayette, M. A., & Norcross, J. C. (2017). Addiction training in clinical

psychology: Are we keeping up with the rising epidemic? *American Psychologist,*
72, 689–695.

Director, L. (2002). The value of relational psychoanalysis in the treatment of chronic
drug and alcohol use. *Psychoanalytic Dialogues, 12,* 551–579.

Dolan, M. P., Black, J. L., Penk, W. E., Robinowitz, R., & DeFord, H. A. (1985). Contracting for treatment termination to reduce illicit drug use among methadone
maintenance treatment failures. *Journal of Consulting and Clinical Psychology,*
53(4), 549–551.

Domjan, M. (2015). *The principles of learning and behavior* (7th ed.). Stamford, CT:
Cengage Learning.

Donovan, D. M., Ingalsbe, M. H., Benbow, J., & Daley, D. C. (2013). 12-step interventions and mutual support programs for substance use disorders: An overview.
Social Work in Public Health, 28, 313–332.

Drake, R. E., Luciano, A. E., Mueser, K. T., Covell, N. H., Essock, S. M., Xie, H., et al.
(2016). Longitudinal course of clients with co-occurring schizophrenia-spectrum
and substance use disorders in urban mental health centers: A 7-year prospective
study. *Schizophrenia Bulletin, 42,* 202–211.

Drake, R. E., Mercer-McFadden, C., Mueser, K. T., McHugo, G. J., & Bond, G. R.
(1998). Review of integrated mental health and substance abuse—treatment for
patients with dual disorders. *Schizophrenia Bulletin, 24,* 589–608.

Drake, R. E., & Mueser, K. T. (2000). Psychosocial approaches to dual diagnosis.
Schizophrenia Bulletin, 26, 105–118.

Drake, R. E., & Mueser, K. T. (2001). Managing comorbid schizophrenia and substance
abuse. *Current Psychiatry Reports, 3,* 418–422.

Drake, R. E., Mueser, K. T., & Brunette, M. F. (2007). Management of persons with co-
occurring severe mental illness and substance use disorder: Program implications.
World Psychiatry, 6, 131–136.

Drake, R. E., & Wallach, M. A. (1999). Homelessness and mental illness: A story of
failure. *Psychiatric Services, 50,* 589.

Drake, R. E., Wallach, M. A., Alverson, H. S., & Mueser, K. T. (2002). Psychosocial
aspects of substance abuse by clients with severe mental illness. *Journal of Nervous*
and Mental Disease, 190, 100–106.

Draycott, S. (2007). Hunting the snark: The concept of motivation. *Issues in Forensic*
Psychology, 7, 26–33.

Drossel, C., Rummel, C., & Fisher, J. E. (2009). Assessment and cognitive behavior therapy: Functional analysis as key process. In W. T. O'Donohue & J. E. Fisher (Eds.),
General principles and empirically supported techniques of cognitive behavior
therapy (pp. 15–41). Hoboken, NJ: Wiley.

Drug Abuse Resistance Education (DARE). (2017). Teaching student decision making
for safe and healthy living. Retrieved June 28, 2017, from *www.dare.org.*

Dube, S. R., Anda, R. F., Felitti, V. J., Croft, J. B., Edwards, V. J., & Giles, W. H. (2001).
Growing up with parental alcohol abuse: Exposure to childhood abuse, neglect,
and household dysfunction. *Child Abuse and Neglect, 25,* 1627–1640.

Duffy, J. (1992). *The sanitarians: A history of American public health.* Urbana: University of Illinois Press.

Dukes, R. L., Stein, J. A., & Ullman, J. B. (1997). Long-term impact of Drug Abuse
Resistance Education (D.A.R.E.). Results of a 6-year follow-up. *Evaluation*
Review, 21, 483–500.

Dunn, M. G., Mezzich, A., Janiszewski, S., Kirisci, L., & Tarter, R. E. (2001). Transmission of neglect in substance abuse families: The role of child dysregulation and

parental SUD. *Journal of Child and Adolescent Substance Abuse* [Special Issue: Etiology of Substance Use Disorder in Children and Adolescents], *10*, 123–132.

Eaton, N. R. (2015). Latent variable and network models of comorbidity: Toward an empirically derived nosology. *Social Psychiatry and Psychiatric Epidemiology, 50*, 845–849.

Edwards, G. (2010). The trouble with drink: Why ideas matter. *Addiction, 105*, 797–804.

Ellickson, P. L., Bell, R. M., & McGuigan, K. (1993). Preventing adolescent drug use: Long-term results of a junior high program. *American Journal of Public Health, 83*, 856–861.

Elliot, A. J., McGregor, H. A., & Thrash, T. M. (2002). The need for competence. In E. L. Deci & R. M. Ryan (Eds.), *Handbook of self-determination research* (pp. 361–387). Rochester, NY: University of Rochester Press.

Elliot, J. (1995, March). Drug prevention placebo: How DARE wastes time money, and police. *Reason, 26*, 14–21.

Ellul, J. (1965). *Propaganda: The formation of men's attitudes.* New York: Vintage.

Emery, S., Gilpin, E. A., Ake, C., Farkas, A. J., & Pierce, J. P. (2000). Characterizing and identifying "hard-core" smokers: Implications for further reducing smoking prevalence. *American Journal of Public Health, 90*(3), 387–394.

Ennett, S. T., Ringwalt, C. L., Thorne, J., Rohrbach, L. A., Vincus, A., Simons-Rudolph, A., et al. (2003). A comparison of current practice in school-based substance use prevention programs with meta-analytic findings. *Prevention Science, 4*, 1–14.

Faggiano, F., Minozzi, S., Versino, E., & Buscemi, D. (2014). Universal school-based prevention for illicit drug use. *Cochrane Database of Systematic Reviews, 12*, Article No. CD003020.

Falloon, I. R. H. (2003). Behavioral family therapy. In G. P. Sholevar (Ed.), *Textbook of family and couples therapy: Clinical applications* (pp. 147–172). Washington, DC: American Psychiatric Publishing.

Fals-Stewart, W., Birchler, G. R., & Kelley, M. L. (2006). Learning sobriety together: A randomized clinical trial examining behavioral couples therapy with alcoholic female patients. *Journal of Consulting and Clinical Psychology, 74*, 579–591.

Fals-Stewart, W., Kashdan, T. B., O'Farrell, T. J., & Birchler, G. R. (2002). Behavioral couples therapy for drug-abusing patients: Effects on partner violence. *Journal of Substance Abuse Treatment, 22*, 87–96.

Fals-Stewart, W., Klosterman, K., Yates, B. T., O'Farrell, T. J., & Birchler, G. R. (2005). Brief relationship therapy for alcoholism: A randomized clinical trial examining clinical efficacy and cost-effectiveness. *Psychology of Addictive Behaviors, 19*, 363–371.

Fals-Stewart, W., Lam, W. K. K., & Kelley, M. L. (2009). Behavioral couple therapy: Partner-involved treatment for substance-abusing women. In K. T. Brady, S. E. Back, & S. F. Greenfield (Eds.), *Women and addiction: A comprehensive hand-book* (pp. 323–338). New York: Guilford Press.

Fals-Stewart, W., O'Farrell, T. J., & Birchler, G. R. (2001). Behavioral couples therapy for male methadone maintenance patients: Effects on drug-abusing behavior and relational adjustment. *Behavior Therapy, 32*, 391–411.

Fals-Stewart, W., O'Farrell, T. J., Feehan, M., Birchler, G. R., Tiller, S., & McFarlin, S. K. (2000). Behavioral couples therapy versus individual-based treatment for male substance-abusing patients: An evaluation of significant individual change and comparison of improvement rates. *Journal of Substance Abuse Treatment, 18*, 249–254.

Fang, L., Barnes-Ceeney, K., & Schinke, S. P. (2011). Substance use behavior among early-adolescent Asian American girls: The impact of psychological and family factors. *Women and Health, 51,* 623–642.

Faraone, S. V., Tsuang, M. T., & Tsuang, D. W. (1999). *Genetics of mental disorders: A guide for students, clinicians, and researchers.* New York: Guilford Press.

Fauth-Bühler, M., Mann, K., & Potenza, M. N. (2017). Pathological gambling: A review of the neurobiological evidence relevant for its classification as an addictive disorder. *Addiction Biology, 22,* 885–897.

Feather, N. T. (1987). Gender differences in values: Implications of the expectancy-value model. In F. Halisch & J. Kuhl (Eds.), *Motivation, intention, and volition* (pp. 31–45). Berlin: Springer-Verlag.

Feist, J., & Feist, G. J. (2009). *Theories of personality* (7th ed.). Boston: McGraw-Hill.

Fenton, M. C., Keyes, K., Geier, T., Greenstein, E., Skodol, A., Krueger, B., et al. (2012). Psychiatric comorbidity and the persistence of drug use disorders in the United States. *Addiction, 107,* 599–609.

Ferri, M., Amato, L., & Davoli, M. (2006). Alcoholics Anonymous and other 12-step programmes for alcohol dependence (review). *Cochrane Database of Systematic Reviews, 3,* Article No. CD005032.

Fife, J. E., McCreary, M., Brewer, T., & Adegoke, A. A. (2011). Family rituals, family involvement, and drug attitudes among recovering substance abusers. *North American Journal of Psychology, 13,* 87–98.

Fillmore, K. M. (1987a). Prevalence, incidence and chronicity of drinking patterns and problems among men as a function of age: A longitudinal and cohort analysis. *British Journal of Addiction, 82,* 77–83.

Fillmore, K. M. (1987b). Women's drinking across the adult life course as compared to men's. *British Journal of Addiction, 82,* 801–811.

Fillmore, K. M., & Midanik, L. (1984). Chronicity of drinking problems among men: A longitudinal study. *Journal of Studies on Alcohol, 45,* 228–236.

Fingarette, H. (1988). *Heavy drinking: The myth of alcoholism as a disease.* Berkeley: University of California Press.

Finlay, A. K., Ram, N., Maggs, J. L., & Caldwell, L. L. (2012). Leisure activities, the social weekend, and alcohol use: Evidence from a daily study of first-year college students. *Journal of Studies on Alcohol and Drugs, 73,* 250–259.

Fischer, J. L., Spann, L., & Crawford, D. (1991). Measuring codependency. *Alcoholism Treatment Quarterly, 8*(1), 87–100.

Fish, J., Osberg, T. M., & Syed, M. (2017). "This is the way we were raised": Alcohol beliefs and acculturation in relation to alcohol consumption among Native Americans. *Journal of Ethnicity in Substance Abuse, 16*(2), 219–245.

Fisher, E. B., Auslander, W. F., Munro, J. F., Arfken, C. L., Brownson, R. C., & Owens, N. W. (1998). Neighbors for a smoke-free north side: Evaluation of a community organization approach to promoting smoking cessation among African-Americans. *American Journal of Public Health, 88,* 1658–1663.

Fisher, L. (2008, August 29). Duchovny: Sex addict onscreen and off. *ABC News.* Retrieved April 22, 2018, from *http://abcnews.go.com/Entertainment/ story?id=5686632&page=1.*

Fitzsimmons, R., Amin, N., & Uversky, V. N. (2016). Understanding the roles of intrinsic disorder in subunits of hemoglobin and the disease process of sickle cell anemia. *Intrinsically Disordered Proteins, 4*(1), e1248273.

Flanagan, E. H., Buck, T., Gamble, A., Hunter, C., Sewell, I., & Davidson, L. (2016). "Recovery Speaks": A photovoice intervention to reduce stigma among primary care providers. *Psychiatric Services, 67,* 566–569.

Flay, B. R., & Allred, C. G. (2003). Long-term effects of the Positive Action Program. *American Journal of Health Behavior, 27*(Suppl. 1), S6–S21.

Fletcher, J. B., & Reback, C. J. (2017). Mental health disorders among homeless, sub-stance-dependent men who have sex with men. *Drug and Alcohol Review, 36,* 555–559.

Flynn, P. M., & Brown, B. S. (2008). Co-occurring disorders in substance abuse treatment: Issues and prospects. *Journal of Substance Abuse Treatment, 34,* 36–47.

Flynn, P. M., & Simpson, D. D. (2009). Adoption and implementation of evidence-based treatment. In P. M. Miller (Ed.), *Evidence-based addiction treatment* (pp. 419–437). New York: Academic Press.

Forster, J. L., Murray, D. M., Wolfson, M., Blaine, T. M., Wagenaar, A. C., & Hennrikus, D. J. (1998). The effects of community policies to reduce youth access to tobacco. *American Journal of Public Health, 88*(8), 1193–1198.

Foster, D. W., Ye, F., Chung, T., Hipwell, A. E., & Sartor, C. E. (2018). Longitudinal associations between marijuana-related cognitions and marijuana use in African-American and European-American girls from early to late adolescence. *Psychology of Addictive Behaviors, 32,* 104–114.

Frances, A. J. (2010, March 24). DSM5 suggests opening the door to behavioral addictions: Behavioral addictions are a slippery slope. *Psychology Today.* Retrieved April 22, 2018, from *www.psychologytoday.com/us/blog/dsm5-in-distress/201003/dsm5-suggests-opening-the-door-behavioral-addictions.*

Frances, A. (2017, May 17). Behavioral addictions: A dangerous and slippery slope. *Huffington Post.* Retrieved February 23, 2018, from *www.huffingtonpost.com/allen-frances/behavioral-addictions-a-d_b_9959140.html.*

Frankish, C. J., George, A., Daniel, M., Doyle-Waters, M., Walker, M., & Members of the BC Consortium for Health Promotion Research. (1997). *Participatory health promotion research in Canada: A community guidebook.* Ottawa, ON, Canada: Minister of Public Works and Government Services.

Frascella, J., Potenza, M. N., Brown, L. L., & Childress, A. R. (2010). Shared brain vulnerabilities open the way for nonsubstance addictions: Carving addiction at a new joint. *Annals of the New York Academy of Sciences, 1187,* 294–315.

Freud, S. (1953). The interpretation of dreams. In J. Strachey (Ed. & Trans.), *The standard edition of the complete psychological works of Sigmund Freud* (Vols. 4 and 5). London: Hogarth Press. (Original work published 1900)

Freyer-Adam, J., Baumann, S., Schnuerer, I., Haberecht, K., Bischof, G., John, U., et al. (2014). Does stage tailoring matter in brief alcohol interventions for job-seekers?: A randomized controlled trial. *Addiction, 109,* 1845–1856.

Friederichs, S. A. H., Oenema, A., Bolman, C., Guyaux, J., van Keulen, H. M., & Lechner, L. (2014). I Move: Systematic development of a web-based computer tailored physical activity intervention, based on motivational interviewing and self-determination theory. *BMC Public Health, 14*(1), 1–29.

Friedman, G. D. (2004). *Primer of epidemiology* (5th ed.). New York: McGraw-Hill.

Friedman, S. R., Maslow, C., Bolyard, M., Sandoval, M., Mateu-Gelabert, P., & Neaigus, A. (2004). Urging others to be healthy: "Intravention" by injection drug users as a community prevention goal. *AIDS Education and Prevention, 16*(3), 250–263.

Frost, R., & McNaughton, N. (2017). The neural basis of delay discounting: A review and preliminary model. *Neuroscience and Biobehavioral Reviews, 79,* 48–65.

Fuller, T. L., & Wells, S. J. (2003). Predicting maltreatment recurrence among CPS cases with alcohol and other drug involvement. *Children and Youth Services Review 25,* 553–569.

Fuller-Thomson, E., Roane, J. L., & Brennenstuhl, S. (2016). Three types of adverse childhood experiences, and alcohol and drug dependence among adults: An investigation using population-based data. *Substance Use and Misuse, 51*(11), 1451–1461.

Galea, S., Riddle, M., & Kaplan, G. A. (2010). Causal thinking and complex system approaches in epidemiology. *International Journal of Epidemiology, 39,* 97–106.

Gambrill, E. (2010). Evidence-informed practice: Antidote to propaganda in the helping professions. *Research on Social Work Practice, 20*(3), 302–320.

Garcia-Fernandez, G., Secades-Villa, R., Garcia-Rodriguez, O., Alvarez-Lopez, H., Fernandez-Hermida, J. R., Fernandez-Artamendi, S., et al. (2011). Long-term benefits of adding incentives to the community reinforcement approach for cocaine dependence. *European Addiction Research, 17,* 139–145.

Garcia-Rodriguez, O., Secades-Villa, R., Higgins, S. T., Fernandez-Hermida, J. R., Carballo, J. L., Errasti Perez, J. M., et al. (2009). Effects of voucher-based intervention on abstinence and retention in an outpatient treatment for cocaine addiction: A randomized controlled trial. *Experimental and Clinical Psychopharmacology, 17,* 131–138.

Garland, E. L., Bryan, C. J., Finan, P. H., Thomas, E. A., Priddy, S. E., Riquino, M. R., et al. (2017). Pain, hedonic regulation, and opioid misuse: Modulation of momentary experience by Mindfulness-Oriented Recovery Enhancement in opioid-treated chronic pain patients. *Drug and Alcohol Dependence, 173,* S65–S72.

Gately, I. (2008). *Drink: A cultural history of alcohol.* New York: Gotham Books.

Gaume, J., Gmel, G., & Daeppen, J. (2008). Brief alcohol interventions: Do counsellors' and patients' communication characteristics predict change? *Alcohol and Alcoholism, 43,* 62–69.

Gaume, J., Longabaugh, R., Magill, M., Bertholet, N., Gmel, G., & Daeppen, J. (2016). Under what conditions?: Therapist and client characteristics moderate the role of change talk in brief motivational intervention. *Journal of Consulting and Clinical Psychology, 84*(3), 211–220.

Gay, P. (1988). *Freud: A life for our time.* New York: Norton.

Gemson, D. H., Moats, H. L., Watkins, B. X., Ganz, M. L., Robinson, S., & Healton, E. (1998). Laying down the law: Reducing illegal tobacco sales to minors in central Harlem. *American Journal of Public Health, 88,* 936–939.

General Accountability Office. (2015, February). Drug shortages: Better management of the quota process for controlled substances needed: Coordination between DEA and FDA should be improved (GAO-15-202). Retrieved December 11, 2017 from *www.gao.gov/assets/670/668252.pdf.*

George, R. L. (1990). *Counseling the chemically dependent: Theory and practice.* Englewood Cliffs, NJ: Prentice-Hall.

George, R. L., & Cristiani, T. S. (1995). *Counseling: Theory and practice.* Needham Heights, MA: Allyn & Bacon.

Gerst, K. R., Gunn, R. L., & Finn, P. R. (2017). Delay discounting of losses in alcohol use disorders and antisocial psychopathology: Effects of a working memory load. *Alcoholism: Clinical and Experimental Research, 41,* 1768–1774.

Gifford, E. V., Kohlenberg, B. S., Hayes, S. C., Pierson, H. M., Piasecki, M. P., Antonuccio, D. O., et al. (2011). Does acceptance and relationship focused behavior therapy contribute to bupropion outcomes?: A randomized controlled trial of functional analytic psychotherapy and acceptance and commitment therapy for smoking cessation. *Behavior Therapy, 42,* 700–715.

Godley, M. D., Passetti, L. L., Subramanian, G. A., Funk, R. R., Smith, J. E., & Meyers, R. J. (2017). Adolescent Community Reinforcement Approach implementation and treatment outcomes for youth with opioid problem use. *Drug and Alcohol Dependence, 174,* 9–16.

Godley, S. H., Hunter, B. D., Fernández-Artamendi, S., Smith, J. E., Meyers, R. J., & Godley, M. D. (2014). A comparison of treatment outcomes for adolescent community reinforcement approach participants with and without co-occurring problems. *Journal of Substance Abuse Treatment, 46,* 463–471.

Gola, M., Wordecha, M., Sescousse, G., Lew-Starowicz, M., Kossowski, B., Wypych, M., et al. (2017). Can pornography be addictive?: An fMRI study of men seeking treatment for problematic pornography use. *Neuropsychopharmacology, 42,* 2021–2031.

Goldbach, J. T., Tanner-Smith, E. E., Bagwell, M., & Dunlap, S. (2014). Minority stress and substance use in sexual minority adolescents: A meta-analysis. *Prevention Science, 15,* 350–363.

Goldman, M. S. (2002). Expectancy and risk for alcoholism: The unfortunate exploitation of a fundamental characteristic of neurobehavioral adaptation. *Alcoholism: Clinical and Experimental Research, 26,* 737–746.

Goldman, M. S., Brown, S. A., & Christiansen, B. A. (1987). Expectancy theory: Thinking about drinking. In H. T. Blane & K. E. Leonard (Eds.), *Psychological theories of drinking and alcoholism.* New York: Guilford Press.

Goode, E. (1993). *Drugs in American society* (4th ed.). New York: McGraw-Hill.

Gordon, A. A. (1898). *The beautiful life of Frances E. Willard: A memorial volume.* Chicago: Woman's Temperance Publishing Association.

Gorman, D. M. (2017). Has the National Registry of Evidence-based Programs and Practices (NREPP) lost its way? *International Journal of Drug Policy, 45,* 40–41.

Gorsky, E. (2016, updated May 8). Haggard says he is "completely heterosexual." *Denver Post.* Retrieved November 16, 2018, from *www.denverpost.com/2007/02/05/haggard-says-he-is-completely-heterosexual.*

Gotham, H. J., Sher, K. J., & Wood, P. K. (1997). Predicting stability and change in frequency of intoxication from the college years to beyond: Individual-difference and role transition variables. *Journal of Abnormal Psychology, 106,* 619–629.

Gough, J. B. (1881). *Sunlight and shadow.* Hartford, CT: Worthington.

Grant, B. F., & Dawson, D. A. (1997). Age of onset of alcohol use and its association with DSM-IV alcohol abuse and dependence: Results from the National Longitudinal Alcohol Epidemiologic Survey. *Journal of Substance Abuse, 9,* 103–110.

Grant, B. F., Goldstein, R. B., Saha, T. D., Chou, S. P., Jung, J., Zhang, H., et al. (2015). Epidemiology of DSM-5 alcohol use disorder: Results from the National Epidemiologic Survey on Alcohol and Related Conditions-III. *JAMA Psychiatry, 72,* 757–766.

Grant, B. F., Saha, T. D., Ruan, W. J., Goldstein, R. B., Chou, S. P., Jung, J., et al. (2016). Epidemiology of DSM-5 drug use disorder: Results from the National Epidemiologic Survey on Alcohol and Related Conditions-III. *JAMA Psychiatry, 73,* 39–47.

Grant, B. F., Stinson, F. S., Dawson, D. A., Chou, S. P., Dufour, M. C., Compton, W., et al. (2006). Prevalence and co-occurrence of substance use disorders and independent mood and anxiety disorders: Results from the National Epidemiologic Survey on Alcohol and Related Conditions. *Alcohol Research and Health, 29,* 107–120.

Grant, J. E., Potenza, M. N., Weinstein, A., & Gorelick, D. A. (2010). Introduction to behavioral addictions. *American Journal of Drug and Alcohol Abuse, 36,* 233–241.

Green, L. W. (1992). Promoting comprehensive interventions. In H. D. Holder & J. M. Howard (Eds.), *Community prevention trials for alcohol problems: Methodological issues* (pp. 247–250). Westport, CT: Praeger.

Green, L. W., George, M. A., Daniel, M., Frankish, C. J., Herbert, C. J., Bowie, W. R., et al. (1995). *Study of participatory research in health promotion: Review and recommendations for the development of participatory research in health promotion in Canada.* Ottawa, ON: Royal Society of Canada.

Green, L. W., & Kreuter, M. W. (2002). Fighting back or fighting themselves?: Community coalitions against substance abuse and their use of best practices. *American Journal of Preventive Medicine, 23,* 303–306.

Green, L. W., & Mercer, S. L. (2001). Can public health researchers and agencies reconcile the push from funding bodies and the pull from communities? *American Journal of Public Health, 91*(12), 1926–1929.

Greenberg, G. A., & Rosenheck, R. A. (2008). Jail incarceration, homelessness, and mental health: A national study. *Psychiatric Services, 59,* 170–177.

Greenberg, G. A., & Rosenheck, R. A. (2010). Mental health correlates of past homelessness in the National Comorbidity Study Replication. *Journal of Health Care for the Poor and Underserved, 21,* 1234–1249.

Greenblatt, J. C. (1998). Practitioners should be aware of co-occurring marijuana use and delinquent/depressive behaviors among youth (Data from the Substance Abuse and Mental Health Services Administration, Office of Applied Studies) (University of Maryland–Center for Substance Abuse Research). *CESAR FAX, 7*(45), 1.

Greenleaf, J. (1984). Co-alcoholic/para-alcoholic: Who's who and what's the difference? In S. Wegscheider-Cruse (Ed.), *Co-dependency: An emerging issue* (pp. 5–17). Pompano Beach, FL: Health Communications.

Griffin, K. W., Botvin, G. J., Nichols, T. R., & Doyle, M. (2003). Effectiveness of a universal drug abuse prevention approach for youth at high risk for substance use initiation. *Preventive Medicine, 36,* 1–7.

Gullo, M. J., Matveeva, M., Feeney, G. F., Young, R. M., & Connor J. P. (2017). Social cognitive predictors of treatment outcome in cannabis dependence. *Drug and Alcohol Dependence, 170,* 74–81.

Guo, G., Roettger, M. E., & Cai, T. (2008). The integration of genetic propensities into social-control models of delinquency and violence in male youths. *American Sociological Review, 73,* 543–568.

Gurman, A. S. (2011). Couple therapies. In S. B. Messer & A. S. Gurman (Eds.), *Essential psychotherapies: Theory and practice* (3rd ed., pp. 345–383). New York: Guilford Press.

Guy, G. P., Watson, M., Seidenberg, A. B., Hartman, A. M., Holman, D. M., & Perna, F. (2017). Trends in indoor tanning and its association with sunburn among US adults. *Journal of the American Academy of Dermatology, 76,* 1191–1993.

Haaga, J. G., & Reuter, P. H. (1995). Prevention: The (lauded) orphan of drug policy. In R. H. Coombs & D. M. Ziedonis (Eds.), *Handbook on drug abuse prevention: A comprehensive strategy to prevent the abuse of alcohol and other drugs.* Boston: Allyn & Bacon.

Hadland, S. E., Krieger, M. S., & Marshall, B. D. L. (2017). Industry payments to physicians for opioid products, 2013–2015. *American Journal of Public Health, 107,* 1493–1495.

Hagger, M. S., Lonsdale, A. J., Hein, V., Koka, A., Lintunen, T., Pasi, H., et al. (2012). Predicting alcohol consumption and binge drinking in company employees: An application of planned behaviour and self-determination theories. *British Journal of Health Psychology, 17,* 379–407.

Hall, C. S., Lindzey, G., & Campbell, J. B. (1998). *Theories of personality* (4th ed.). New York: Wiley.

Hallfors, D., Cho, H., Livert, D., & Kadushin, C. (2002). Fighting back against substance abuse—Are community coalitions winning? *American Journal of Preventive Medicine, 23,* 237–245.

Hallgren, K. A., & Moyers, T. B. (2011). Does readiness to change predict in-session motivational language?: Correspondence between two conceptualizations of client motivation. *Addiction, 106,* 1261–1269.

Hamilton, K., & Hagger, M. S. (2018). Effects of self-efficacy on healthy eating depends on normative support: A prospective study of long-haul truck drivers. *International Journal of Behavioral Medicine, 25,* 265–270.

Hardon, A., & Hymans, T. D. (2014). Ethnographies of youth drug use in Asia. *International Journal of Drug Policy, 25,* 749–754.

Harned, M. S., Chapman, A. L., Dexter-Mazza, E. T., Murray, A., Comtois, K. A., & Linehan, M. M. (2009). Treating co-occurring Axis I disorders in recurrently suicidal women with borderline personality disorder: A 2-year randomized trial of dialectical behavior therapy versus community treatment by experts. *Personality Disorders: Theory, Research, and Treatment, 5*(1), 35–45.

Harris, J. S., Stewart, D. G., & Stanton, B. C. (2017). Urge surfing as aftercare in adolescent alcohol use: A randomized control trial. *Mindfulness, 8,* 144–149.

Harris, K. B., & Miller, W. R. (1990). Behavioral self-control training for problem drinkers: Components of efficacy. *Psychology of Addictive Behaviors, 4*(2), 82–90.

Harrison, B. (1971). *Drink and the Victorians: The temperance question in England, 1815–1872.* Pittsburgh, PA: University of Pittsburgh Press.

Hart, A. B., Lynch, K. G., Farrer, L., Gelernter, J., & Kranzler, H. R. (2016). Which alcohol use disorder criteria contribute to the association of ADH1B with alcohol dependence? *Addiction Biology, 21,* 924–938.

Hart, C. L., & Ksir, C. J. (2018). *Drugs, society and human behavior* (17th ed.). New York: McGraw-Hill Education.

Hartnett, D., Carr, A., Hamilton, E., & O'Reilly, G. (2017). The effectiveness of functional family therapy for adolescent behavioral and substance misuse problems: A meta-analysis. *Family Process, 56,* 607–619.

Hartzler, B., Lash, S. J., & Roll, J. M. (2012). Contingency management in substance abuse treatment: A structured review of the evidence for its transportability. *Drug and Alcohol Dependence, 112,* 1–10.

Hasan, A., Falkai, P., Wobrock, T., Lieberman, J., Glenthøj, B., Gattaz, W. F., et al. (2015). World Federation of Societies of Biological Psychiatry (WFSBP) Guidelines for Biological Treatment of Schizophrenia: Part 3. Update 2015 Management of special circumstances: Depression, suicidality, substance use disorders and pregnancy and lactation. *World Journal of Biological Psychiatry, 16,* 142–170.

Hasin, D. S., & Grant, B. F. (2015). The National Epidemiologic Survey on Alcohol and Related Conditions (NESARC) waves 1 and 2: Review and summary of findings. *Social Psychiatry and Psychiatric Epidemiology, 50,* 1609–1640.

Hawkins, E. H. (2009). A tale of two systems: Co-occurring mental health and substance abuse disorders treatment for adolescents. *Annual Review of Psychology, 60,* 197–227.

Hawkins, J. D., Catalano, R. F., & Kent, L. A. (1991). Combining broadcast media and parent education to prevent teenage drug abuse. In I. Donohew, H. E. Sypher, & W. J. Bukowski (Eds.), *Persuasive communication and drug abuse prevention.* Hillsdale, NJ: Erlbaum.

Hayes, S. C., Follette, V. M., & Linehan, M. M. (Eds.). (2004). *Mindfulness and acceptance: Expanding the cognitive-behavioral tradition.* New York: Guilford Press.

Hayes, S. C., Strosahl, K. D., & Wilson, K. G. (2012). *Acceptance and commitment therapy: The process and practice of mindful change* (2nd ed.). New York: Guilford Press.

Heath, D. B. (1988). Emerging anthropological theory and models of alcohol use and alcoholism. In C. D. Chaudron & D. A. Wilkinson (Eds.), *Theories on alcoholism*. Toronto, ON, Canada: Addiction Research Foundation.

Heather, N. (2005). Motivational interviewing: Is it all our clients need? *Addiction Research and Theory, 13*(1), 1–18.

Heather, N., Adamson, S. J., Raistrick, D., Slegg, G. P., & UKATT Research Team. (2010). Initial preference for drinking goal in the treatment of alcohol problems: I. Baseline differences between abstinence and non-abstinence groups. *Alcohol and Alcoholism, 45*, 128–135.

Heather, N., & Robertson, I. (1983). *Controlled drinking*. London: Methuen.

Hecht, M. L., Colby, M., & Miller-Day, M. (2010). The dissemination of keepin' it REAL through D.A.R.E. America: A lesson in disseminating health messages. *Health Communication, 25*, 585–586.

Hedegaard, H., Warner, M., & Miniño A. M. (2017). *Drug overdose deaths in the United States, 1999–2016* (NCHS Data Brief, No. 294). Hyattsville, MD: National Center for Health Statistics. Retreived July 25, 2018, from *www.cdc.gov/nchs/data/databriefs/db294.pdf*.

Heilig, M. (2015). *The thirteenth step: Addiction in the age of brain science*. New York: Columbia University Press.

Heintzelman, S. J., & King, L. A. (2014). Life is pretty meaningful. *American Psychologist, 69*, 561–574.

Heller, D. (2011, June 14). End Pete Rose's ban, let him enter hall. *Washington Times*. Retrieved April 22, 2018, from *www.washingtontimes.com/news/2011/jun/14/end-roses-ban-let-him-enter-hall*.

Henderson, C. E., Dakof, G. A., Greenbaum, P. E., & Liddle, H. A. (2010). Effectiveness of multidimensional family therapy with higher severity substance-abusing adolescents: Report from two randomized controlled trials. *Journal of Consulting and Clinical Psychology, 78*(1), 885–897.

Henderson, C. E., Wevodau, A. L., Henderson, S. E., Colbourn, L., Gharagozloo, L., North, L. W., et al. (2016). An independent replication of the Adolescent-Community Reinforcement Approach with justice-involved youth. *American Journal on Addictions, 25*, 233–240.

Hendricks, P. S., Reich, R. R., & Westmaas, J. L. (2009). Expectancies. In G. L. Fisher & N. A. Roget (Eds.), *Encyclopedia of substance abuse prevention, treatment, and recovery* (Vol. 1, pp. 386–389). Thousand Oaks, CA: SAGE.

Hendriks, V., van der Schee, E., & Blanken, P. (2012). Matching adolescents with a cannabis use disorder to multidimensional family therapy or cognitive behavioral therapy: Treatment effect moderators in a randomized controlled trial. *Drug and Alcohol Dependence, 125*, 119–126.

Henggeler, S. W. (2011). Efficacy studies to large-scale transport: The development and validation of multisystemic therapy programs. *Annual Review of Clinical Psychology, 7*, 351–381.

Henggeler, S. W., & Schaeffer, C. M. (2016). Multisystemic therapy®: Clinical overview, outcomes, and implementation research. *Family Process, 55*, 514–528.

Henggeler, S. W., Schoenwald, S. K., Borduin, C. M., Rowland, M. D., & Cunningham, P. B. (2009). *Multisystemic therapy for antisocial behavior in children and adolescents* (2nd ed.). New York: Guilford Press.

Hernandez-Lopez, M., Luciano, M. C., Bricker, J. B., Roales-Nieto, J. G., & Montesinos, F. (2009). Acceptance and commitment therapy for smoking cessation: A preliminary study of its effectiveness in comparison with cognitive behavioral therapy. *Psychology of Addictive Behaviors, 23*, 723–730.

Herzog, T. A., Abrams, D. B., Emmons, K. M., Linnan, L. A., & Shadel, W. G. (1999).

Do processes of change predict smoking stage movements?: A prospective analysis of the transtheoretical model. *Health Psychology, 18*(4), 369–375.

Hester, R. K. (1995). Behavioral self-control training. In R. K. Hester & W. R. Miller (Eds.), *Handbook of alcoholism treatment approaches: Effective alternatives* (2nd ed., pp. 148–159). Needham Heights, MA: Allyn & Bacon.

Hettema, J. E., & Hendricks, P. S. (2010). Motivational interviewing for smoking cessation: A meta-analytic review. *Journal of Consulting and Clinical Psychology, 78*(6), 868–884.

Hettema, J., Steele, J., & Miller, W. R. (2005). Motivational interviewing. *Annual Review of Clinical Psychology, 1,* 91–111.

Heuser, J. P. (1990). *A preliminary evaluation of short-term impact of the Preparing for Drug-Free Years community service program in Oregon.* Salem: Oregon Department of Justice, Crime Analysis Center.

Higgins, S. T., Alessi, S. M., & Dantona, R. L. (2002). Voucher-based incentives: A substance abuse treatment innovation. *Addictive Behaviors, 27,* 887–910.

Higgins, S. T., Budney, A. J., Bickel, W. K., Foerg, F. E., Donham, R., & Badger, G. J. (1994). Incentives improve treatment retention and cocaine abstinence in ambulatory cocaine-dependent patients. *Archives of General Psychiatry, 51,* 568–576.

Higgins, S. T., Budney, A. J., Bickel, W. K., Foerg, F. E., Ogden, D., & Badger, G. J. (1995). Outpatient behavioral treatment for cocaine dependence. *Experimental and Clinical Psychopharmacology, 3,* 205–212.

Higgins, S. T., Budney, A. J., Bickel, W. K., Hughes, J. R., Foerg, F., & Badger, G. (1993). Achieving cocaine abstinence with a behavioral approach. *American Journal of Psychiatry, 150,* 763–769.

Higgins, S. T., Delaney, D. D., Budney, A. J., Bickel, W. K., Hughes, J. R., Foerg, F., et al. (1991). A behavioral approach to achieving initial cocaine abstinence. *American Journal of Psychiatry, 148*(9), 1218–1224.

Higgins, S. T., Heil, S. H., Dantona, R., Donham, R., Matthews, M., & Badger, G. J. (2007). Effects of varying the monetary value of voucher-based incentives on abstinence achieved during and following treatment among cocaine-dependent outpatients. *Addiction, 102,* 271–281.

Higgins, S. T., Heil, S. H., & Lussier, J. P. (2004). Clinical implications of reinforcement as a determinant of substance use disorders. *Annual Review of Psychology, 55,* 431–461.

Higgins, S. T., Sigmon, S. C., Wong, C. J., Heil, S. H., Badger, G. J., Donham, R., et al. (2003). Community reinforcement therapy for cocaine-dependent outpatients. *Archives of General Psychiatry, 60,* 1043–1052.

Higgins, S. T., Wong, C. J., Badger, G. J., Haug-Ogden, D. E., & Dantona, R. L. (2000). Contingent reinforcement increases cocaine abstinence during outpatient treatment and one year of follow-up. *Journal of Consulting and Clinical Psychology, 68,* 64–72.

Higham, S., & Bernstein, L. (2017, October 15). The drug industry's triumph over the DEA. *Washington Post.* Retrieved December 23, 2017, from *www.washingtonpost.com/graphics/2017/investigations/dea-drug-industry_congress/?utm_term=.5331e25ae198.*

Hill, T. D., & Jorgenson, A. (2018). Bring out your dead!: A study of income inequality and life expectancy in the United States, 2000–2010. *Health and Place, 49,* 1–6.

Hill, P. F., Yi, R., Spreng, R. N., & Diana R. A. (2017). Neural congruence between intertemporal and interpersonal self-control: Evidence from delay and social discounting. *NeuroImage, 162,* 186–198.

Hingson, R. W., & Howland, J. (2002). Comprehensive community interventions to promote health: Implications for college-age drinking problems. *Journal of Studies on Alcohol, 2002*(Suppl. 14), 226–240.

Hingson, R., McGovern, T., Howland, J., & Hereen, T. (1996). Reducing alcohol-impaired driving in Massachusetts. *American Journal of Public Health, 86,* 791–797.

Hodgins, D. C., Ching, L. E., & McEwen, J. (2009). Strength of commitment language in motivational interviewing and gambling outcomes. *Psychology of Addictive Behaviors, 23,* 122–130.

Holdcraft, L. C., Iacono, W. G., & McGue, M. K. (1998). Antisocial personality disorder and depression in relation to alcoholism: A community-based sample. *Journal of Studies on Alcohol, 59,* 222–226.

Holder, H. (Ed.). (1997). A community prevention trial to reduce alcohol-involved trauma. *Addiction, 92*(Suppl. 2), S155–S301.

Holder, H., Gruenewald, P. J., Ponicki, W. R., Treno, A. J., Grube, J. W., Saltz, R. F., et al. (2000). Effects of community-based interventions on high-risk driving and alcohol-related injuries. *Journal of the American Medical Association, 284,* 2341–2347.

Hollingsworth, A., Ruhm, C. J., & Simon, K. (2017). Macroeconomic conditions and opioid abuse. *Journal of Health Economics, 56,* 222–233.

Hong, J. S., Huang, H., Sabri, B., & Kim, J. S. (2011). Substance abuse among Asian American youth: An ecological review of the literature. *Children and Youth Services Review, 33,* 669–677.

Horgan, J. (2011, September 16). Are psychiatric medications making us sicker? *Chronicle of Higher Education.* Retrieved April 22, 2018, from *http://chronicle.com/article/Are-Psychiatric-medications/128976/?sid=at&utm_source=at&utm_medium=en.*

Houck, J. M., & Moyers, T. B. (2015). Within-session communication patterns predict alcohol treatment outcomes. *Drug and Alcohol Dependence, 157,* 205–209.

Hove, M. C., Parkhill, M. R., Neighbors, C., McConchie, J. M., & Fossos, N. (2010). Alcohol consumption and intimate partner violence perpetration among college students: The role of self-determination. *Journal of Studies on Alcohol and Drugs, 71,* 78–85.

Hser, Y. I., Li, J., Jiang, H., Zhang, R., Du, J., Zhang, et al. (2011). Effects of a randomized contingency management intervention on opiate abstinence and retention in methadone maintenance treatment in China. *Addiction, 106,* 1801–1809.

Hu, H., Eaton, W. W., Anthony, J. C., Wu, L. T., & Cottler, L. B. (2017). Age of first drunkenness and risks for all-cause mortality: A 27-year follow-up from the epidemiologic catchment area study. *Drug and Alcohol Dependence, 176,* 148–153.

Huang, T. T., Drewnowski, A., Kumanyika, S. K., & Glass, T. A. (2009). A systems-oriented multilevel framework for addressing obesity in the 21st century. *Preventing Chronic Disease, 6,* 1–10.

Hulvershorn, L. A., Quinn, P. D., & Scott, E. L. (2015). Treatment of adolescent substance use disorders and co-occurring internalizing disorders: A critical review and proposed model. *Current Drug Abuse Reviews, 8,* 41–49.

Humphreys, K., & McLellan, A. T. (2011). A policy-oriented review of strategies for improving the outcomes of services for substance use disorder patients. *Addiction, 106,* 2058–2066.

Hunt, G. E., Siegfried, N., Morley, K., Sitharthan, T., & Cleary, M. (2013). Psychosocial interventions for people with both severe mental illness and substance misuse. *Cochrane Database of Systematic Reviews, 10,* Article No. CD001088.

Hunt, G. H., & Azrin, N. H. (1973). The community-reinforcement approach to alcoholism. *Behaviour Research and Therapy, 11,* 91–104.

Hunt, G. P., & Evans, K. (2008). "The great unmentionable": Exploring the pleasures and benefits of ecstasy from the perspectives of drug users. *Drugs: Education, Prevention and Policy, 15*(4), 329–349.

Hunter-Reel, D., McCrady, B. S., Hildebrandt, T., & Epstein, E. E. (2010). Indirect effect of social support for drinking on drinking outcomes: The role of motivation. *Journal of Studies on Alcohol and Drugs, 71,* 930–970.

Hussaarts, P., Roozen, H. G., Meyers, R. J., van de Wetering, B. J. M., & McCrady, B. S. (2011). Problem areas reported by substance abusing individuals and their concerned significant others. *American Journal on Addictions, 21,* 38–46.

IBIS World. (2017, April). Tanning salons—US market research report. Retrieved April 1, 2018, from *www.ibisworld.com/industry-trends/market-research-reports/other-services-except-public-administration/personal-laundry/tanning-salons.html.*

Institute of Medicine. (1994). *Reducing risks for mental disorders: Frontiers for preventive intervention research.* Washington, DC: National Academy Press.

Ioannidis, K., Treder, M. S., Chamberlain, S. R., Kiraly, F., Redden, S. A., Stein, D. J., et al. (2018). Problematic internet use as an age-related multifaceted problem: Evidence from a two-site survey. *Addictive Behaviors, 81,* 157–166.

Jackson, J. K. (1954). The adjustment of the family to the crisis of alcoholism. *Quarterly Journal of Studies on Alcohol, 15*(4), 562–586.

Jackson, J. K. (1962). Alcoholism and the family. In D. J. Pittman & C. R. Snyder (Eds.), *Society, culture, and drinking patterns* (pp. 472–492). New York: Wiley.

Janssen, T., Treloar Padovano, H., Merrill, J. E., & Jackson, K. M. (2018). Developmental relations between alcohol expectancies and social norms in predicting alcohol onset. *Developmental Psychology, 54,* 281–292.

Jellinek, E. M. (1955). The "craving" for alcohol. *Quarterly Journal of Studies on Alcohol, 16,* 35–38.

Jessor, R., Donovan, J. E., & Costa, F. M. (1991). *Beyond adolescence: Problem behavior and young adult development.* New York: Cambridge University Press.

Jessor, R., & Jessor, S. L. (1977). *Problem behavior and psychosocial development: A longitudinal study of youth.* New York: Academic Press.

Jiang, Z., Hu, X., & Wang, Z. (2018). Career adaptability and plateaus: The moderating effects of tenure and job self-efficacy. *Journal of Vocational Behavior, 104,* 59–71.

Johnides, B. D., Borduin, C. M., Wagner, D. V., & Dopp, A. R. (2017). Effects of multisystemic therapy on caregivers of serious juvenile offenders: A 20-year follow-up to a randomized clinical trial. *Journal of Consulting and Clinical Psychology, 85,* 323–334.

Johnson, B. A. (2010). Medication treatment of different types of alcoholism. *American Journal of Psychiatry, 167,* 630–639.

Johnson, V. E. (1980). *I'll quit tomorrow* (rev. ed.). San Francisco: Harper & Row.

Johnson Institute. (1987). *How to use intervention in your professional practice: A guide for helping-professionals who work with chemical dependents and their families.* Minneapolis, MN: Author.

Judd, P. H., Thomas, N., Schwartz, T., Outcalt, A., & Hough, R. (2003). A dual diagnosis demonstration project: Treatment outcomes and costs analysis. *Journal of Psychoactive Drugs, 23*(SARC Suppl. 1), 181–192.

Kabat-Zinn, J. (1994). *Wherever you go, there you are: Mindfulness meditation in everyday life.* New York: Hyperion.

Kalant, H. (2009). What neurobiology cannot tell us about addiction. *Addiction, 105,* 780–789.

Kandel, D. B. (2003). Does marijuana use cause use of other drugs? *Journal of the American Medical Association, 289,* 482–483.

Kandel, D., & Faust, R. (1975). Sequence and stages in patterns of adolescent drug use. *Archives of General Psychiatry, 32*(7), 923–932.

Kandel, D. B., Huang, F. Y., & Davies, M. (2001). Comorbidity between patterns of substance dependence and psychiatric syndromes. *Drug and Alcohol Dependence, 64,* 233–241.

Kandel, D. B., Yamaguchi, K., & Chen, K. (1992). Stages of progression in drug involvement from adolescence to adulthood: Further evidence for the gateway theory. *Journal of Studies on Alcohol, 53*(5), 447–457.

Kaslow, N. J., Bhaju, J., & Celano, M. (2011). Family therapies. In S. B. Messer & A. S. Gurman (Eds.), *Essential psychotherapies: Theory and practice* (3rd ed., pp. 297–344). New York: Guilford Press.

Kasser, T. (2002). Sketches for a self-determination theory of values. In E. L. Deci & R. M. Ryan (Eds.). *Handbook of self-determination research* (pp. 123–140). Rochester, NY: University of Rochester Press.

Kaymaz, N., Drukker, M., Lieb, R., Wittchen, H. U., Werbeloff, N., Weiser, M., et al. (2012). Do subthreshold psychotic experiences predict clinical outcomes in unselected non-help-seeking population-based samples?: A systematic review and meta-analysis, enriched with new results. *Psychological Medicine, 42,* 2239–2253.

Kearney, R. (1999). On the good of marriage. In *Marriage and virginity: Works of Saint Augustine: A translation for the 21st century.* New York: New York City Press.

Keefe, P. R. (2017, October 30). The family that built an empire of pain: The Sackler dynasty's ruthless marketing of painkillers has generated billions of dollars—and millions of addicts. *The New Yorker.* Retrieved December 20, 2017, from *www. newyorker.com/magazine/2017/10/30/the-family-that-built-an-empire-of-pain.*

Kelley, M. L., & Fals-Stewart, W. (2007). Treating paternal drug abuse with learning sobriety together: Effects on adolescents versus children. *Drug and Alcohol Dependence, 92,* 228–238.

Kelley, M. L., & Fals-Stewart, W. (2008). Treating paternal alcoholism with learning sobriety together: Effects on adolescents versus preadolescents. *Journal of Family Psychology, 21,* 435–444.

Kellogg, S. H. (2003). On "gradualism" and the building of the harm reduction-abstinence continuum. *Journal of Substance Abuse Treatment, 25,* 241–247.

Kelly, B. C., Trimarco, J., LeClair, A., Pawson, M., Parsons, J. T., & Golub, S. A. (2015). Symbolic boundaries, subcultural capital and prescription drug misuse across youth cultures. *Sociology of Health and Illness, 37*(3), 325–339.

Kelly, J. F., Stout, R. L., Tonigan, J. S., Magill, M., & Pagano, M. E. (2010). Negative affect, relapse, and Alcoholics Anonymous (AA): Does AA work by reducing anger? *Journal of Studies on Alcohol and Drugs, 71,* 434–444.

Kelly, J. F., & Urbanoski, K. (2012). Youth recovery contexts: The incremental effects of 12-step attendance and involvement on adolescent outpatient outcomes. *Alcoholism: Clinical and Experimental Research, 36,* 1219–1229.

Kelly, J. F., & Westerhoff, C. M. (2010). Does it matter how we refer to individuals with substance-related conditions?: A randomized study of two commonly used terms. *International Journal of Drug Policy, 21,* 202–207.

Kelly, J. F., & Yeterian, J. D. (2012). Empirical awakening: The new science on mutual help and implications for cost containment under health care reform. *Substance Abuse, 33,* 85–91.

Kendler, K. S., Ji, J., Edwards, A. C., Ohlsson, H., Sundquist, J., & Sundquist, K. (2015). An extended Swedish national adoption study of alcohol use disorder. *JAMA Psychiatry, 72*(3), 211–218.

Kendler, K. S., Sundquist, K., Ohlsson, H., Palmér, K., Maes, H., Winkleby, M. A., et al. (2012). Genetic and familial environmental influences on the risk for drug abuse: A national Swedish adoption study. *Archives of General Psychiatry, 69,* 690–697.

Kennedy, K., & Gregoire, T. K. (2009). Theories of motivation in addiction treatment: Testing the relationship of the transtheoretical model of change and self-determination theory. *Journal of Social Work Practice in the Addictions, 9,* 163–183.

Kerr, D. C. R., Bae, H., Phibbs, S., & Kern, A. C. (2017). Changes in undergraduates' marijuana, heavy alcohol and cigarette use following legalization of recreational marijuana use in Oregon. *Addiction, 112,* 1992–2001.

Khantzian, E. J. (1980). An ego/self theory of substance dependence: A contemporary psychoanalytic perspective. In D. J. Lettieri, M. Sayers, & H. W. Pearson (Eds.), *Theories on drug abuse: Selected contemporary perspectives* (DHHS Publication No. ADM 8-967). Washington, DC: U.S. Government Printing Office.

Khantzian, E. J. (2012). Reflections on treating addictive disorders: A psychodynamic perspective. *American Journal of Addictions, 21,* 274–279.

Khantzian, E. J., Halliday, K. S., & McAuliffe, W. E. (1990). *Addiction and the vulnerable self: Modified dynamic group therapy for substance abusers.* New York: Guilford Press.

Kidorf, M., & Stitzer, M. L. (1993). Contingent access to methadone maintenance treatment: Effects on cocaine use of mixed opiate-cocaine abusers. *Experimental and Clinical Psychopharmacology, 1*(1–4), 200–206.

Kidorf, M., & Stitzer, M. L. (1996). Contingent use of take-homes and split-dosing to reduce illicit drug use of methadone patients. *Behavior Therapy, 27,* 41–51.

Kikkert, M., Goudriaan, A., de Waal, M., Peen, J., & Dekker, J. (2018). Effectiveness of Integrated Dual Diagnosis Treatment (IDDT) in severe mental illness outpatients with a co-occurring substance use disorder. *Journal of Substance Abuse Treatment, 95,* 35–42.

Kim, H., & Eaton, N. R. (2015). The hierarchical structure of common mental disorders: Connecting multiple levels of comorbidity, bifactor models, and predictive validity. *Journal of Abnormal Psychology, 124,* 1064–1078.

King, L. W. (Trans.). (2005). *Hammurabi's Code of Laws Ancient History Sourcebook.* New York: Fordham University. Retrieved July 20, 2012, from *www.fordham.edu/ halsall/ancient/hamcode.asp.*

King, S. M., Keyes, M., Winters, K. C., McGue, M., & Iacono, W. G. (2017). Genetic and environmental origins of gambling behaviors from ages 18 to 25: A longitudinal twin family study. *Psychology of Addictive Behaviors, 31*(3), 367–374.

Kirby, K. C., Benishek, L. A., Kerwin, M. E., Dugosh, K. L., Carpenedo, C. M., Bresani, E., et al. (2017). Analyzing components of Community Reinforcement and Family Training (CRAFT): Is treatment entry training sufficient? *Psychology of Addictive Behaviors, 31*(7), 818–827.

Kirst, M., Zerger, S., Misir, V., Hwang, S., & Stergiopoulos, V. (2015). The impact of a Housing First randomized controlled trial on substance use problems among homeless individuals with mental illness. *Drug and Alcohol Dependence, 146,* 24–29.

Klag, S. M., Creed, P., & O'Callaghan, F. (2010). Early motivation, well-being, and treatment engagement of chronic substance users undergoing treatment in a therapeutic community setting. *Substance Use and Misuse, 45,* 1112–1130.

Klein, D. N., & Riso, L. P. (1993). Psychiatric disorders: Problems of boundaries and comorbidity. In C. G. Costello (Ed.), *Basic issues in psychopathology*. New York: Guilford Press.

Knee, C. R., & Neighbors, C. (2002). Self-determination, perception of peer pressure, and drinking among college students. *Journal of Applied Social Psychology, 32*(3), 522–543.

Knudson, T. M., & Terrell, H. K. (2012). Codependency, perceived interparental conflict, and substance abuse in the family of origin. *American Journal of Family Therapy, 40,* 245–257.

Koffarnus, M. N., & Kaplan, B. A. (2018). Clinical models of decision making in addiction. *Pharmacology, Biochemistry, and Behavior, 164,* 71–83.

Kohatsu, N. D., Robinson, J. G., & Torner, J. C. (2004). Evidence-based public health: An evolving concept. *American Journal of Preventive Medicine, 27*(5), 417–421.

Kolb, L. (1928). Drug addiction. *Archives of Neurology and Psychiatry, 20,* 171–183.

Kolodny, A., Courtwright, D. T., Hwang, C. S., Kreiner, P., Eadies, J. L., Clark, T. W., et al. (2015). The prescription opioid and heroin crisis: A public health approach to an epidemic of addiction. *Annual Review of Public Health, 36, 559–574.*

Koob, G. F., & Le Moal, M. (2001). Drug addiction, dysregulation of reward, and allostasis. *Neuropsychopharmacology 24,* 97–129.

Kopak, A. M., Chen, A. C., Haas, S. A., & Gillmore, M. R. (2012). The importance of family factors to protect against substance use related problems among Mexican heritage and White youth. *Drug and Alcohol Dependence, 124,* 34–41.

Kosovski, J. R., & Smith, D. C. (2011). Everybody hurts: Addiction, drama, and the family in the reality television show *Intervention. Substance Use and Misuse, 46,* 852–858.

Krammer, J., Pinker-Domenig, K., Robson, M. E., Gönen, M., Bernard-Davila, B., Morris, E. A., et al. (2017). Breast cancer detection and tumor characteristics in BRCA1 and BRCA2 mutation carriers. *Breast Cancer Research and Treatment, 163,* 565–571.

Krawczyk, N., Feder, K. A., Saloner, B., Crum, R. M., Kealhofer, M., & Mojtabai, R. (2017). The association of psychiatric comorbidity with treatment completion among clients admitted to substance use treatment programs in a U.S. national sample. *Drug and Alcohol Dependence, 175,* 157–163.

Kreuter, M. W., Lezin, N. A., & Young, L. A. (2000). Evaluating community-based collaborative mechanisms: Implications for practitioners. *Health Promotion Practice, 1,* 49–63.

Kristjansson, S. D., Pergadia, M. L., Agrawal, A., Lessov-Schlaggar, C. N., McCarthy, D. M., Piasecki, T. M., et al. (2011). Smoking outcome expectancies in young adult female smokers: Individual differences and associations with nicotine dependence in a genetically informative sample. *Drug and Alcohol Dependence, 116,* 37–44.

Krmpotich, T., Mikulich-Gilbertson, S., Sakai, J., Thompson, L., Banich, M. T., & Tanabe, J. (2015). Impaired decision-making, higher impulsivity, and drug severity in substance dependence and pathological gambling. *Journal of Addiction Medicine, 9,* 273–280.

Kulesza, M., Hunter, S. B., Shearer, A. L., & Booth, M. (2017). Relationship between provider stigma and predictors of staff turnover among addiction treatment providers. *Alcoholism Treatment Quarterly, 35*(1), 63–70.

Kulesza, M., Matsuda, M., Ramirez, J. J., Werntz, A. J., Teachman, B. A., & Lindgren, K. P. (2016). Towards greater understanding of addiction stigma: Intersectionality with race/ethnicity and gender. *Drug and Alcohol Dependence, 169,* 85–91.

Kumpfer, K. L., Alvarado, R., & Whiteside, H. O. (2003). Family-based interventions for substance use and misuse prevention. *Substance Use and Misuse, 38*(11–13), 1759–1787.

Kuntsche, E., Rossow, I., Simons-Morton, B., Bogt, T. T., Kokkevi, A., & Godeau, E. (2013). Not early drinking but early drunkenness is a risk factor for problem behaviors among adolescents from 38 European and North American countries. *Alcoholism: Clinical and Experimental Research, 37,* 308–314.

Kushner, M. G. (2014). Seventy-five years of comorbidity research. *Journal of Studies on Alcohol and Drugs, 75*(Suppl. 17), 50–58.

Kushnir, V., Godinho, A., Hodgins, D. C., Hendershot, C. S., & Cunningham, J. A. (2016). Motivation to quit or reduce gambling: Associations between Self-Determination Theory and the Transtheoretical Model of Change. *Journal of Addictive Diseases, 35*(1), 58–65.

Kwok, P. Y., Deng, Q., Zakeri, H., Taylor, S. L., & Nickerson, D. A. (1996). Increasing the information content of STS-based genome maps: Identifying polymorphisms in mapped STSs. *Genomics, 31,* 123–126.

Lac, A., & Luk, J. W. (2018). Testing the amotivational syndrome: Marijuana use longitudinally predicts lower self-efficacy even after controlling for demographics, personality, and alcohol and cigarette use. *Prevention Science, 19,* 117–126.

Lamont, M. (1992). *Money, morals, and manners: The culture of the French and American upper-middle class.* Chicago: University of Chicago Press.

Langton, P. A. (Ed.). (1995). *The challenge of participatory research: Preventing alcohol-related problems in ethnic communities.* Washington, DC: Center for Substance Abuse Prevention, U.S. Department of Health and Human Services.

Larimer, M. E., Malone, D. K., Garner, M. D., Atkins, D. C., Burlingham, B., Lonczak, H. S., et al. (2009). Health care and public service use and costs before and after provision of housing for chronically homeless persons with severe alcohol problems. *Journal of the American Medical Association, 301*(13), 1349–1357.

Larrieu, J. A., Heller, S. S., Smyke, A. T., & Zeanah, C. H. (2008). Predictors of permanent loss of custody for mothers of infants and toddlers in foster care. *Infant Mental Health Journal, 29*(1), 48–60.

LaVeist, T. A., Gaskin, D. J., & Richard, P. (2009). *The economic burden of health inequalities in the United States.* Washington, DC: Joint Center for Political and Economic Studies. Retrieved July 24, 2017, from *http://jointcenter.org/sites/default/files/Economic%20Burden%20of%20Health%20Inequalities%20Fact%20Sheet.pdf.*

Lawson, A., & Lawson, G. A. (1998). *Alcoholism and the family: A guide to treatment and prevention* (2nd ed.). Gaithersburg, MD: Aspen.

LeClair, A., Kelly, B. C., Pawson, M., Wells, B. E., & Parsons, J. T. (2015). Motivations for prescription drug misuse among young adults: Considering social and developmental contexts. *Drugs: Education, Prevention and Policy, 22,* 208–216.

Leeds, J., & Morgenstern, J. (1996). Psychoanalytic theories of substance abuse. In F. Rotgers, D. S. Keller, & J. Morgenstern (Eds.), *Treating substance abuse: Theory and technique.* New York: Guilford Press.

Leigh, J., Bowen, S., & Marlatt, G. A. (2005). Spirituality, mindfulness, and substance abuse. *Addictive Behaviors, 30,* 1335–1341.

LeTendre, M. L., & Reed, M. B. (2017). The effect of adverse childhood experience on clinical diagnosis of a substance use disorder: Results of a national representative study. *Substance Use and Misuse, 52*(6), 689–697.

Letourneau, E. J., Henggeler, S. W., Borduin, C. M., Schewe, P. A., McCart, M. R., Chapman, J. E., et al. (2009). Multisystemic therapy for juvenile sexual offenders: 1-year results from a randomized effectiveness trial. *Journal of Family Psychology, 23*(1), 89–102.

Levin, J. (2017). An antipoverty agenda for public health: Background and recommendations. *Public Health Reports, 132,* 431–435.

Levine, H. G. (1978). The discovery of addiction: Changing conceptions of habitual drunkenness in America. *Journal of Studies on Alcohol, 39,* 143–174.

Lewis, J. A., Dana, R. Q., & Blevins, G. A. (1988). *Substance abuse counseling: An individualized approach.* Pacific Grove, CA: Brooks/Cole.

Lewis, M. (2015). *The biology of desire: Why addiction is not a disease.* New York: Public Affairs.

Lewis, M. (2017). Addiction and the brain: Development, not disease. *Neuroethics, 10,* 7–18.

Li, L., Zhu, S., Tse, N., Tse, S., & Wong, P. (2015). Effectiveness of motivational interviewing to reduce illicit drug use in adolescents: A systematic review and meta-analysis. *Addiction, 111,* 795–805.

Liddle, H. A. (2002). *Multidimensional family therapy for adolescent cannabis users, Cannabis Youth Treatment Series, Volume 5* (DHHS Pub. No. 05-4011). Rockville, MD: Center for Substance Abuse Treatment, Substance Abuse and Mental Health Services Administration.

Liddle, H. A. (2016). Multidimensional family therapy: Evidence base for transdiagnostic treatment outcomes, change mechanisms, and implementation in community settings. *Family Process, 55,* 558–576.

Liddle, H. A., Rowe, C. L., Dakof, G. A., Henderson, C. E., & Greenbaum, P. E. (2009). Multidimensional family therapy for young adolescent substance abuse: Twelve-month outcomes of a randomized clinical trial. *Journal of Consulting and Clinical Psychology, 77*(1), 12–25.

Linden, D. J. (2011). *The compass of pleasure.* New York: Viking.

Lindqvist, H., Forsberg, L., Enebrink, P., Andersson, G., & Rosendahl, I. (2017). The relationship between counselors' technical skills, clients' in-session verbal responses and outcome in smoking cessation treatment. *Journal of Substance Abuse Treatment, 77,* 141–149.

Linehan, M. M. (2015). *DBT® skills training manual* (2nd ed.). New York: Guilford Press.

Linehan, M. M., Dimeff, L. A., Reynolds, S. K., Comtois, K. A., Welch, S. S., Heagerty, P., et al. (2002). Dialectical behavior therapy versus comprehensive validation therapy plus 12-step for the treatment of opioid dependent women meeting criteria for borderline personality disorder. *Drug and Alcohol Dependence, 67,* 13–26.

Lingford-Hughes, A., Watson, B., Kalk, N., & Reid, A. (2010). Neuropharmacology of addiction and how it informs treatment. *British Medical Bulletin, 96,* 93–110.

Link, B. G., & Phelan, J. C. (2001). Conceptualizing stigma. *Annual Review of Sociology, 27,* 363–385.

Lipari, R. N., Park-Lee, E., & Van Horn, S. (2016). *America's need for and receipt of substance use treatment in 2015: The CBHSQ Report: September 29.* Rockville, MD: Center for Behavioral Health Statistics and Quality, Substance Abuse and Mental Health Services Administration. Retrieved June 25, 2017, from *www.samhsa.gov/data/sites/default/files/report_2716/ShortReport-2716.html.*

Littell, J. H., & Girvin, H. (2002). Stages of change: A critique. *Behavior Modification, 26*(2), 223–273.

Littell, J. H., & Girvin, H. (2004). Ready or not: Uses of the stages of change model in child welfare. *Child Welfare, 83*(4), 341–366.

Lloyd, M. H., Akin, B. A., & Brook, J. (2017). Parental drug use and permanency for young children in foster care: A competing risks analysis of reunification, guardianship, and adoption. *Children and Youth Services Review, 77,* 177–187.

Loflin, M. J. E., Earleywine, M., Farmer, S., Slavin, M., Luba, R., & Bonn-Miller,

M. (2017). Placebo effects of edible cannabis: Reported intoxication effects at a 30-minute delay. *Journal of Psychoactive Drugs, 49,* 393–397.

Loton, D. J., & Waters, L. E. (2017). The mediating effect of self-efficacy in the connections between strength-based parenting, happiness and psychological distress in teens. *Frontiers in Psychology, 8,* 1707.

Lundahl, B. W., Kunz, C., Brownell, C., Tollefson, D., & Burke, B. L. (2010). A meta-analysis of motivational interviewing: Twenty-five years of empirical studies. *Research on Social Work Practice, 20*(2), 137–160.

Lundahl, B., Moleni, T., Burke, B. L., Butters, R., Tollefson, D., Butler, C., et al. (2013). Motivational interviewing in medical care settings: A systematic review and meta-analysis of randomized controlled trials. *Patient Education and Counseling, 93,* 157–168.

Luoma, J. B., Kohlenberg, B. S., Hayes, S. C., & Fletcher, L. (2012). Slow and steady wins the race: A randomized clinical trial of acceptance and commitment therapy targeting shame in substance use disorders. *Journal of Consulting and Clinical Psychology, 80,* 43–53.

Lydall, G. J., Bass, N. J., McQuillin A., Lawrence, J., Anjorin, A., Kandaswamy, R., et al. (2011). Confirmation of prior evidence of genetic susceptibility to alcoholism in a genome-wide association study of comorbid alcoholism and bipolar disorder. *Psychiatric Genetics, 21,* 294–306.

Lynskey, M. T., Heath, A. C., Bucholz, K. K., Slutske, W. S., Madden, P. A. F., Nelson, E. C., et al. (2003). Escalation of drug use in early-onset cannabis users vs co-twin controls. *Journal of the American Medical Association, 289,* 427–433.

MacAndrew, C., & Edgerton, R. B. (1969). *Drunken comportment: A social explanation.* Chicago: Aldine de Gruyter.

MacGregor, S. (2000, July 2). Art Schlichter: Bad bets and wasted talent. *Cincinnati Enquirer.* Retrieved April 22, 2018, from *www.enquirer.com/editions/2000/07/02/ spt_art_schlichter_bad.html.*

Mack, A. H., Frances, R. J., & Miller, S. I. (2005). Addiction and the law. In R. J. Frances, S. I. Miller, & A. H. Mack (Eds.), *Clinical textbook of addictive disorders* (3rd ed., pp. 355–366). New York: Guilford Press.

MacKillop, J., Amlung, M. T., Few, L. R., Ray, L. A., Sweet, L. H., & Munafò, M. R. (2011). Delayed reward discounting and addictive behavior: A meta-analysis. *Psychopharmacology, 216,* 305–321.

Madden, G. J., & Johnson, P. S. (2010). A delay-discounting primer. In G. J. Madden & W. K. Bickel (Eds.), *Impulsivity: The behavioral and neurological science of discounting* (pp. 11–37). Washington, DC: American Psychological Association.

Maffetone, P. B., Rivera-Dominguez, I., & Laursen, P. B. (2017). Overfat adults and children in developed countries: The public health importance of identifying excess body fat. *Frontiers of Public Health, 5,* 190.

Magill, M., Apodaca, T. R., Barnett, N. P., & Monti, P. M. (2010). The route to change: Within-session predictors of change plan completion in a motivational interview. *Journal of Substance Abuse Treatment, 38,* 299–305.

Magill, M., Apodaca, T. R., Borsari, B., Gaume, J., Hoadley, A., Gordon, R. E. F., et al. (2018). A meta-analysis of motivational interviewing process: Technical, relational, and conditional process models of change. *Journal of Consulting and Clinical Psychology, 86*(2), 140–157.

Manderscheid, R. (2014). The Affordable Care Act: Overview and implications for county and city behavioral health and intellectual/developmental disability programs. *Journal of Social Work in Disability and Rehabilitation, 13,* 87–96.

Mangelsdorf, S. C., & Schoppe-Sullivan, S. J. (2007). Introduction: Emergent family systems. *Infant Behavior and Development, 30,* 60–62.

Mann, C. C. (1994). Behavioral genetics in transition. *Science, 264*, 1686–1689.

Manuel, J. K., Austin, J. L., Miller, W. R., McCrady, B. S., Tonigan, J. S., Meyers, R. J., et al. (2012). Community reinforcement and family training: A pilot comparison of group and self-directed delivery. *Journal of Substance Abuse Treatment, 43*, 129–136.

Marikar, S. (2011, July 1). Can David Duchovny recover from sex addiction? *ABC News/ Entertainment.* Retrieved April 22, 2018, from *http://abcnews.go.com/Entertainment/david-duchovny-tea-leoni-sex-addiction-blame-strife/story?id=13970246.*

Marinchak, J. S., & Morgan, T. J. (2012). Behavioral treatment techniques for psychoactive substance use disorders. In S. T. Walters & F. Rotgers (Eds.), *Treating substance abuse: Theory and technique* (3rd ed., pp. 138–166). New York: Guilford Press.

Marion, T. R., & Coleman, K. (1990). Recovery issues and treatment resources. In D. C. Daley & M. S. Raskin (Eds.), *Treating the chemically dependent and their families.* Newbury Park, CA: Sage.

Marlatt, G. A. (1985). Cognitive factors in the relapse process. In G. A. Marlatt & J. R. Gordon (Eds.), *Relapse prevention* (pp. 128–200). New York: Guilford Press.

Marlatt, G. A., Baer, J. S., & Quigley, L. A. (1995). Self-efficacy and addictive behavior. In A. Bandura (Ed.), *Self-efficacy in changing societies.* New York: Cambridge University Press.

Marlatt, G. A., Demming, B., & Reid, J. B. (1973). Loss of control drinking in alcoholics: An experimental analogue. *Journal of Abnormal Psychology, 81*, 233–241.

Marlatt, G. A., & Gordon, J. R. (1979). Determinants of relapse: Implications for the maintenance of behavior change. In P. A. Davidson & S. M. Davidson (Eds.), *Behavioral medicine: Changing health lifestyles.* New York: Brunner/Mazel.

Marlatt, G. A., & Gordon, J. R. (Eds.). (1985). *Relapse prevention: Maintenance strategies in the treatment of addictive behaviors.* New York: Guilford Press.

Marlatt, G. A., & Witkiewitz, K. (2010). Update on harm reduction policy and intervention research. *Annual Review of Clinical Psychology, 6*, 591–606.

Marlatt, G. A., Witkiewitz, K., Dillworth, T. M., Bowen, S. W., Parks, G. A., Macpherson, L. M., et al. (2004). Vipassana meditation as a treatment for alcohol and drug use disorders. In S. C. Hayes, V. M. Follette, & M. M. Linehan (Eds.), *Mindfulness and acceptance: Expanding the cognitive-behavioral tradition* (pp. 261–287). New York: Guilford Press.

Martins, S. S., Sarvet, A., Santaella-Tenorio, J., Saha, T., Grant, B. F., & Hasin, D. S. (2017). Changes in US lifetime heroin use and heroin use disorder prevalence from the 2001–2002 to 2012–2013 National Epidemiologic Survey on Alcohol and Related Conditions. *JAMA Psychiatry, 74*(5), 445–455.

Massella, J. D. (1990). Intervention: Breaking the addiction cycle. In D. C. Daley & M. S. Raskin (Eds.), *Treating the chemically dependent and their families.* Newbury Park, CA: SAGE.

Massey, J., Kilkenny, M., Batdorf, S., Sanders, S. K., Ellison, D., Halpin, J., et al. (2017). Opioid overdose outbreak—West Virginia, August, 2016. *Morbidity and Mortality Weekly Report, 66*, 975–980.

Mather, C. (1708). *Sober considerations on a growing flood of iniquity.* Boston.

Matthews, J. I., Doerr, L., & Dworatzek, P. D. N. (2016). University students intend to eat better but lack coping self-efficacy and knowledge of dietary recommendations. *Journal of Nutrition Education and Behavior, 48*, 12–19.

Matusow, H., & Rosenblum, A. (2013). The most critical unresolved issue associated with psychoanalytic theories of addiction: Can the talking cure tell us anything about substance use and misuse? *Substance Use and Misuse, 48*, 239–247.

McAfee, T., Babb, S., McNabb, S., & Fiore, M. C. (2015). Helping smokers quit—Opportunities created by the Affordable Care Act. *New England Journal of Medicine, 372*(1), 5–7.

McAuliffe, W. E., & Gordon, R. A. (1980). Reinforcement and the combination of effects: Summary of a theory of opiate addiction. In D. J. Lettieri, M. Sayers, & H. Wallenstein-Pearson (Eds.), *Theories on drug abuse: Selected contemporary perspectives* (DHHS Publication No. ADM 84-967). Washington, DC: U.S. Government Printing Office.

McCabe, S. E., West, B. T., Jutkiewicz, E. M., & Boyd, C. J. (2017). Multiple DSM-5 substance use disorders: A national study of US adults. *Human Psychopharmacology, 32*, e2625.

McCarty, D., Perrin, N. A., Green, C. A., Polen, M. R., Leo, M. C., & Lynch, F. (2010). Methadone maintenance and the cost and utilization of health care among individuals dependent on opioids in a commercial health plan. *Drug and Alcohol Dependence, 111*, 235–240.

McComb, J. L., & Sabiston, C. M. (2010). Family influences on adolescent gambling behavior: A review of the literature. *Journal of Gambling Studies, 26*, 503–520.

McConnaughy, E. A., DiClemente, C. C., Prochaska, J. O., & Velicer, W. F. (1989). Stages of change in psychotherapy: A follow-up report. *Psychotherapy, 26*(4), 494–503.

McCrady, B. S. (2006). Family and other close relationships. In W. R. Miller & K. M. Carroll (Eds.), *Rethinking substance abuse: What the science shows, and what we should do about it* (pp. 166–181). New York: Guilford Press.

McCrady, B. S., Ladd, B. O., & Hallgren, K. A. (2012). Theoretical bases of family approaches to substance abuse treatment. In S. T. Walters & F. Rotgers (Eds.), *Treating substance abuse: Theory and technique* (3rd ed., pp. 224–255). New York: Guilford Press.

McCrady, B. S., Owens, M. D., Borders, A. Z., & Brovko, J. M. (2014). Psychosocial approaches to alcohol use disorders since 1940: A review. *Journal of Studies on Alcohol and Drugs, 75*(Suppl. 17), 68–78.

McCutcheon, V. V., Scherrer, J. F., Grant, J. D., Xian, H., Haber, J. R., Jacob, T., et al. (2013). Parent, sibling and peer associations with subtypes of psychiatric and substance use disorder comorbidity in offspring. *Drug and Alcohol Dependence, 128*, 20–29.

McGovern, M. P., Xie, H., Segal, S. R., Siembab, L., & Drake, R. E. (2006). Addiction treatment services and co-occurring disorders: Prevalence estimates, treatment practices, and barriers. *Journal of Substance Abuse Treatment, 31*, 267–275.

McGreal, C. (2017, October 19). How big pharma's money—and it politicians—feed the US opioid crisis. *The Guardian*. Retrieved December 7, 2017, from *www.theguardian.com/us-news/2017/oct/19/big-pharma-money-lobbying-us-opioid-crisis*.

McKee, S. A., Carroll, K. M., Sinha, R., Robinson, C. N., Cavallo, D., & O'Malley, S. (2007). Enhancing brief cognitive-behavioral therapy with motivational enhancement techniques in cocaine users. *Drug and Alcohol Dependence, 91*(1), 97–101.

McKeon, A., Frye, M. A., & Delanty, N. (2008). The alcohol withdrawal syndrome. *Journal of Neurology, Neurosurgery, and Psychiatry, 79*, 854–862.

McKim, W. A. (1986). *Drugs and behavior: An introduction to behavioral pharmacology*. Englewood Cliffs, NJ: Prentice-Hall.

McKinlay, J. B., & Marceau, L. D. (2000). To boldly go . . . *American Journal of Public Health, 90*, 25–33.

McLellan, A. T. (2011). Considerations on performance contracting: A purchaser's perspective. *Addiction, 106*, 1731–1732.

McLellan, A. T., Kemp, J., Brooks, A., & Carise, D. (2008). Improving public addiction treatment through performance contracting: The Delaware experiment. *Health Policy, 87,* 296–308.

McLellan, A. T., Lewis, D. C., O'Brien, C. P., & Kleber, H. D. (2000). Drug dependence, a chronic medical illness: Implications for treatment, insurance, and outcome evaluation. *Journal of the American Medical Association, 284,* 1689–1695.

McLellan, A. T., & Woodworth, A. M. (2014). The affordable care act and treatment for "Substance Use Disorders": Implications of ending segregated behavioral healthcare. *Journal of Substance Abuse Treatment, 46,* 541–545.

McNeil, R., Guirguis-Younger, M., Dilley, L. B., Aubry, T. D., Turnbull, J., & Hwang, S. W. (2012). Harm reduction services as a point-of-entry to and source of end-of-life care and support for homeless and marginally housed persons who use alcohol and/or illicit drugs: A qualitative analysis. *BMC Public Health, 12,* 312.

Mee-Lee, D., Shulman, G. D., Fishman, M., Gastfriend, D. R., & Miller, M. M. (Eds.). (2013). *The ASAM Criteria: Treatment criteria for addictive, substance-related, and co-occurring conditions* (3rd ed.). Carson City, NV: The Change Companies.

Meier, B. (2007, May 10). In guilty plea, OxyContin maker to pay $600 million. *New York Times.* Retrieved December 20, 2017, from *www.nytimes.com/2007/05/10/business/11drug-web.html.*

Meier, P. S., Warde, A., & Holmes, J. (2018). All drinking is not equal: How a social practice theory lens could enhance public health research on alcohol and other health behaviours. *Addiction, 113,* 206–213.

Mercer, C. G., Mueser, K. T., & Drake, R. E. (1998). Organizational guidelines for dual disorders programs. *Psychiatric Quarterly, 69,* 145–168.

Mercer, S. L., MacDonald, G., & Green, L. W. (2004, July). Participatory research and evaluation: From best practices for all states to achievable practices within each state in the context of the Master Settlement Agreement. *Health Promotion Practice, 5*(3, Suppl.), 167S–178S.

Merry, J. (1966). The "loss of control" myth. *Lancet, 1,* 1257–1258.

Merton, R. K. (1968). *Social theory and social structure.* New York: Free Press.

Messina, N., & Jeter, K. (2012). Parental methamphetamine use and manufacture: Child and familial outcomes. *Journal of Public Child Welfare, 6,* 296–312.

Meyer, I. H. (2003). Prejudice, social stress, and mental health in lesbian, gay, and bisexual populations: Conceptual issues and research evidence. *Psychological Bulletin, 129,* 674–697.

Meyers, R. J., Villanueva, M., & Smith, J. E. (2005). The community reinforcement approach: History and new directions. *Journal of Cognitive Psychotherapy, 19*(3), 247–260.

Miguel, C. S., Martins, P. A., Moleda, N., Klein, M., Chaim-Avancini, T., Gobbo, M. A., et al. (2016). Cognition and impulsivity in adults with attention deficit hyperactivity disorder with and without cocaine and/or crack dependence. *Drug and Alcohol Dependence, 160,* 97–104.

Milam, J. R., & Ketcham, K. (1983). *Under the influence.* New York: Bantam.

Milkman, H. B., & Sunderwirth, S. G. (1987). *Craving for ecstasy: The consciousness and chemistry of escape.* Lexington, MA: D. C. Heath.

Miller, G. C., & Holden, C. (2010, February 12). Proposed revisions to psychiatry's canon unveiled. *Science, 327,* 770–771.

Miller, L. K. (1980). *Principles of everyday behavior analysis.* Monterey, CA: Brooks/Cole.

Miller, P. M. (Ed.). (2009). *Evidence-based addiction treatment.* New York: Academic Press/Elsevier.

Miller, P. M., Smith, G. T., & Goldman, M. S. (1990). Emergence of alcohol expectancies in childhood: A possible critical period. *Journal of Studies on Alcohol, 51,* 343–349.

Miller, W. R. (1982). Treating problem drinkers: What works. *The Behavior Therapist, 5,* 15–19.

Miller, W. R. (2004). The phenomenon of quantum change. *Journal of Clinical Psychology/In Session, 60,* 453–460.

Miller, W. R. (2006). Motivational factors in addictive behaviors. In W. R. Miller & K. M. Carroll (Eds.), *Rethinking substance abuse: What the science shows, and what we should do about it* (pp. 134–150). New York: Guilford Press.

Miller, W. R., & C'de Baca, J. (2001). *Quantum change: When epiphanies and sudden insights transform ordinary lives.* New York: Guilford Press.

Miller, W. R., Forcehimes, A. A., & Zweben, A. (2011). *Treating addiction: A guide for professionals.* New York: Guilford Press.

Miller, W. R., & Hester, R. K. (1980). Treating the problem drinker. In W. R. Miller (Ed.), *The addictive behaviors: Treatment of alcoholism, drug abuse, smoking, and obesity.* Elmsford, NY: Pergamon Press.

Miller, W. R., Meyers, R. J., & Tonigan, J. S. (1999). Engaging the unmotivated in treatment for alcohol problems: A comparison of three strategies for intervention through family members. *Journal of Consulting and Clinical Psychology, 67,* 688–697.

Miller, W. R., & Moyers, T. B. (2017). Motivational interviewing and the clinical science of Carl Rogers. *Journal of Consulting and Clinical Psychology, 85,* 757–766.

Miller, W. R., & Page, A. C. (1991). Warm turkey: Other routes to abstinence. *Journal of Substance Abuse Treatment, 8,* 227–232.

Miller, W. R., & Rollnick, S. (2009). Ten things that motivational interviewing is not. *Behavioural and Cognitive Psychotherapy, 37,* 129–140.

Miller, W. R., & Rollnick, S. (2012). Meeting in the middle: Motivational interviewing and self-determination theory. *International Journal of Behavioral Nutrition and Physical Activity, 9,* 25.

Miller, W. R., & Rollnick, S. (2013). *Motivational interviewing: Preparing people for change* (3rd ed.). New York: Guilford Press.

Miller, W. R., & Tonigan, J. S. (1996). Assessing drinkers' motivation for change: The Stages of Change Readiness and Treatment Eagerness Scale (SOCRATES). *Psychology of Addictive Behaviors 10,* 81–89.

Miller-Tutzauer, C., Leonard, K. E., & Windle, M. (1991). Marriage and alcohol use: A longitudinal study of "maturing out." *Journal of Studies on Alcohol, 52(5),* 434–440.

Mills, B., Caetano, R., Ramisetty-Mikler, S., & Bernstein, I. H. (2012). The dimensionality and measurement properties of alcohol outcome expectancies across Hispanic national groups. *Addictive Behaviors, 37,* 327–330.

Miltenberger, R. G. (2016). *Behavior modification: Principles and procedures* (6th ed.). Boston: Cengage Learning.

Minkler, M., & Wallerstein, N. (Eds.). (2003). *Community-based participatory research in health.* San Francisco: Jossey-Bass.

Misra, R. K. (1980). Achievement, anxiety, and addiction. In D. J. Lettieri, M. Sayers, & H. W. Pearson (Eds.), *Theories on drug abuse: Selected contemporary perspectives* (DHHS Publication No. ADM 84-967). Washington, DC: U.S. Government Printing Office.

Monk, R. L., & Heim, D. (2013). A critical systematic review of alcohol-related outcome expectancies. *Substance Use and Misuse, 48,* 539–557.

Monte, C. F. (1980). *Beneath the mask: An introduction to theories of personality.* New York: Holt, Rinehart & Winston.

Montgomery, A. J., Lingford-Hughes, A. R., Egerton, A., Nutt, D. J., & Grasby, P. M. (2007). The effect of nicotine on striatal dopamine release in man: A [11C]raclopride PET study. *Synapse, 61,* 637–645.

Moody, L., Franck, C., Hatz, L., & Bickel, W. K. (2016). Impulsivity and polysubstance use: A systematic comparison of delay discounting in mono-, dual-, and trisubstance use. *Experimental and Clinical Psychopharmacology, 24,* 30–37.

Moos, R. H. (2008). Active ingredients of substance use-focused self-help groups. *Addiction, 103,* 387–396.

Moos, R. H., & Moos, B. S. (2006). Participation in treatment and Alcoholics Anonymous: A 16-year follow-up of initially untreated individuals. *Journal of Clinical Psychology, 62*(6), 735–750.

Moos, R. H., & Timko, C. (2008). Outcome research on 12-step and other self-help programs. In M. Galanter, & H. D. Kleber (Eds.), *The American Psychiatric Publishing textbook of substance abuse treatment* (4th ed., pp. 511–521). Washington, DC: American Psychiatric Publishing.

Morgenstern, J., & McKay, J. R. (2007). Rethinking the paradigms that inform behavioral treatment research for substance use disorders. *Addiction, 102,* 1377–1389.

Moriarty, H., Stubbe, M., Bradford, S., Tapper, S., & Lim, B. T. (2011). Exploring resilience in families living with addiction. *Journal of Primary Health Care, 3*(3), 210–217.

Moyers, T. B., Houck, J., Glynn, L. H., Hallgren, K. A., & Manuel, J. K. (2017). A randomized controlled trial to influence client language in substance use disorder treatment. *Drug and Alcohol Dependence, 172,* 43–50.

Moyers, T. B., Martin, T., Christopher, P. J., Houck, J. M., & Tonigan, J. S. (2007). Client language as a mediator of motivational interviewing efficacy: Where is the evidence? *Alcoholism, Clinical and Experimental Research, 31*(Suppl. 3), 40S–47S.

Moyers, T. B., Martin, T., Houck, J. M., Christopher, P. J., & Tonigan, J. S. (2009). From in-session behaviors to drinking outcomes: A causal chain for motivational interviewing. *Journal of Consulting and Clinical Psychology, 77,* 1113–1124.

Moynihan, R., Heath, I., & Henry, D. (2002). Selling sickness: The pharmaceutical industry and disease mongering. *British Medical Journal, 324,* 886–891.

Mueller, M. D., & Wyman, J. R. (1997). Study sheds light on the state of drug abuse treatment nationwide. *NIDA Notes, 12*(5), 1, 4–8.

Mueser, K. T., Drake, R. E., & Wallach, M. A. (1998). Dual diagnosis: A review of etiological theories. *Addictive Behaviors, 23,* 717–734.

Mueser, K. T., & Gingerich, S. (2013). Treatment of co-occurring psychotic and substance use disorders. *Social Work in Public Health, 28,* 424–439.

Mueser, K. T., Noordsy, D. L., Drake, R. E., & Fox, L. (2003). *Integrated treatment for dual disorders: A guide to effective treatment.* New York: Guilford Press.

Murphy, S. L., & Khantzian, E. J. (1995). Addiction as a "self-medication" disorder: Application of ego psychology to the treatment of substance abuse. In A. M. Washton (Ed.), *Psychotherapy and substance abuse: A practitioner's handbook.* New York: Guilford Press.

Musto, D. F. (1999). *The American disease: Origins of narcotic control* (2nd ed.). New York: Oxford University Press.

Nace, E. P., Birkmayer, F., Sullivan, M. A., Galanter, M., Fromson, J. A., Frances, R. J., et al. (2007). Socially sanctioned coercion mechanisms for addiction treatment. *American Journal on Addictions, 16,* 15–23.

Nadelmann, E., & LaSalle, L. (2017). Two steps forward, one step back: Current harm reduction policy and politics in the United States. *Harm Reduction Journal, 14*(1), 1–7.

Náfrádi, L., Nakamoto, K., & Schulz, P. J. (2017). Is patient empowerment the key to promote adherence?: A systematic review of the relationship between self-efficacy, health locus of control and medication adherence. *PLOS ONE, 12*(10), e0186458.

Nasim, A., Fernander, A., Townsend, T. G., Corona, R., & Belgrave, F. C. (2011). Cultural protective factors for community risks and substance use among rural African American adolescents. *Journal of Ethnicity in Substance Abuse, 10,* 316–336.

Nathan, P. E., Conrad, M., & Skinstad, A. H. (2016). History of the concept of addiction. *Annual Review of Clinical Psychology, 12,* 29–51.

National Baseball Hall of Fame. (2018). Hall of famers. Retrieved April 22, 2018, from *http://baseballhall.org/hall-famers.*

National Health Promotion Associates. (2017). LifeSkills® Training. Retrieved July 1, 2017, from *www.lifeskillstraining.com.*

National Institute on Alcohol Abuse and Alcoholism. (1990). *Alcohol and health: Seventh special report to the U.S. Congress* (DHHS Publication No. ADM 90-1656). Washington, DC: U.S. Government Printing Office.

National Institute on Alcohol Abuse and Alcoholism. (1994). *Alcohol and health: Eighth special report to the U.S. Congress* (NIH Publication No. 94-3699). Bethesda, MD: National Institutes of Health.

National Institute on Alcohol Abuse and Alcoholism. (1997). *Ninth special report to the U.S. Congress on alcohol and health.* Bethesda, MD: National Institutes of Health.

National Institute on Drug Abuse. (2003). *Preventing drug use among children and adolescents: A research-based guide for parents, educators, and community leaders* (2nd ed.) (NIH Publication No. 04-4212[A]). Bethesda, MD: National Institutes of Health.

National Institutes of Health. (2017). Genetics home reference. Retrieved June 18, 2017, from *https://ghr.nlm.nih.gov.*

Neale, M. C., & Kendler, K. S. (1995). Models of comorbidity for multifactorial disorders. *American Journal of Human Genetics, 57,* 935–953.

Neighbors, C. J., Barnett, N. P., Rohsenow, D. J., Colby, S. M., & Monti, P. (2010). Cost-effectiveness of a motivational intervention for alcohol-involved youth in a hospital emergency department. *Journal of Studies on Alcohol and Drugs, 71,* 384–394.

Nestler, E. J. (2014). Epigenetic mechanisms of drug addiction. *Neuropharmacology 76,* 259–268.

Netherland, J., & Hansen, H. B. (2016). The war on drugs that wasn't: Wasted whiteness, "dirty doctors," and race in media coverage of prescription opioid misuse. *Culture, Medicine and Psychiatry, 40,* 664–686.

Niemiec, C. P., Ryan, R. M., Patrick, H., Deci, E. L., & Williams, G. C. (2010). The energization of health-behavior change: Examining the associations among autonomous self-regulation, subjective vitality, depressive symptoms, and tobacco abstinence. *Journal of Positive Psychology, 5*(2), 122–138.

Nijhuis, H. G. J., & van der Maesen, L. J. G. (1994). The philosophical foundations of public health: An invitation to debate. *Journal of Epidemiology and Community Health, 48,* 1–3.

Nisbett, R. E., Aronson, J., Blair, C., Dickens, W., Flynn, J., Halpern, D. F., et al. (2012). Intelligence: New findings and theoretical developments. *American Psychologist, 67,* 130–159.

Norcross, J. C., Krebs, P. M., & Prochaska, J. O. (2011). Stages of change. *Journal of Clinical Psychology: In Session, 67,* 143–154.

Nordrum, A. (2014, September 10). The new D.A.R.E. program: This one works. *Scientific American.* Retrieved July 1, 2017, from *www.scientificamerican.com/article/the-new-d-a-r-e-program-this-one-works.*

Nowinski, J. (2012). Facilitating 12-step recovery from substance abuse. In S. T. Walters

& F. Rotgers (Eds.), *Treating substance abuse: Theory and technique* (3rd ed., pp. 191–223). New York: Guilford Press.

Nowinski, J., & Baker, S. (2003). *The twelve-step facilitation handbook: A systematic approach to recovery from substance dependence.* Center City, MN: Hazelden.

Nuttin, J. R. (1987). The respective roles of cognition and motivation in behavioral dynamics, intention, and volition. In F. Halisch & J. Kuhl (Eds.), *Motivation, intention, and volition* (pp. 309–320). Berlin: Springer-Verlag.

O'Farrell, T. J., Choquette, K. A., & Cutter, H. S. G. (1998). Couples relapse prevention sessions after behavioral marital therapy for alcoholics and their wives: Outcomes during three years after starting treatment. *Journal of Studies on Alcohol, 59,* 357–370.

O'Farrell, T. J., Choquette, K. A., Cutter, H. S. G., Brown, E., & McCourt, W. F. (1993). Behavioral marital therapy with and without additional couples relapse prevention sessions for alcoholics and their wives. *Journal of Studies on Alcohol, 54,* 652–666.

O'Farrell, T. J., & Clements, K. (2012). Review of outcome research on marital and family therapy in treatment for alcoholism. *Journal of Marital and Family, 38,* 122–144.

O'Farrell, T. J., & Fals-Stewart, W. (2006). *Behavioral couples therapy for alcoholism and drug abuse.* New York: Guilford Press.

O'Farrell, T. J., & Fals-Stewart, W. (2008). Family therapy. In M. Galanter & H. D. Kleber (Eds.), *Textbook of substance abuse treatment* (4th ed., pp. 429–441). Arlington, VA: American Psychiatric Publishing.

O'Farrell, T. J., & Murphy, C. M. (1995). Marital violence before and after alcoholism treatment. *Journal of Consulting and Clinical Psychology, 63,* 256–262.

O'Farrell, T. J., Schumm, J. A., Murphy, M. M., & Muchowski, P. M. (2017). A randomized clinical trial of behavioral couples therapy versus individually-based treatment for drug-abusing women. *Journal of Consulting and Clinical Psychology, 85,* 309–322.

Ogden, C. L., Carroll, M. D., Fryar, C. D., & Flegal, K. M. (2015). *Prevalence of obesity among adults and youth: United States, 2011–2014* (NCHS Data Brief, No. 219) Hyattsville, MD: National Center for Health Statistics. Retrieved March 6, 2018, from *www.cdc.gov/nchs/data/databriefs/db219.pdf.*

Okrent, D. (2010). *Last call: The rise and fall of prohibition.* New York: Scribner.

Oksanen, A. (2014). Affect and addiction in *Celebrity Rehab* reality television show. *Addiction Research and Theory, 22,* 137–146.

Olds, R. S., Thombs, D. L., & Ray-Tomasek, J. (2005). Relations between normative beliefs and initiation intentions toward cigarettes, alcohol and marijuana. *Journal of Adolescent Health, 37,* 75.e7–75e.13.

Olmstead, T. A., Ostrow, C. D., & Carroll, K. M. (2010). Cost-effectiveness of computer-assisted training in cognitive-behavioral therapy as an adjunct to standard care for addiction. *Drug and Alcohol Dependence, 110,* 200–207.

Orford, J., Copello, A., Velleman, R., & Templeton, L. (2010). Family members affected by a close relative's addiction: The stress-strain-coping-support model. *Drugs: Education, Prevention and Policy, 17*(Suppl. 1), 36–43.

Orford, J., Velleman, R., Copello, A., Templeton, L., & Ibanga, A. (2010). The experiences of affected family members: A summary of two decades of qualitative research. *Drugs: Education, Prevention and Policy, 17*(Suppl. 1), 44–62.

Owens, M. M., Amlung, M. T., Beach, S. R. H., Sweet, L. H., & MacKillop, J. (2017). Delay discounting differences in brain activation, connectivity, and structure in individuals with addiction: A systematic review protocol. *Systematic Reviews, 6,* 138.

Oxford Economics. (2014, September). Economic impact of the US gaming industry. Retrieved April 22, 2018, from *www.multivu.com/players/English/7338051-american-gaming-association-releases-oxford-economics-gaming-industry-impact-study/links/7338051-Economic-Impact-of-US-Gaming-Industry.pdf.*

Padgett, D. K., Stanhope, V., Henwood, B. F., & Stefancic, A. (2011). Substance use outcomes among homeless clients with serious mental illness: Comparing Housing First with Treatment First programs. *Community Mental Health Journal, 47,* 227–232.

Padwa, H., Guerrero, E. G., Braslow, J. T., & Fenwick, K. M. (2015). Barriers to serving clients with co-occurring disorders in a transformed mental health system. *Psychiatric Services, 66,* 547–550.

Painter, J. E., Borba, C. P. C., Hynes, M., Mays, D., & Glanz, K. (2008). The use of theory in health behavior research from 2000 to 2005: A systematic review. *Annals of Behavioral Medicine, 35,* 358–362.

Palamar, J. J., Griffin-Tomas, M., & Kamboukos, D. (2015). Reasons for recent marijuana use in relation to use of other illicit drugs among high school seniors in the United States. *American Journal of Drug and Alcohol Abuse, 41,* 323–331.

Parker, A., Scantlebury, A., Booth, A., MacBryde, J. C., Scott, W. J., Wright, K., et al. (2018). Interagency collaboration models for people with mental ill health in contact with the police: A systematic scoping review. *BMJ Open, 8*(3), e019312.

Patnode, S. (2007). "Their lack of masculine security and aggression was obvious": Gender and the medicalization of inebriety in the United States, 1930–50. *Canadian Bulletin of Medical History, 24,* 67–92.

Patrick, H., & Williams, G. C. (2012). Self-determination theory: Its application to health behavior and complementarity with motivational intviewing. *International Journal of Behavioral Nutrition and Physical Activity, 9,* 1–12.

Patterson, G. R. (1996). Some characteristics of a developmental theory for early-onset delinquency. In M. F. Lenzenweger & J. J. Haugaard (Eds.), *Frontiers of developmental psychopathology.* New York: Oxford University Press.

Pattison, E. M., Sobell, M. B., & Sobell, L. C. (1977). *Emerging concepts of alcohol dependence.* New York: Springer.

Pavey, L., & Sparks, P. (2009). Reactance, autonomy and paths to persuasion: Examining perceptions of threats to freedom and informational value. *Motivation and Emotion, 33,* 277–290.

Payer, L. (1992). *Disease-mongers.* New York: Wiley.

Peavy, K. M., Cochran, B. N., & Wax, J. (2010). What they want: Motivation and treatment choice in nontreatment-seeking substance abusers. *Addictive Disorders and Their Treatment, 9*(4), 150–157.

Peele, S. (1985). *The meaning of addiction: Compulsive experience and its interpretation.* Lexington, MA: D. C. Heath.

Peele, S. (1989). *Diseasing of America: Addiction treatment out of control.* Lexington, MA: Lexington Books.

Peele, S. (1996). Assumptions about drugs and the marketing of drug policies. In W. K. Bickel & R. J. DeGrandpre (Eds.), *Drug policy and human nature: Psychological perspectives on the prevention, management, and treatment of illicit drug abuse.* New York: Plenum Press.

Peele, S. (2016). People control their addictions: No matter how much the "chronic" brain disease model of addiction indicates otherwise, we know that people can quit addictions—with special reference to harm reduction and mindfulness. *Addictive Behaviors Reports, 4,* 97–101.

Pentz, M. A., Dwyer, J. H., MacKinnon, D. P., Flay, B. R., Hansen, W. B., Wang, E. Y., et al. (1989). A multicommunity trial for primary prevention of adolescent drug abuse: Effects on drug use prevalence. *Journal of the American Medical Association, 261*(22), 3259–3266.

Perrone, M., & Weider, B. (2016, December 15). Pro-painkiller echo chamber shaped policy amid drug epidemic (Center for Public Integrity). Retrieved December 7, 2017, from *www.publicintegrity.org/2016/09/19/20201/pro-painkiller-echo-chamber-shaped-policy-amid-drug-epidemic.*

Perry, C. L., Williams, C. L., Veblen-Mortenson, S., Toomey, T. L., Komro, K. A., Anstine, P. S., et al. (1996). Project Northland: Outcomes of a communitywide alcohol use prevention program during early adolescence. *American Journal of Public Health, 86,* 956–965.

Pesis-Katz, I., Williams, G. C., Niemiec, C. P., & Fiscella, K. (2011). Cost-effectiveness of intensive tobacco dependence intervention based on self-determination theory. *American Journal of Managed Care, 17*(10), e393–e398.

Petersen, C. L., & Zettle, R. D. (2009). Treating inpatients with comorbid depression and alcohol use disorders: A comparison of acceptance and commitment therapy versus treatment as usual. *Psychological Record, 59,* 521–536.

Petry, N. M. (2002). Discounting of delayed rewards in substance abusers: Relationship to antisocial personality disorder. *Psychopharmacology 162,* 425–432.

Petry, N. M., Peirce, J. M., Stitzer, M. L., Blaine, J., Roll, J. M., Cohen, A., et al. (2005). Effect of prize-based incentives on outcomes in stimulant abusers in outpatient psychosocial treatment programs: A National Drug Abuse Treatment Clinical Trials Network Study. *Archives of General Psychiatry, 62,* 1148–1156.

Pierce, R. C., & Kumaresan, V. (2006). The mesolimbic dopamine system: The final common pathway for the reinforcing effect of drugs of abuse? *Neuroscience and Biobehavioral Reviews, 30,* 215–238.

Pilowsky, D. J., Keyes, K. M., & Hasin, D. S. (2009). Adverse childhood events and lifetime alcohol dependence. *American Journal of Public Health, 99,* 258–263.

Portenoy, R. K. (1996). Opioid therapy for chronic nonmalignant pain: Clinician's perspective. *Journal of Law, Medicine, and Ethics, 24,* 296–309.

Portenoy, R. K., & Foley, K. M. (1986). Chronic use of opioid analgesics in non-malignant pain: Report of 38 cases. *Pain, 25,* 171–186.

Porter, R. (1985). The drinking man's disease: The "pre-history" of alcoholism in Georgian Britain. *British Journal of Addiction, 80,* 385–396.

Powers, M. B., Vedel, E., & Emmelkamp, P. M. G. (2008). Behavioral couples therapy (BCT) for alcohol and drug use disorders: A meta-analysis. *Clinical Psychology Review, 28,* 952–962.

Priester, M. A., Browne, T., Iachini, A., Clone, S., DeHart, D., & Seay K. D. (2016). Treatment access barriers and disparities among individuals with co-occurring mental health and substance use disorders: An integrative literature review. *Journal of Substance Abuse Treatment, 61,* 47–59.

Pringle, J., Grasso, K., & Lederer L. (2017). Integrating the integrated: Merging integrated dual diagnosis treatment (IDDT) with housing first. *Community Mental Health Journal, 53,* 672–678.

Prochaska, J. O., & DiClemente, C. C. (1982). Transtheoretical therapy: Toward a more integrative model of change. *Psychotherapy: Theory, Research and Practice, 20,* 161–173.

Prochaska, J. O., DiClemente, C. C., & Norcross, J. C. (1992). In search of how people change: Application to addictive behavior. *American Psychologist, 47,* 1102–1114.

Prochaska, J. O., & Norcross, J. C. (2018). *Systems of psychotherapy: A transtheoretical analysis* (9th ed.). New York: Oxford University Press.

Project MATCH Research Group. (1997). Matching alcoholism treatments to client heterogeneity: Project MATCH posttreatment drinking outcomes. *Journal of Studies on Alcohol, 58,* 7–29.

Putwain, D., Remedios, R., & Symes, W. (2015). Experiencing fear appeals as a challenge or a threat influences attainment value and academic self-efficacy. *Learning and Instruction, 40,* 21–28.

Quinnipiac University Poll. (2017, February 23). Republicans out of step with U.S. voters on key issues, Quinnipiac University national poll finds: Most voters support legalized marijuana. Retrieved August 3, 2017, from *https://poll.qu.edu/images/polling/us/us02232017_U68mdxwa.pdf.*

Rand Corporation. (1994). *Controlling cocaine: Supply versus demand programs.* Santa Monica, CA: Author.

Rannazzisi, J. T. (2014, December 29). *Comments from the Drug Enforcement Administration: A letter to Marcia Crosse, Director of Health Care, U.S. General Accountability Office.* Washington, DC: U.S. Department of Justice, Drug Enforcement Administration. Retrieved December 11, 2017, from *www.gao.gov/assets/670/668252.pdf.*

Rash, C. J., & Copeland, A. L. (2008). The Brief Smoking Consequences Questionnaire-Adult (BSCQ-A): Development of a short form of the SCQ-A. *Nicotine and Tobacco Research, 10,* 1633–1643.

Rasmussen, K. G. (2008). Antidepressants and manic symptoms. *American Journal of Psychiatry, 165,* 263–264.

Redvers, A. (2007). Review of *Theory of addiction. British Journal of Psychiatry, 191,* 273–274.

Reese, F. L., Chassin, L., & Molina, B. S. (1994). Alcohol expectancies in early adolescence: Predicting drinking behavior from alcohol expectancies and paternal alcoholism. *Journal of Studies on Alcohol, 55,* 276–284.

Reynolds, B. (2006). A review of delay-discounting research with humans: Relations to drug use and gambling. *Behavioural Pharmacology, 17,* 651–667.

Richter, L., & Foster, S. E. (2014). Effectively addressing addiction requires changing the language of addiction. *Journal of Public Health Policy, 35,* 60–64.

Rieckmann, T. R., Abraham, A. J., & Bride, B. E. (2016). Implementation of motivational interviewing in substance use disorder treatment: Research network participation and organizational compatibility. *Journal of Addiction Medicine, 10,* 402–407.

Ries, R. K., Galanter, M., & Tonigan, J. S. (2008). Twelve-step facilitation: An adaptation for psychiatric practitioners and patients. In M. Galanter & H. D. Kleber (Eds), *Textbook of substance abuse treatment* (4th ed., pp. 373–386). Washington, DC: American Psychiatric Publishing.

Rigotti, N. A., DiFranza, J. R., Chang, Y., Tisdale, T., Kemp, B., & Singer, D. E. (1997). The effect of enforcing tobacco-sales laws on adolescents, access to tobacco and smoking behavior. *New England Journal of Medicine, 337,* 1044–1051.

Ringwalt, C., Ennett, S. T., & Holt, K. D. (1991). An outcome evaluation of Project DARE (Drug Abuse Resistance Education). *Health Education Research, 6,* 327–337.

Robbins, M. S., Feaster, D. J., Horigian, V. E., Rohrbaugh, M., Shoham, V., Bachrach, K., et al. (2011). Brief strategic family therapy versus treatment as usual: Results of a multisite randomized trial for substance using adolescents. *Journal of Consulting and Clinical Psychology, 79,* 713–727.

Roberts W., & Fillmore, M. T. (2017). Curbing the DUI offender's self-efficacy to drink and drive: A laboratory study. *Drug and Alcohol Dependence, 172,* 73–79.

Robertson, I., Heather, N., Dzialdowski, A., Crawford, J., & Winton, M. (1986). A comparison of minimal versus intensive controlled drinking treatment interventions for problem drinkers. *British Journal of Clinical Psychology, 25,* 185–194.

Rogers, E. M. (1995). *Diffusion of innovations* (4th ed.). New York: Free Press.

Rollnick, S., Heather, N., Gold, R., & Hall, W. (1992). Development of a short "readiness to change" questionnaire for use in brief, opportunistic interventions among excessive drinkers. *British Journal of Addiction, 87,* 743–754.

Roos, C. R., Bowen, S., & Witkiewitz, K. (2017). Baseline patterns of substance use disorder severity and depression and anxiety symptoms moderate the efficacy of mindfulness-based relapse prevention. *Journal of Consulting and Clinical Psychology, 85*(11), 1041–1051.

Roozen, H. G., de Waart, R., & van der Kroft, P. (2010). Community reinforcement and family training: An effective option to engage treatment-resistant substance-abusing individuals in treatment. *Addiction, 105,* 1729–1738.

Rorabaugh, W. J. (1976). *The alcoholic republic: America, 1790–1840.* Unpublished doctoral dissertation, University of California, Berkeley, CA.

Rose, G. S., & Walters, S. T. (2012). Theories of motivation and addictive behavior. In S. T. Walters & F. Rotgers (Eds.), *Treating substance abuse: Theory and technique* (3rd ed., pp. 9–27). New York: Guilford Press.

Rose, P. (2004, January 12). Exclusive: Pete Rose's confession. *Sports Illustrated, 100*(1).

Rosenbaum, D. P., & Hanson, G. S. (1998). Assessing the effects of school-based drug education: A six-year multilevel analysis of Project DARE. *Journal of Research in Crime and Delinquency, 35,* 381–412.

Rosenberg, H., Melville, J., Levell, D., & Hodge, J. E. (1992). A 10-year follow-up survey of acceptability of controlled drinking in Britain. *Journal of Studies on Alcohol, 53,* 441–446.

Rotgers, F. (2012). Cognitive-behavioral theories of substance abuse. In S.T. Walters & F. Rotgers (Eds.), *Treating substance abuse: Theory and technique* (3rd ed., pp. 113–137). New York: Guilford Press.

Rothschild, D. (2010). Partners in treatment: Relational psychoanalysis and harm reduction therapy. *Journal of Clinical Psychology, 66,* 136–149.

Rothschild, D., & Gellman, M. (2009). Finding the common ground: Contemporary psychoanalysis and substance abuse treatment. *Journal of Addictive Diseases, 28,* 28–38.

Rowe, C. L. (2012). Family therapy for drug abuse: Review and updates 2003–2010. *Journal of Marital and Family Therapy, 38,* 59–81.

Rowe, C. L., & Liddle, H. A. (2008). Multidimensional family therapy for adolescent alcohol abusers. *Alcoholism Treatment Quarterly, 26,* 105–123.

Ruan, H., Bullock, C. L., & Reger, G. M. (2017). Implementation of contingency management at a large VA addiction treatment center. *Psychiatric Services, 68,* 1207–1209.

Rudd, R. A., Seth, P., David, F., & Scholl, L. (2016). Increases in drug and opioid-involved overdose deaths—United States, 2010–2015. *Morbidity and Mortality Weekly Report, 65,* 1445–1452.

Ruff, S., McComb, J. L., Coker, C. J., & Sprenkle, D. H. (2010). Behavioral couples therapy for the treatment of substance abuse: A substantive and methodological review of O'Farrell, Fals-Stewart, and colleagues' program of research. *Family Process, 49,* 439–456.

Rush, B. (1943). An inquiry into the effects of ardent spirits on the human body and mind, with an account of the means for preventing and of the remedies for curing them. *Quarterly Journal of Studies on Alcohol, 4,* 325–341. (Original work published 1790)

Rush, B., Urbanoski, K., Bassani, D., Castel, S., Wild, T. C., Strike, C., et al. (2008). Prevalence of co-occurring substance use and other mental disorders in the Canadian population. *Canadian Journal of Psychiatry, 53*, 800–809.

Ryan, C., & Lewis, J. M. (2017). *Computer and Internet use in the United States: 2015* (American Community Survey Reports, ACS-37). Washington, DC: U.S. Census Bureau. Retrieved December 6, 2017, from *www.census.gov/content/dam/Census/library/publications/2017/acs/acs-37.pdf.*

Ryan, H., Girion, L., & Glover, S. (2016, July 10). More than 1 million Oxycontin pills ended up in the hands of criminals and addicts: What the drugmaker knew. *Los Angeles Times.* Retrieved December 6, 2017, from *www.latimes.com/projects/la-me-oxycontin-part2.*

Ryan, R. M. (1992). Agency and organization: Intrinsic motivation, autonomy, and the self in psychological development. In R. Dienstbier (Series Ed.) & J. E. Jacobs (Vol. Ed.), *Nebraska Symposium on Motivation: Vol. 40. Developmental perspectives on motivation* (pp. 1–56). Lincoln: University of Nebraska Press.

Ryan, R. M. (1995). Psychological needs and the facilitation of integrative processes. *Journal of Personality, 63*, 397–427.

Ryan, R. M., & Deci, E. L. (2002). An overview of self-determination theory: An organismic dialectical perspective. In E. L. Deci & R. M. Ryan (Eds.), *Handbook of self-determination research* (pp. 3–33). Rochester, NY: University of Rochester Press.

Ryan, R. M., & Deci, E. L. (2008). A self-determination theory approach to psychotherapy: The motivational basis for effective change. *Canadian Psychology, 49*, 186–193.

Ryan, R. M., & Deci, E. L. (2017). *Self-determination theory: Basic psychological needs in motivation, development, and wellness.* New York: Guilford Press.

Ryan, R. M., Lynch, M. F., Vansteenkiste, M., & Deci, E. L. (2011). Motivation and autonomy in counseling, psychotherapy, and behavior change: A look at theory and practice. *The Counseling Psychologist, 39*, 193–260.

Samson, J. E., & Tanner-Smith, E. E. (2015). Single-session alcohol interventions for heavy-drinking college students: A systematic review and meta-analysis. *Journal of Studies on Alcohol and Drugs, 76*, 530–543.

Sanchez-Craig, M., & Lei, H. (1986). Disadvantages to imposing the goal of abstinence on problem drinkers: An empirical study. *British Journal of Addiction, 81*(4), 505–512.

Sandoz, J. (2004). Codependency? *Annals of the American Psychotherapy Association, 7*(2), 37.

Sankar, P., & Cho, M. K. (2002). Toward a new vocabulary of human genetic variation. *Science, 298*, 1337–1339.

Santisteban, D. A., Coatsworth, J. D., Perez-Vidal, A., Kurtines, W. M., Schwartz, S. J., LaPerriere, A., et al. (2003). Efficacy of brief strategic family therapy in modifying Hispanic adolescent behavior problems and substance use. *Journal of Family Psychology, 17*, 121–133.

Saunders, J. B. (2006). Substance dependence and non-dependence in the *Diagnostic and Statistical Manual of Mental Disorders* (DSM) and the *International Classification of Diseases* (ICD): Can an identical conceptualization be achieved? *Addiction, 101*(Suppl. 1), 48–58.

Sawyer, A. M., & Borduin, C. M. (2011). Effects of multisystemic therapy through midlife: A 21.9-year follow-up to a randomized clinical trial with serious and violent juvenile offenders. *Journal of Consulting and Clinical Psychology, 79*, 643–652.

Scannapieco, M., & Connell-Carrick, K. (2007). Assessment of families who have substance abuse issues: Those who maltreat their infants and toddlers and those who do not. *Substance Use and Misuse, 42,* 1545–1553.

Scaturo, D. J., Hayes, T., Sagula, D., & Walter, T. (2000). The concept of codependency and its context within family systems theory. *Family Therapy, 27,* 63–70.

Schmidt, L. A., Rieckmann, T., Abraham, A., Molfenter, T., Capoccia, V., Roman, P., et al. (2012). Advancing recovery: Implementing evidence-based treatment for substance use disorders at the systems level. *Journal of Studies on Alcohol and Drugs, 73,* 413–422.

Schneider, M., & Preckel, F. (2017). Variables associated with achievement in higher education: A systematic review of meta-analyses. *Psychological Bulletin, 143,* 565–600.

Schuckit, M. A. (1989). Familial alcoholism. *Drug Abuse and Alcoholism Newsletter, 18(9),* 1–3.

Schultz, W. (2015). The chemical imbalance hypothesis: An evaluation of the evidence. *Ethical Human Psychology and Psychiatry, 17,* 60–75.

Schumm, J. A., O'Farrell, T. J., & Andreas, J. B. (2012). Behavioral couples therapy when both partners have a current alcohol use disorder. *Alcoholism Treatment Quarterly, 30,* 407–421.

Schumm, J. A., O'Farrell, T. J., Kahler, C. W., Murphy, M. M., & Muchowski, P. (2014). A randomized clinical trial of behavioral couples therapy versus individually based treatment for women with alcohol dependence. *Journal of Consulting and Clinical Psychology, 82,* 993–1004.

Scutchfield, F. D., & Keck, C. W. (2017). Deaths of despair: Why? What to do? *American Journal of Public Health, 107,* 1564–1565.

Sellman, D. (2009). The 10 most important things known about addiction. *Addiction, 105,* 6–13.

Sessions, J. (2017, May 10). *Memorandum for all federal prosecutors: Subject: Department charging and sentencing policy.* Washington, DC: United States Office of the Attorney General. Retrieved March 21, 2018, from *www.justice.gov/opa/press-release/file/965896/download.*

Sexton, T. L. (2011). *Functional family therapy in clinical practice: An evidence-based treatment model for working with troubled adolescents.* New York: Routledge.

Sexton, T., & Turner, C. W. (2011). The effectiveness of functional family therapy for youth with behavioral problems in a community practice setting. *Couple and Family Psychology: Research and Practice, 1(S),* 3–15.

Shaffer, H. J. (2015). What is addiction?: A perspective. Retrieved April 22, 2018, from *www.divisiononaddiction.org/html/whatisaddiction.htm.*

Sharp, S. I., McQuillin, A., Marks, M., Hunt, S. P., Stanford, S. C., Lydall, G. J., et al. (2014). Genetic association of the tachykinin receptor 1 TACR1 gene in bipolar disorder, attention deficit hyperactivity disorder, and the alcohol dependence syndrome. *American Journal of Medical Genetics, Part B, Neuropsychiatric Genetics, 165B,* 373–380.

Shaw, D. (1996). *The pleasure police.* New York: Doubleday.

Shaw, M. A., & DiClemente, C. C. (2016). Temptation minus self-efficacy in alcohol relapse: A Project MATCH follow-up. *Journal of Studies on Alcohol and Drugs, 77,* 521–525.

Sheeran, P., Maki, A., Montanaro, E., Avishai-Yitshak, A., Bryan, A., Klein, W. P., et al. (2016). The impact of changing attitudes, norms, and self-efficacy on health-related intentions and behavior: A meta-analysis. *Health Psychology, 35,* 1178–1188.

Sheidow, A. J., & Henggeler, S. W. (2008). Multisystemic therapy for alcohol and other drug abuse in delinquent adolescents. *Alcoholism Treatment Quarterly, 26,* 125–145.

Sher, K. J. (1997). Psychological characteristics of children of alcoholics. *Alcohol, Health and Research World, 21*(3), 247–254.

Shiffrin, R. M., & Schneider, W. (1977). Controlled and automatic human information processing: II. Perceptual learning, automatic attending, and a general theory. *Psychological Review, 84,* 127–190.

Siegel, S. (1982). Drug dissociation in the nineteenth century. In F. C. Colpaert & J. L. Slangen (Eds.), *Drug discrimination: Applications in CNS pharmacology.* Amsterdam: Elsevier.

Simons, J., Correia, C. J., Carey, K. B., & Borsari, B. E. (1998). Validating a five-factor marijuana motives measure: Relations with use, problems, and alcohol motives. *Journal of Counseling Psychology, 45,* 265–273.

Sitzmann, T., & Ely, K. (2011). A meta-analysis of self-regulated learning in work-related training and educational attainment: What we know and where we need to go. *Psychological Bulletin, 137,* 421–442.

Skog, O. J., & Duckert, F. (1993). The development of alcoholics' and heavy drinkers' consumption: A longitudinal study. *Journal of Studies on Alcohol, 54,* 178–188.

Sloboda, Z., Stephens, R. C., Stephens, P. C., Grey, S. F., Teasdale, B., Hawthorne, R. D., et al. (2009). The Adolescent Substance Abuse Prevention Study: A randomized field trial of a universal substance abuse prevention program. *Drug and Alcohol Dependence, 102,* 1–10.

Slutske, W. S., Zhu, G., Meier, M. H., & Martin, N. G. (2010). Genetic and environmental influences on disordered gambling in men and women. *Archives of General Psychiatry, 67,* 624–630.

Small, E., & Kohl, P. L. (2012). African American caregivers and substance abuse in child welfare: Identification of multiple risk profiles. *Journal of Family Violence, 27,* 415–426.

Smeets, E., Roefs, A., & Jansen, A. (2009). Experimentally induced chocolate craving leads to an attentional bias in increased distraction but not in speeded detection. *Appetite, 53,* 370–375.

Smith, A., & Anderson, M. (2018, March 1). Social media use in 2018 (Pew Research Center). Retrieved March 6, 2018, from *file:///C:/Users/dlt0119/Downloads/PI_2018.03.01_Social-Media_FINAL.pdf.*

Smith, G. T., Goldman, M. S., Greenbaum, P. E., & Christiansen, B. A. (1995). Expectancy for social facilitation from drinking: The divergent paths of high-expectancy and low-expectancy adolescents. *Journal of Studies on Alcohol, 104*(1), 32–40.

Smith, J. E., & Meyers, R. J. (2004). *Motivating substance abusers to enter treatment: Working with family members.* New York: Guilford Press.

Smith, J. E., Meyers, R. J., & Austin, J. L. (2008). Working with family members to engage treatment-refusing drinkers: The CRAFT program. *Alcoholism Treatment Quarterly, 26,* 169–193.

Smith, J. L. (2009). War on drugs. In G. L. Fisher & N. A. Roget (Eds.), *Encyclopedia of substance abuse prevention, treatment, and recovery* (Vol. 2, pp. 997–1000). Thousand Oaks, CA: SAGE.

Smout, M. F., Longo, M., Harrison, S., Minniti, R., Wickes, W., & White, J. M. (2010). Psychosocial treatment for methamphetamine use disorders: A preliminary randomized controlled trial of cognitive behavior therapy and acceptance and commitment therapy. *Substance Abuse, 31,* 98–107.

Sobell, M. B., & Sobell, L. C. (1976). Second year treatment outcome of alcoholics treated by individualized behavior therapy: Results. *Behaviour Research and Therapy, 14,* 195–215.

Sobell, M. B., & Sobell, L. C. (2006). Obstacles to the adoption of low risk drinking goals in the treatment of alcohol problems in the United States: A commentary. *Addiction Research and Theory, 14,* 19–24.

Sobell, M. B., Wilkinson, D. A., & Sobell, L. C. (1990). Alcohol and drug problems. In A. S. Bellack, M. Hersen, & A. E. Kazdin (Eds.), *International handbook of behavior modification* (2nd ed., pp. 415–435). New York: Plenum Press.

Sporting News. (1998). Baseball's 100 greatest players. Retrieved August 8, 2011, from *www.baseball-almanac.com.*

Spoth, R. L., Redmond, C., & Shin, C. (2001). Randomized trial of brief family interventions for general populations: Adolescent substance use outcomes 4 years after baseline. *Journal of Consulting and Clinical Psychology, 69,* 627–642.

Stacy, A. W., Newcomb, M. D., & Bentler, P. M. (1991). Cognitive motivation and drug use: A 9-year longitudinal study. *Journal of Abnormal Psychology, 100,* 502–515.

Stanton, D., & Shadish, W. R. (1997). Outcome, attrition, and family-couples treatment for drug abuse: A meta-analysis and review of the controlled, comparative studies. *Psychological Bulletin, 122,* 170–191.

Stefflre, B., & Burks, H. M. (1979). Function of theory in counseling. In H. M. Burks & B. Stefflre (Eds.), *Theories of counseling.* New York: McGraw-Hill.

Steinglass, P. (1981). The alcoholic at home: Patterns of interaction in dry, wet, and transitional stages of alcoholism. *Archives of General Psychiatry, 38,* 578–584.

Steinglass, P. (1987). *The alcoholic family.* New York: Basic Books.

Steinglass, P., Weiner, S., & Mendelson, J. H. (1971). A systems approach to alcoholism: A model and its clinical application. *Archives of General Psychiatry, 24,* 401–408.

Stitzer, M., & Bigelow, G. (1978). Contingency management in a methadone maintenance program: Availability of reinforcers. *International Journal of the Addictions, 13*(5), 737–746.

Stitzer, M. L., Bigelow, G. E., & Liebson, I. (1980). Reducing drug use among methadone maintenance clients: Contingent reinforcement for morphine-free urines. *Addictive Behaviors, 5,* 333–340.

Stockwell, T., Pauly, B., Chow, C., Erickson, R. A., Krysowaty, B., Roemer, A., et al. (2018). Does managing the consumption of people with severe alcohol dependence reduce harm?: A comparison of participants in six Canadian managed alcohol programs with locally recruited controls. *Drug and Alcohol Review, 37*(Suppl. 1), S159–S166.

Stone, D. B., Armstrong, R. W., Macrina, D. M., & Pankau, J. W. (1996). *Introduction to epidemiology.* Boston: McGraw-Hill.

Storbjörk, J. (2017). Commentary on Witkiewitz et al. (2017): Abstinence or moderation-a choice for whom and why? *Addiction, 112,* 2122–2123.

Straus, S. E., Glasziou, P., Richardson, W. S., & Haynes, R. B. (2011). *Evidence-based medicine: How to practice and teach it* (4th ed.). Edinburgh, UK: Elsevier.

Strine, T. W., Dube, S. R., Edwards, V. J., Prehn, A. W., Rasmussen, S., Wagenfeld, M., et al. (2012). Associations between adverse childhood experiences, psychological distress, and adult alcohol problems. *American Journal of Health Behavior, 36,* 408–423.

Substance Abuse and Mental Health Services Administration (SAMHSA). (2002). Report to Congress on the prevention and treatment of co-occurring substance abuse and mental disorders. Retrieved April 21, 2018, from *www.ct.gov/dmhas/lib/dmhas/cosig/cooccurringreport.pdf.*

Substance Abuse and Mental Health Services Administration (SAMHSA). (2011). *Results from the 2010 National Survey on Drug Use and Health: Summary of national findings* (HHS Publication No. SMA 11-4658, NSDUH Series H-41). Rockville, MD: Author.

Substance Abuse and Mental Health Services Administration (SAMHSA). (2017). *Key substance use and mental health indicators in the United States: Results from the 2016 National Survey on Drug Use and Health* (HHS Publication No. SMA 17-5044, NSDUH Series H-52). Rockville, MD: Author. Retrieved May 25, 2018, from *https://store.samhsa.gov/product/Key-Substance-Use-and-Mental-Health-Indicators-in-the-United-States-/SMA17-5044*.

Substance Abuse and Mental Health Services Administration (SAMHSA). (2018, January). Statement of Elinore F. McCance-Katz, MD, PhD, Assistant Secretary for Mental Health and Substance Use regarding the National Registry of Evidence-based Programs and Practices and SAMHSA's new approach to implementation of evidence-based practices (EBPs). Retrieved May 3, 2018, from *www.samhsa.gov/newsroom/press-announcements/201801110330*.

Suh, H. N., & Flores, L. Y. (2017). Relative deprivation and career decision self-efficacy: Influences of self-regulation and parental educational attainment. *Career Development Quarterly, 65*, 145–158.

Sullivan, S. G., & Wu, Z. (2007). Rapid scale up of harm reduction in China. *International Journal of Drug Policy, 18*, 118–128.

Sun, W., Skara, S., Sun, P., Dent, C. W., & Sussman, S. (2006). Project Towards No Drug Abuse: Long-term substance use outcomes evaluation. *Preventive Medicine, 42*, 188–192.

Sunderland, M., Slade, T., & Krueger R. F. (2015). Examining the shared and unique relationships among substance use and mental disorders. *Psychological Medicine, 45*, 1103–1113.

Sussman, S. (1996). Development of a school-based drug abuse prevention curriculum for high risk youth. *Journal of Psychoactive Drugs, 26*, 214–267.

Sussman, S., Dent, C. W., & Stacy, A. W. (2002). Project Towards No Drug Abuse: A review of the findings and future directions. *American Journal of Health Behavior, 26*, 354–365.

Sussman, S., Dent, C. W., Stacy, A. W., & Craig, S. (1998). One-year outcomes of Project Towards No Drug Abuse. *Preventive Medicine, 27*, 632–642.

Sussman, S., Lisha, N., & Griffiths, M. (2011). Prevalence of the addictions: A problem of the majority or the minority? *Evaluation and the Health Professions, 34*, 3–56.

Sussman, S., Rohrbach, L. A., Patel, R., & Holiday, K. (2003). A look at an interactive classroom-based drug abuse prevention program: Interactive contents and suggestions for research. *Journal of Drug Education, 33*, 355–368.

Sussman, S., Sun, P., McCuller, W. J., & Dent, C. W. (2003). Project Towards No Drug Abuse: Two-year outcomes of a trial that compares health educator delivery to self-instruction. *Preventive Medicine, 37*, 155–162.

Swensen, I. D. (2015). Substance-abuse treatment and mortality. *Journal of Public Economics, 122*, 13–30.

Swift, E. M. (1989, March 6). Facing the music: Wade Boggs of the Red Sox stayed cool in spring training despite his erstwhile lover's steamy revelations. *Sports Illustrated, 70*(10), 38–45. Retrieved April 22, 2018, from *www.si.com/vault/issue/702486/1/1*.

Swinburn, B. A., Sacks, G., Hall, K. D., McPherson, K., Finegood, D. T., Moodie, M. L., et al. (2011). The global obesity pandemic: Shaped by global drivers and local environments. *Lancet, 378*, 804–814.

Sylla, M., Harawa, N., & Reznick, O. G. (2010). The first condom machine in a U.S. jail: The challenge of harm reduction in a law and order environment. *American Journal of Public Health, 100*(6), 982–985.

Szapocznik, J., Hervis, O., & Schwartz, S. (2003). *Brief strategic family therapy for adolescent drug abuse* (NIH Pub. No. 03-4751). Bethesda, MD: National Institute on Drug Abuse.

Szapocznik, J., Muir, J. A., Duff, J. H., Schwartz, S. J., & Brown, C. H. (2015). Brief Strategic Family Therapy: Implementing evidence-based models in community settings. *Psychotherapy Research, 25,* 121–133.

Takamatsu, S. K., Martens, M. P., & Arterberry, B. J. (2016). Depressive symptoms and gambling behavior: Mediating role of coping motivation and gambling refusal self-efficacy. *Journal of Gambling Studies, 32,* 535–546.

Talbott, G. D. (1989). Alcoholism should be treated as a disease. In B. Leone (Ed.), *Chemical dependency: Opposing viewpoints.* San Diego, CA: Greenhaven.

Taleff, M. J. (1997). *A handbook to assess and treat resistance in chemical dependency.* Dubuque, IA: Kendall/Hunt.

Tang, Y., Posner, M. I., Rothbart, M. K., & Volkow, N. D. (2015). Circuitry of self-control and its role in reducing addiction. *Trends in Cognitive Sciences, 19,* 439–444.

Tang, Y., Tang, R., & Posner, M. I. (2016). Mindfulness meditation improves emotion regulation and reduces drug abuse. *Drug and Alcohol Dependence, 163*(Suppl. 1), S13–S18.

Tanner-Smith, E. E., Wilson, S. J., & Lipsey, M. W. (2013). The comparative effectiveness of outpatient treatment for adolescent substance abuse: A meta-analysis. *Journal of Substance Abuse Treatment, 44,* 145–158.

Tatarsky, A., & Kellogg, S. (2012). Harm reduction psychotherapy. In G. A. Marlatt, M. E. Larimer, & K. Witkiewitz (Eds.), *Harm reduction: Pragmatic strategies for managing high-risk behaviors* (2nd ed., pp. 36–60). New York: Guilford Press.

Templeton, L. (2012). Dilemmas facing grandparents with grandchildren affected by parental substance misuse. *Drugs: Education, Prevention and Policy, 19,* 11–18.

Thombs, D. L. (1991). Expectancies versus demographics in discriminating between college drinkers: Implications for alcohol abuse prevention. *Health Education Research, 6*(4), 491–495.

Thombs, D. L. (1993). The differentially discriminating properties of alcohol expectancies for female and male drinkers. *Journal of Counseling and Development, 71,* 321–325.

Thombs, D. L., & Ray-Tomasek, J. (2001). Superintendents' intentions toward DARE: Results from a statewide survey. *American Journal of Health Education, 32,* 267–274.

Thompson, A. B., Goodman, M. S., & Kwate, N. O. A. (2016). Does learning about race prevent substance abuse?: Racial discrimination, racial socialization and substance use among African Americans. *Addictive Behaviors, 61,* 1–7.

Tiet, Q. Q., & Mausbach, B. (2007). Treatments for patients with dual diagnosis: A review. *Alcoholism: Clinical and Experimental Review, 31,* 1–24.

Tiffany, S. T. (1990). A cognitive model of drug urges and drug-use behavior: Role of automatic and nonautomatic processes. *Psychological Review, 97,* 147–168.

Tiffany, S. T., & Conklin, C. A. (2000). A cognitive processing model of alcohol craving and compulsive alcohol use. *Addiction, 95*(Suppl. 2), S145–S153.

Tiffany, S. T., & Wray, J. (2009). The continuing conundrum of craving. *Addiction, 104,* 1618–1619.

Tooley, E. M., & Moyers, T. B. (2012). Motivational interviewing in practice. In S. T. Walters & F. Rotgers (Eds.), *Treating substance abuse: Theory and technique* (3rd ed., pp. 28–47). New York: Guilford Press.

Townshend, T., & Lake, A. (2017). Obesogenic environments: Current evidence of the built and food environments. *Perspectives in Public Health, 137,* 38–44.

Tracy, S. W. (2005). *Alcoholism in America: From Reconstruction to Prohibition*. Baltimore: Johns Hopkins University Press.

Tracy. S. W. (2007). Medicalizing alcoholism one hundred years ago. *Harvard Review of Psychiatry, 15,* 86–91.

Transparency Market Research. (2016, August). Sun care market: ToC. Retrieved April 1, 2018, from *www.transparencymarketresearch.com/report-toc/13910.*

Troesch, L. M., & Bauer, C. E. (2017). Second career teachers: Job satisfaction, job stress, and the role of self-efficacy. *Teaching and Teacher Education, 67,* 389–398.

Tsai, J., Kasprow, W. J., & Rosenheck, R. A. (2013). Latent homeless risk profiles of a national sample of homeless veterans and their relation to program referral and admission patterns. *American Journal of Public Health, 103*(Suppl. 2), S239–S247.

Tsuang, M. T., Lyons, M. J., Meyer, J. M., Doyle, T., Eisen, S. A., Goldberg, J., et al. (1998). Co-occurrence of abuse of different drugs in men: The role of drug-specific and shared vulnerabilities. *Archives of General Psychiatry, 55,* 967–972.

Turney, K., & Wildeman, C. (2017). Adverse childhood experiences among children placed in and adopted from foster care: Evidence from a nationally representative survey. *Child Abuse and Neglect, 64,* 117–129.

Twohig, M. P., & Crosby, J. M. (2010). Acceptance and commitment therapy as a treatment for problematic Internet pornography viewing. *Behavior Therapy, 41,* 285–295.

United Nations Office on Drugs and Crime. (2017). *Afghanistan opium survey 2017: Cultivation and production.* Vienna: United Nations Office on Drugs and Crime and Islamic Republic of Afghanistan Ministry of Counter Narcotics. Retrieved December 7, 2017, from *https://reliefweb.int/sites/reliefweb.int/files/resources/Afghan_opium_survey_2017_cult_prod_web.pdf.*

Unrod, M., Gironda, R. J., Clark, M. E., White, K. E., Simmons, V. N., Sutton, S. K., et al. (2014). Smoking behavior and motivation to quit among chronic pain patients initiating multidisciplinary pain treatment: A prospective study. *Pain Medicine, 15,* 1294–1303.

Urbanoski, K. A. (2010). Coerced addiction treatment: Client perspectives and the implications of their neglect. *Harm Reduction Journal, 7*(1), 13.

U.S. Bureau of Labor Statistics. (2012, February). The recession of 2007–2009. Retrieved December 12, 2017, from *www.bls.gov/spotlight/2012/recession/pdf/recession_bls_spotlight.pdf.*

U.S. Census Bureau. (2012). U.S. Census Bureau projections show a slower growing, older, more diverse nation a half century from now. Retrieved July 24, 2017, from *www.census.gov/newsroom/releases/archives/population/cb12-243.html.*

U.S. Department of Health and Human Services. (2011). HHS action plan to reduce racial and ethnic health disparities: A nation free of disparities in health and health care. Retrieved April 15, 2017, from *https://minorityhealth.hhs.gov/npa/files/plans/hhs/hhs.plancomplete.pdf.*

U.S. Department of Health and Human Services. (2017). *HealthyPeople.gov. Office of Disease Prevention and Health Promotion.* Washington, DC. Retrieved June 23, 2017, from *www.healthypeople.gov.*

U.S. Department of Health and Human Services, Administration for Children and Families, Administration on Children, Youth and Families, Children's Bureau. (2017). Child Maltreatment 2015. Retrieved March 26, 2018, from *www.acf.hhs.gov/programs/cb/research-data-technology/statistics-research/child-maltreatment.*

U.S. Drug Enforcement Administration. (2016a). Counterfeit prescription pills containing Fentanyls: A global threat (DEA Intelligence Brief [unclassified],

DEA-DCT-DIB-021-16). Retrieved December 10, 2017, from *www.dea.gov/docs/ Counterfeit%20Prescription%20Pills.pdf.*

U.S. Drug Enforcement Administration. (2016b). DEA reduces amount of opioid controlled substances to be manufactured in 2017. Retrieved December 11, 2017, from *www.dea.gov/divisions/hq/2016/hq100416.shtml.*

U.S. Drug Enforcement Administration. (2017a). Diversion control division. Retrieved December 20, 2017, from *www.deadiversion.usdoj.gov/21cfr/cfr/1301/1301_74. htm.*

U.S. Drug Enforcement Administration. (2017b). 2017 National drug threat assessment (unclassified), DEA-DCT-DIR-040-17. Retrieved December 10, 2017, from *www. dea.gov/docs/DIR-040-17_2017-NDTA.pdf.*

U.S. General Accounting Office. (2003a). *Prescription drugs: OxyContin abuse and diversion and efforts to address the problem* (GAO-04-110). Washington, DC: Author.

U.S. General Accounting Office. (2003b). *Youth illicit drug use prevention: DARE long-term evaluations and federal efforts to identify effective programs.* Washington, DC: Author.

U.S. General Accounting Office. (2015). *Better management of the quota process for controlled substances needed: Coordination between DEA and FDA should be improved* (GAO-15-202). Washington, DC: Author.

U.S. Office of National Drug Control Policy. (2016). FY 2017 budget and performance summary: A companion to the National Drug Control Strategy. Retrieved June 30, 2017, from *https://obamawhitehouse.archives.gov/sites/default/files/ondcp/ policy-and-research/fy2017_budget_summary-final.pdf.*

U.S. Preventive Services Task Force, Grossman, D. C., Curry, S. J., Owens, D. K., Barry, M. J., Caughey, A. B., et al. (2018). Behavioral counseling to prevent skin cancer: U.S. Preventive Services Task Force Recommendation Statement. *Journal of the American Medical Association, 319,* 1134–1142.

Vader, A. M., Walters, S. T., Prabhu, G. C., Houck, J. M., & Field, C. A. (2010). The language of motivational interviewing and feedback: Counselor language, client language, and client drinking outcomes. *Psychology of Addictive Behaviors, 24*(2), 190–197.

Vaillant, G. E. (1990). We should retain the disease concept of alcoholism. *Harvard Medical School Mental Health Letter, 6*(9), 4–6.

Vaillant, G. E. (1995). *The natural history of alcoholism revisited.* Cambridge, MA: Harvard University Press.

Vaillant, G. (2005). Conversation with George Vaillant. *Addiction, 100,* 274–280.

Vale, B., & Edwards, G. (2011). *Physician to the fleet: The life and times of Thomas Trotter, 1760–1832.* Woodbridge, Suffolk, UK: Boydell Press.

Vallance, K., Stockwell, T., Pauly, B., Chow, C., Gray, E., Krysowaty, B., et al. (2016). Do managed alcohol programs change patterns of alcohol consumption and reduce related harm?: A pilot study. *Harm Reduction Journal, 13,* 1–12.

van Boekel, L. C., Brouwers, E. P. M., van Weeghel, J., & Garretsen, H. F. L. (2014). Healthcare professionals' regard towards working with patients with substance use disorders: Comparisons of primary care, general psychiatry and specialist addiction services. *Drug and Alcohol Dependence, 134,* 92–98.

van der Pol, T. M., Haeve, M., Noom, M. J., Stams, G. J. J. M., Doreleijers, T. A. H., van Domburgh, L., et al. (2017). The effectiveness of multidimensional family therapy in treating adolescents with multiple problem behaviors—a meta-analysis. *Journal of Child Psychology and Psychiatry, 58,* 532–545.

van Wormer, K., & Davis, D. R. (2013). *Addiction treatment: A strengths perspective* (3rd ed.). Belmont, CA: Brooks/Cole-Cengage Learning.

Van Zee, A. (2009). The promotion and marketing of OxyContin: Commercial triumph, public health tragedy. *American Journal of Public Health, 99,* 221–227.

Vanderploeg, J. J., Connell, C. M., Caron, C., Saunders, L., Katz, K. H., & Kraemer Tebes, J. (2007). The impact of parental alcohol or drug removals on foster care placement experiences: A matched comparison group study. *Child Maltreatment, 12,* 125–136.

Vansteenkiste, M., & Sheldon, K. M. (2006). There's nothing more practical than a good theory: Integrating motivational interviewing and self-determination theory. *British Journal of Clinical Psychology, 45,* 63–82.

Vanyukov, M. (2009). Genetic aspects of addiction. In G. L. Fisher & N. A. Roget (Eds.), *Encyclopedia of substance abuse prevention, treatment, and recovery* (Vol. 1, pp. 427–430). Thousand Oaks, CA: SAGE.

Vanyukov, M. M., Tarter, R. E., Kirillova, G. P., Kirisci, L., Reynolds, M. D., Kreek, M. J., et al. (2012). Common liability to addiction and "gateway hypothesis": Theoretical, empirical and evolutionary perspective. *Drug and Alcohol Dependence, 123*(Suppl. 1), S3–S17.

Verhulst, B., Neale, M. C., & Kendler, K. S. (2015). The heritability of alcohol use disorders: A meta-analysis of twin and adoption studies. *Psychological Medicine, 45,* 1061–1072.

Vernig, P. M. (2011). Family roles in homes with alcohol-dependent parents: An evidence-based review. *Substance Use and Misuse, 46,* 535–542.

Vidrine, J. I., Spears, C. A., Heppner, W. L., Reitzel, L. R., Marcus, M. T., Cinciripini, P. M., et al. (2016). Efficacy of mindfulness-based addiction treatment (MBAT) for smoking cessation and lapse recovery: A randomized clinical trial. *Journal of Consulting and Clinical Psychology, 84*(9), 824–838.

Vink, J. M. (2016). Genetics of addiction: Future focus on gene × environment interaction? *Journal of Studies on Alcohol and Drugs, 77,* 684–687.

Volkow, N. D., & Baler, R. D. (2014). Addiction science: Uncovering neurobiological complexity. *Neuropharmacology, 76,* 235–249.

Volkow, N. D., Fowler, J. S., & Wang, G. J. (2003). The addicted human brain: Insights from imaging studies. *Journal of Clinical Investigation, 111,* 1444–1451.

Volkow, N. D., Wise, R. A., & Baler R. (2017). The dopamine motive system: Implications for drug and food addiction. *Nature Reviews Neuroscience, 18,* 741–752.

von Bertalanffy, L. (1968). *General system theory: Foundations, development, applications* (rev. ed.). New York: George Braziller.

Wagenaar, A. C., Gehan, J. P., Jones-Webb, R., Toomey, T. L., & Forster, J. (1999). Communities mobilizing for change on alcohol: Lessons and results from a 15-community randomized trial. *Journal of Community Psychology, 27,* 315–326.

Wagenaar, A. C., Murray, D. M., Gehan, J. P., Wolfson, M., Forster, J., Toomey, T. L., et al. (2000). Communities mobilizing for change on alcohol: Outcomes from a randomized community trial. *Journal of Studies on Alcohol, 61,* 85–94.

Wagenaar, A. C., Murray, D. M., & Toomey, T. L. (2000). Communities mobilizing for change on alcohol (CMCA): Effects of a randomized trial on arrests and traffic crashes. *Addiction, 95,* 209–217.

Wagner, M. (2011, March 6). Schlichter blames addiction but never says "gambling" in jail interview. *Columbus Dispatch.* Retrieved April 22, 2018, from *www.dispatch. com/content/stories/local/2011/03/06/schlichter-blames-addiction-but-never-says-gambling-in-jail-interview.html.*

Wahlberg, L., Nirenberg, A., & Capezuti, E. (2016). Distress and coping self-efficacy in inpatient oncology nurses. *Oncology Nursing Forum, 43,* 738–746.

Wain, R. M., Wilbourne, P. L., Harris, K. W., Pierson, H., Teleki, J., Burling, T. A., et al. (2011). Motivational interview improves treatment entry in homeless veterans. *Drug and Alcohol Dependence, 115,* 113–119.

Waldron, H. B., Kern-Jones, S., Turner, C. W., Peterson, T. R., & Ozechowski, T. J. (2007). Engaging resistant adolescents in drug abuse treatment. *Journal of Substance Abuse Treatment, 32,* 133–142.

Waldron, H. B., Slesnick, N., Brody, J. L., Turner, C. W., & Peterson, T. R. (2001). Treatment outcomes for adolescent substance abuse at 4- and 7-month assessments. *Journal of Consulting and Clinical Psychology, 69,* 802–813.

Waldron, H. B., & Turner, C. W. (2008). Evidence-based psychosocial treatments for adolescent substance abuse. *Journal of Clinical Child and Adolescent Psychology, 37,* 238–261.

Wall, J. D., & Przeworski, M. (2000). When did the human population size start increasing? *Genetics, 155,* 1865–1874.

Walsh, Z., & Stuart, G. (2009). Moderation in use. In G. L. Fisher & N. A. Roget (Eds.), *Encyclopedia of substance abuse prevention, treatment, and recovery* (Vol. 1, pp. 554–555). Thousand Oaks, CA: SAGE.

Wang, J. C., Hinrichs, A. L., Stock, H., Budde, J. P., Allen, R., Bertelsen, S., et al. (2004). Evidence of common and specific genetic effects: Association of the muscarinic acetylcholine receptor M2 (*CHRM2*) gene with alcohol dependence and major depressive syndrome. *Human Molecular Genetics, 13*(17), 1903–1911.

Warner, J. (2003). *Craze: Gin and debauchery in the age of reason.* New York: Random House.

Watkins, K. E., Hunter, S. B., Burnam, M. A., Pincus, H. A., & Nicholson, G. (2005). Review of treatment recommendations for persons with a co-occurring affective or anxiety and substance use disorder. *Psychiatric Services, 56,* 913–926.

Webb, A., Lind, P. A., Kalmijn, J., Feiler, H. S., Smith, T. L., Schuckit, M. A., et al. (2011). The investigation into CYP2E1 in relation to the level of response to alcohol through a combination of linkage and association analysis. *Alchololism: Clinical and Experimental Research, 35,* 20–18.

Webb, T. L., Sniehotta, F. F., & Michie, S. (2010). Using theories of behavior change to inform interventions for addictive behaviours. *Addiction, 105,* 1879–1892.

Wegscheider-Cruse, S. (1989). *Another chance: Hope and health for the alcoholic family* (2nd ed.). Palo Alto, CA: Science and Behavior Books.

Weinberg, D. (2005). *Of others inside: Insanity, addiction and belonging in America.* Philadelphia: Temple University Press.

Weinberger, A. H., McKee, S. A., & George, T. P. (2010). Changes in smoking expectancies in abstinent, reducing, and non-abstinent participants during a pharmacological trial for smoking cessation. *Nicotine and Tobacco Research, 12,* 937–943.

Weinstein, N., Przybylski, A. K., & Ryan, R. M. (2012). The index of autonomous functioning: Development of a scale of human autonomy. *Journal of Research in Personality, 46,* 397–413.

Weiss, R. (2006). Behavioral genetics and the media. In E. Parens, A. R. Chapman, & N. Press (Eds.), *Wrestling with behavioral genetics* (pp. 307–326). Baltimore: Johns Hopkins University Press.

Wessell, M. T., Martino-McAllister, J. M., & Gallon, E. C. (2009). Tolerance. In G. L. Fisher & N. A. Roget (Eds.), *Encyclopedia of substance abuse prevention, treatment, and recovery* (Vol. 2, pp. 921–924). Thousand Oaks, CA: SAGE.

West, R. T. (2005). Time for a change: Putting the transtheoretical (stages of change) model to rest. *Addiction, 100,* 1036–1039.

West, R. (2006). *Theory of addiction.* Oxford, UK: Blackwell.

West, R., & Brown, J. (2013). *Theory of addiction* (2nd ed.). Hoboken, NJ: Wiley.

White, W. L. (2014). *Slaying the dragon: The history of addiction treatment and recovery in America* (2nd ed.). Bloomington, IL: Chestnut Health Systems/Lighthouse Institute.

White, W. L., & Kelly, J. F. (2011). Alcohol/drug/substance "abuse": The history and (hopeful) demise of a pernicious label. *Alcoholism Treatment Quarterly, 29,* 317–321.

Whiteside, U., Cronce, J. M., Pedersen, E. R., & Larimer, M. E. (2010). Brief motivational feedback for college students and adolescents: A harm reduction approach. *Journal of Clinical Psychology: In Session, 66*(2), 150–163.

Wild, T. C., Cunningham, J. A., & Ryan, R. M. (2006). Social pressure, coercion, and client engagement at treatment entry: A self-determination theory perspective. *Addictive Behaviors, 31,* 1858–1872.

Wilde, A., Bonfiglioli, C., Meiser, B., Mitchell, P. B., & Schofield, P. R. (2011). Portrayal of psychiatric genetics in Australian print news media, 1996–2009. *Medical Journal of Australia, 195,* 401–404.

Williams, G. C., Minicucci, D. S., Kouides, R. W., Levesque, C. S., Chirkov, V. I., Ryan, R. M., et al. (2002). Self-determination, smoking, diet and health. *Health Education Research, 17*(5), 512–521.

Wilson, G. T. (1988). Alcohol use and abuse: A social learning theory analysis. In C. D. Chaudron & D. A. Wilkinson (Eds.), *Theories on alcoholism.* Toronto, ON, Canada: Addiction Research Foundation.

Winick, C. (1962). Maturing out of narcotic addiction. *Bulletin on Narcotics, 14,* 1–7.

Winters, J., Fals-Stewart, W., O'Farrell, T. J., Birchler, G. R., & Kelley, M. L. (2002). Behavioral couples therapy for female substance-abusing patients: Effects on substance use and relationship adjustment. *Journal of Consulting and Clinical Psychology, 70,* 344–355.

Witkiewitz, K., Bowen, S., Douglas, H., & Hsu, S. H. (2013). Mindfulness-based relapse prevention for substance craving. *Addictive Behaviors, 38,* 1563–1571.

Witkiewitz, K., Pearson, M. R., Hallgren, K. A., Maisto, S. A., Roos, C. R., Kirouac, M., et al. (2017). Who achieves low risk drinking during alcohol treatment?: An analysis of patients in three alcohol clinical trials. *Addiction, 112,* 2112–2121.

Wodak, A., & Cooney, A. (2006). Do needle syringe programs reduce HIV infection among injecting drug users: A comprehensive review of the international evidence. *Substance Use and Misuse, 41,* 777–813.

Wolff, T. (2001a). Community coalition building—contemporary practice and research: Introduction. *American Journal of Community Psychology, 29,* 165–172.

Wolff, T. (2001b). A practitioner's guide to successful coalitions. *American Journal of Community Psychology, 29,* 173–191.

Woodworth, A. M., & McLellan, A. T. (2016). Converging advances in science, policy and public awareness: A time of great opportunity and change in addiction treatment. *Brain Research Bulletin, 123,* 110–113.

World Health Organization. (1998). Health promotion glossary. Retrieved April 15, 2018, from *www.who.int/healthpromotion/about/HPR%20Glossary%201998.pdf.*

Wormington, S. V., Anderson, K. G., & Corpus, J. H. (2011). The role of academic motivation in high school students' current and lifetime alcohol consumption: Adopting a self-determination theory perspective. *Journal of Studies on Alcohol and Drugs, 72,* 965–974.

Wright, B. J., Zhang, S. X., & Farabee, D. (2012). A squandered opportunity?: A review of SAMHSA's National Registry of Evidence-based Programs and Practices for offenders. *Crime and Delinquency, 58,* 954–972.

Wu, L., Zhu, H., & Swartz, M. S. (2016). Treatment utilization among persons with opioid use disorder in the United States. *Drug and Alcohol Dependence, 169,* 117–127.

Wurmser, L. (1974). Psychoanalytic considerations of the etiology of compulsive drug use. *Journal of the American Psychoanalytic Association, 22,* 820–843.

Wurmser, L. (1978). *The hidden dimension: Psychodynamics in compulsive drug use.* New York: Jason Aronson.

Wurmser, L. (1980). Drug use as a protective system. In D. J. Lettieri, M. Sayers, & H. W. Pearson (Eds.), *Theories on drug abuse: Selected contemporary perspectives* (DHHS Publication No. ADM 84-967). Washington, DC: U.S. Government Printing Office.

Xu, H., Wang, F., Kranzler, H. R., Gelernter, J., & Zhang, H. (2017). Alcohol and nicotine codependence-associated DNA methylation changes in promoter regions of addiction-related genes. *Scientific Reports, 7,* Article No. 41816.

Xu, X., Ji, H., Liu, G., Wang, Q., Liu, H., Shen, W., et al. (2016). A significant association between BDNF promoter methylation and the risk of drug addiction. *Gene, 584,* 54–59.

Yalisove, D. L. (1989). Psychoanalytic approaches to alcoholism and addiction: Treatment and research. *Psychology of Addictive Behaviors, 3,* 107–113.

Yang, L. H., Wong, L. Y., Grivel, M. M., & Hasin, D. S. (2017). Stigma and substance use disorders: An international phenomenon. *Current Opinion in Psychiatry, 30,* 378–388.

Yau, Y. H. C., & Potenza, M. N. (2015). Gambling disorder and other behavioral addictions: Recognition and treatment. *Harvard Review of Psychiatry, 23,* 134–146.

Yoshimura, A., Komoto, Y., & Higuchi, S. (2016). Exploration of core symptoms for the diagnosis of alcohol dependence in the ICD-10. *Alcoholism: Clinical and Experimental Research, 40,* 2409–2417.

Young, R. M., Connor, J. P., & Feeney, G. F. X. (2011). Alcohol expectancy changes over a 12-week cognitive-behavioral therapy program are predictive of treatment success. *Journal of Substance Abuse Treatment, 40,* 18–25.

Young-Wolff, K. C., Kendler, K. S., Ericson, M. L., & Prescott, C. A. (2011). Accounting for the association between childhood maltreatment and alcohol-use disorders in males: A twin study. *Psychological Medicine, 41,* 59–70.

Zahodne, L., Nowinski, C., Gershon, R., & Manly, J. (2015). Self-efficacy buffers the relationship between educational disadvantage and executive functioning. *Journal of the International Neuropsychological Society, 21,* 297–304.

Zeldman, A., Ryan, R. M., & Fiscella, K. (2004). Motivation, autonomy support, and entity beliefs: Their role in methadone maintenance treatment. *Journal of Social and Clinical Psychology, 23,* 675–696.

Zimberg, S. (1978). Principles of alcoholism psychotherapy. In S. Zimberg, J. Wallace, & S. B. Blume (Eds.), *Practical approaches to alcoholism psychotherapy.* New York: Plenum Press.

Zimić, J. I., & Jukić, V. (2012). Familial risk factors favoring drug addiction onset. *Journal of Psychoactive Drugs, 44,* 173–185.

Zimring, F. E. (1998). *American youth violence.* New York: Oxford University Press.

Author Index

Subject Index